Further acclaim for
THE FALSE FAT DIET

'An awesome contribution to the puzzle of losing weight. I will recommend this to everyone I know. Clear, reflective and easy to use. A real gem!'
Kathleen Desmaisons, Ph.D., author of *Potatoes Not Prozac*

'*The False Fat Diet* works. It is a must read for anyone who wants to lose weight fast and keep it off'
Dharma Singh Khalsa, M.D., author of *Brain Longevity*

'Elson Haas shares a profound insight in *The False Fat Diet*. If you have a hard time losing weight and if a "healthy" diet leaves you feeling just as tired and bloated as no diet, this book can change your life forever!'
Leo Galland, M.D., author of *Power Healing*

'The potential benefits are enormous. Haas and Cameron Stauth tell numerous stories of patients (including Stauth and his sister) who lost weight instantly, looked younger, and felt better by following the diet that makes the most sense for them'
amazon.com

**OTHER BOOKS
BY ELSON M. HAAS, M.D.**

Staying Healthy with the Seasons

Staying Healthy with Nutrition:
The Complete Guide to Diet and Nutritional Medicine

A Cookbook for All Seasons

The Detox Diet: A How-To Guide for
Cleansing the Body of Toxic Substances

The Staying Healthy Shopper's Guide: Feed Your Family Safely

Vitamins for Dummies (*with Christopher Hobbs, L.Ac.*)

BY CAMERON STAUTH

The New Approach to Cancer

Brain Longevity
(*with Dharma Singh Khalsa, M.D.*)

The Pain Cure
(*with Dharma Singh Khalsa, M.D.*)

THE FALSE FAT DIET

**The Revolutionary 21-Day Programme for
Losing the Weight You Think Is Fat**

ELSON M. HAAS, M.D., AND CAMERON STAUTH

BANTAM BOOKS

London • New York • Toronto • Sydney • Auckland

THE FALSE FAT DIET
A BANTAM BOOK: 0553 81348 X

First publication in Great Britain

PRINTING HISTORY
First published by Ballantine Books,
a division of The Random House Group Inc. 2000
Bantam Books edition published 2001

1 3 5 7 9 10 8 6 4 2

Set in 11½/12pt Granjon by Falcon Oast Graphic Art

Bantam Books are published by Transworld Publishers,
61–63 Uxbridge Road, London W5 5SA,
a division of The Random House Group Ltd,
in Australia by Random House Australia (Pty) Ltd,
20 Alfred Street, Milsons Point, Sydney, NSW 2061, Australia,
in New Zealand by Random House New Zealand Ltd,
18 Poland Road, Glenfield, Auckland 10, New Zealand
and in South Africa by Random House (Pty) Ltd,
Endulini, 5a Jubilee Road, Parktown 2193, South Africa.

Reproduced, printed and bound in Great Britain by
Clays Ltd, St Ives plc

To my dear mother, Shirley Haas. For your faithful support through all my years of finding this new path as a doctor and writer, and for your continued love and kindness towards all your family – you are a great blessing to all of us.

—E.M.H.

For Adrienne

—C.S.

CONTENTS

Acknowledgements   9
Introduction   11

PART ONE: WHY THE DIET WORKS   17

1.   It's Not Fat   19
2.   Why You Will Lose False Fat   47
3.   Why You Will Lose True Fat   69
4.   What Women Need to Know   84
5.   The Extraordinary Side Benefits   109

PART TWO: HOW TO DO THE FALSE FAT DIET   143

6.   Finding Out Your Own False Fat Foods   145
      Sample Elimination Diet Menu Plans   164
7.   The Cleansing Phase   185
8.   False Fat Week   213
9.   The Balance Programme   237
      Sample Menu Plan for the Balance Programme   263

PART THREE: WHAT TO EAT   271

Food Reaction Reference Guide   275
Recipes   298

Resources and Referrals   351
Notes   361
Index   367

ACKNOWLEDGEMENTS

THANK YOU TO CAMERON STAUTH, MY EFFICIENT AND professional co-author, whose eloquent and interactive style motivates and enables each reader to make sense out of this important health information.

Special thanks to Leslie Meredith (our editor), Richard Pine (our agent), and Howard Schiffer (our friend).

To my wife, Tara, and our children, Orion and Ishara, for your continued support in allowing me the time to work, and the joy and love that keeps me inspired to share with others.

To Joanne Victoria and the entire staff of the Preventive Medical Center of Marin, my office since 1984, for your support and motivation to continue my writing. Because the office runs so smoothly, it allows me the space and time with peace of mind to work.

To Bethany Argisle, my long-time friend and inspirational co-worker on many of my books.

To Jim Braly, M.D., and Michael Rosenbaum, M.D., for your wisdom and guidance in helping me flush out some of the false fat factors.

To Mary James, N.D., for your thorough and helpful review of the food allergy/reaction testing information.

To Judy Lane, N.P., one of my work associates, for your review and input on the women's chapter.

To Sandra Stahl, for your diligent, professional work on the manuscript and all of its edits and printouts.

To Eleonora Manzolini, for your artistic cuisine input and

your improvement in making our menus even more tasty.

And a special thank-you to Philippe Boulot and Susan Boulot, for your quality recipes and the added tastiness to *The False Fat Diet*.

—Elson Haas, M.D.
San Rafael, California

THANKS ALSO TO LESLIE MEREDITH, OUR ASTUTE AND insightful editor, who helped to shape and focus this book from the very beginning, and who was a pleasure to work with.

Richard Pine, our literary agent, recognized the importance of this work before it even existed as a book, just as he has spotted so many other important innovations and helped integrate them into the fabric of contemporary culture. Thanks once again, Richard.

Howard Schiffer, media wizard extraordinaire, offered wise advice and kind help throughout the arduous process of presenting these concepts to the American public.

My heartfelt appreciation must also be expressed to the modern pioneers of the concept of nutritional individuality, including Dr. William Donald Kelley, Dr. F. Fuller Royal, Dr. Roger Williams, Dr. Lendon Smith, and Dr. William Philpott. It's been almost twenty-five years since I first started working with some of these esteemed doctors, and many of their words are still fresh in my mind.

This book could not have been written without the emotional support of my wife, Shari, and the technical support of my son, Gabriel, who teaches me new things about science almost every day. Thanks, too, to sweet new arrival Adrienne, for sleeping several consecutive hours almost every night.

Final billing goes to Dr. Elson Haas, a true original thinker, who has now made it possible for untold numbers of people to feel better and live longer.

—Cameron Stauth
Portland, Oregon

INTRODUCTION

By Cameron Stauth

MY INVOLVEMENT WITH THIS BOOK BEGAN IN A GRIM WAY: I was afraid my sister might be dying.

In 1996, Kori developed a mild rash near her collarbone. Over the next three months, it turned into a patch of angry red hives that began to spread slowly all over her chest and back. Her doctor had no idea what was causing the hives, so Kori started climbing a ladder of appointments with specialists – a dermatologist, an allergist, an endocrinologist, even a psychiatrist. For about a year, every Friday was Doctor Day for Kori, but nobody could figure out her problem. She was prescribed topical and oral steroids, a slew of industrial-strength antihistamines, various skin medications, and antidepressants. She also went to a naturopath, who tried all manner of natural curatives. Nothing helped. The hives kept spreading. She became increasingly alarmed, and so did her husband.

As every treatment failed, a suspicion began to grow among her crew of specialists that she had a serious autoimmune disorder, probably lupus, the incurable disease that generally starts as a red rash, then causes increasingly severe skin reactions, and eventually destroys the brain and kidneys. Part of the reason lupus was suspected was because Kori also had a number of systemic symptoms. She was often inexplicably tired, had gained about 25 pounds, had pain in her joints, and suffered from depressed immune function – she seemed to catch everything that was going around. Also, she didn't look healthy; she'd just turned 40, but her face was already starting to broaden and fill out, with a puffy double chin. She was beginning to look similar to our grandmother in old pictures in the family album. Her lack of fitness and vitality was puzzling, because she ate nothing but low-fat foods and worked out at a gym almost every night.

On the day the doctor was scheduled to call with the results of her lupus test, she stayed home from work. If it was bad news, she didn't want to hear it at the office. My brother-in-law waited with her.

Just before five p.m., the doctor called. 'I've got good news,' he said. 'It isn't lupus.'

'Great! But do you know what it *is*?'

'Yes, I do. It's urticaria.'

'What's that?'

'Hives.'

Kori was relieved, if unenlightened.

Two more months went by, and the hives kept working their way toward her face.

Then, one afternoon at the University of Oregon medical school library, I was reading *Natural Health* magazine and came across an intriguing reference to a doctor I'd heard about. His name was Elson Haas, and according to the magazine and other sources in the library, he was getting excellent results treating food allergies by using a different diagnostic method and a more broad-based therapy than conventional allergists. He was also solving many intractable problems, including asthma, migraines, irritable bowel syndrome, and hives!

One of Kori's doctors had already given her a conventional allergy scratch test, which hadn't revealed any allergies, but Dr. Haas reportedly considered the scratch test unreliable for food allergies.

I called Dr. Haas's medical clinic in the San Francisco area and talked to him. He told me Kori could find out for sure if she had any allergies by doing a simple elimination diet, in which she reduced her diet to just a few foods, then added back foods one at a time, noting reactions. Another diagnostic method, he said, was a blood test, which he thought was more accurate and comprehensive than the conventional scratch test.

The blood test was covered by Kori's insurance, so that's what she did.

According to her test, Kori was allergic to several foods, including some low-fat foods she'd been eating frequently. Dr. Haas placed her on an anti-allergen diet, free of her reactive foods. He said that he had begun to call this diet his False Fat Diet, because the most noticeable, immediate, and common reaction to it was the quick loss of the 'false fat' of tissue swelling and abdominal bloating. He primarily used the diet, he said, for weight control.

It was easy for Kori to lay off some of her allergenic foods, such as kidney beans and aged cheese, but she was also allergic to wheat and corn, and avoiding them was more difficult. Even so, she started buying baked goods made only from rice flour and rye flour. They were available at her regular grocery store, and she liked how they tasted.

Besides eating these new foods, Kori could now indulge in a number of foods she'd avoided for years, such as steak, roasted cashews, and even brownies (made from rice flour). This diet was not exactly bread and water, and she enjoyed it. On the first weekend of her False Fat Diet, she admitted that she felt sort of strange – mostly because she was eating more foods that were supposedly fattening – but that the overall transition was relatively easy for her. She also started to eat more whole, unprocessed foods instead of mixes filled with wheat gluten, corn syrup, and stuff she couldn't pronounce. She told me that her family's meals tasted more like our mum's cooking and less like Betty Crocker's.

Then the most amazing thing happened.

Kori started the diet on a Thursday, and by Sunday night, when my wife and I went to her house for dinner, her hives had vanished. Even more striking, she looked about 10 pounds lighter and 5 years younger. What a difference! And it happened in only four days! My wife and I were both envious and intrigued. Kori's stomach and waist seemed to have shrunk, and the puffy, marshmallowy look in her face had started to drain away. Kori was thrilled. She'd hoped to lose weight, since Dr. Haas had said she probably would, but she hadn't expected anything nearly so quick or dramatic.

Results kept occurring every day for two more weeks. Kori soon looked 20 pounds lighter and 10 years younger. The swell-ing and bloat in her face and frame totally disappeared. In addition, she felt far more energetic, she didn't feel as if she were starving at night just before dinner, and she said she was in a better mood most of the time – much more cheerful and relaxed.

After about six months on the diet, Kori began to look pretty much the same as she had 15 or 20 years before, and could wear clothes that had not been out of her closet since the birth of her first child. She weighed about 20 pounds less, but looked as if she'd lost more weight than that, without all that puffiness in her face.

Watching this amazing transformation in Kori really changed my attitude about ageing and its effects upon weight. For the couple of years prior to her dietary change, Kori and I had both begun to think, well, 40 is 40, and once you hit that wall your metabolism is going to go to hell, and you're going to start looking older and fatter, so you'd better just get used to it. I don't see it that way anymore, and Kori certainly doesn't either.

As Kori's diet progressed, she kept consulting Dr. Haas, and I bought two more of his books, which were full of original thinking. One of them, *Staying Healthy with the Seasons*, is considered a classic of integrative medicine, or natural health care.

Dr. Haas was familiar with some of my work, particularly *Brain Longevity* – a medical book I wrote with Dharma Singh Khalsa, M.D. – and we began discussing the idea of writing a book together about his diet. I thought that an anti-allergen weight loss diet was a great idea for a book, and was certain that when other people started getting the life-changing results that Kori had, their experiences would have a major impact on the science of weight control.

I was so fascinated by this diet that I tried it myself. I did an elimination diet, instead of the blood test, to ascertain my own food reactions. Within days, I determined that I was reactive to wheat and milk. No big surprise – I'd known for years that they didn't agree with me, but still used to eat almost a litre of yoghurt every day, thinking that in spite of what my body was telling me, it was a health food, so surely it had to be good for me. I also ate two bagels a day, but they were whole wheat — the much-vaunted complex carbohydrate — so of course they were healthy, right?

Wrong: They're healthy for most people, but not for me. The same week I quit eating wheat and milk, I got rid of a 20-year-old condition of severe chronic heartburn — the 50-Tums-a-day kind, the kind TV ads now portentously call acid reflux disease. I also cleared up sinus congestion so severe that I'd often spent months at a time on antibiotics for sinusitis. The icing on the cake, though, was how much trimmer I looked. I'm not in bad shape — I run five miles every day — but I'd never been able to run off my last 10 pounds, which stuck to my stomach like laminate. In addition, after a meal, my belly would often bloat up so badly I'd have to unbuckle my belt. Believe me, it was no fun to *be* fit and *look* fat, and I'd got to the point where I'd just wanted to give up. Now, though, I'm down to my college weight, with a flat stomach. About 5 of my extra 10 pounds were from food-reaction swelling, so they came off instantly, and the rest came off gradually. I wasn't even trying to diet, but on the False Fat Diet I just don't get as hungry as I used to, and my energy is way up.

The diet was so easy, I felt foolish that I hadn't done it earlier. Now it seems so obvious. If you're like me and you swell up instantly when you get stung by a bee, I'm sure you make certain to avoid them. And if you have an allergy to cat hair and dander, you probably avoid cats. If you react to poison ivy, you don't go near it. But so many of us are reactive to certain foods, yet we eat them anyway, as if we couldn't possibly refrain and don't know why we should.

Fortunately, much of the medical profession now realizes the importance of food allergy, but the public lags behind. When my wife and I adopted our baby daughter last year, the baby had some distressing digestive symptoms, so we called the doctor and asked if we should try switching her from a milk-based formula to a low-allergy soya formula. The doctor said, 'Absolutely' (as in 'Duh'). This is apparently the standard approach now, and parents are supposed to know it. But the low-allergy formula we bought our daughter didn't even *exist* seven years ago, when our son suffered similar symptoms for six long months. Even our son, though, recently benefited from what I've learned from Dr. Haas. All last summer and autumn, he had a scaly pink inflammation near his mouth, but it disappeared within a week when I took him off Nutrasweet.

The allergies in our family are not at all uncommon. It's estimated that more than ten million people suffer significant food reactions, often more severe than Kori's, and that about 125 people die every year from food reactions, compared with 50 from bee stings. In fact, because kids die every year from eating peanuts at school, some lunch programmes have banned peanut butter.

A more insidious effect of food reactions, though, is the constant long-term piling on of ounce after ounce, and pound after pound, until one day people are fat and don't know why. At the same time, they keep gobbling reactive foods and fighting their noxious effects with a host of antacids, antihistamines, and diet products. It would be arrogant of me to say that people are overlooking the obvious, however, because I overlooked it myself for about thirty years.

I am professionally and personally pleased to have helped Dr. Haas introduce this breakthrough diet to the American public. Dr. Haas is convinced that food reactions are the crucial missing piece in the puzzle of weight control. These individual sensitivities finally explain why two people can be on almost identical diets, with very different results.

After spending a year interviewing Dr. Haas, his patients, and other experts – as well as poring over volumes of medical literature – I am certain that Dr. Haas is correct: *This is a medical breakthrough that can change lives*.

In the past, millions of people suffered from difficult diets while sabotaging their own success by unknowingly eating reactive foods.

The days of making that mistake are over.

A new era of weight control has begun.

Dr. Haas's diet is changing the way the world loses weight.

PART ONE

WHY THE DIET WORKS

1
IT'S NOT FAT

I HAVE EXCELLENT NEWS. IT'S SOMETHING YOU HAVEN'T heard before. It's very important.

- **You're not nearly as overweight as you may think.** Much of your weight isn't even fat. It's <u>false fat</u> – the bloating and swelling caused by allergy-like food reactions – and you can shed it almost immediately.
- **This false fat is not your fault.** You are not a glutton. You're not lazy. You just have a very common metabolic problem: food reactions.
- **You can solve this metabolic problem.** The problem is not permanent, and it's not hard to correct. You can solve it over the next few days. It need never return.
- **When you do solve this problem, you'll regain your power over food.** As your false fat fades, so will your food cravings and certain metabolic disorders (such as hormone imbalances). Without these food cravings and metabolic disorders, you'll begin to lose your true fat, steadily and surely. Even if you now lack full control over your eating habits, you can take charge again by correcting your food reactions. You can start taking charge today.

I urge you to carefully consider this great news. It will be your key to having complete power over what you eat, and over the biochemical reactions that foods cause in your body. When you have this power, you will have an entirely new way to solve your weight problem.

You have nothing to gain but knowledge, and nothing to lose but the false fat that's hurting your appearance and the true fat that's hurting your health.

When you conquer your food reactions, your appearance, your health, and your zest for life will improve immeasurably. Things will get better because you will *make* them get better. You will finally have that power. It's true: Knowledge is power.

You really *must* use the power that this knowledge provides. You owe it to yourself. You're worth it.

And here is why you probably *will* use this power: using it will be more pleasant than not using it. For the first time in your life, you are going to enjoy being on a diet. In fact, like most of my patients, you will almost forget that you are on a diet, because the False Fat Diet is quite different from every other diet you've ever been on. It is not based on reducing the quantity of your food. It is based on improving the *quality* of your food.

This diet is not even ultimately intended to make you thin – it is intended to make you *healthy*. As I often tell my patients, 'If you strive for thin, you'll never win. Strive for health and thin will follow.'

Thus, in the conventional sense of the word, this is not even a diet. It is an *eating strategy*. It's a scientifically designed method of giving you power over food, so that you can make smart food choices.

No one else can make these choices for you, because each of your food choices must be carefully individualized. Every person reacts differently to different foods. You are a unique being with your own special biochemistry and your own one-of-a-kind environment and activities. There is only one you, doing what you do, eating what you eat, and meeting the demands that you meet.

Nonetheless, every other diet you've ever been on has been designed *for* other people *by* other people. They have been one-size-fits-all-diets, and that approach simply doesn't work. This time, with The False Fat Diet, you'll help design your own <u>personalized</u> diet, free of your own reactive foods. This diet will be *your* diet. Yours alone. That's why it *will* work.

With the help of this book, you'll learn about the qualities and chemistries of various foods. More important, though, you'll learn about your own unique body. You'll learn which foods are good for you and which aren't – and I promise some surprises.

Right now, you may know which foods are healthy for most people. But if you're basing your own food choices on just this knowledge, you may be doing yourself more harm than good – because you are not most people. You're *you*, and the only diet you'll ever fully succeed on will be your own individualized diet, free of the particular foods that are healthy for most people, but harmful for you.

After years of trying unsuccessfully to lose weight, you may be feeling confused, powerless, frustrated – and hungry. Don't despair! Many of my patients felt like that before they tried this approach. But most of them have succeeded beyond their dreams.

Now it's your turn.

It has taken me approximately 20 years to develop and refine the False Fat Diet. During this time, I have placed hundreds of overweight patients on the diet and have consistently achieved good, and often remarkable, results.

The False Fat Diet is based upon a simple, inarguable medical fact: when people regularly eat foods to which they are reactive, they invariably suffer (1) tissue swelling, (2) abdominal bloating, and (3) metabolic disturbances that cause weight gain.

The tissue swelling and abdominal bloating create a false fat that looks exactly like fat, but is not 'true fat', or adipose tissue. This false fat often adds the appearance of an extra 10 to 25 pounds. The food reactions that cause false fat *are almost never corrected by conventional weight loss diets*.

In addition, metabolic disturbances caused by food reactions create not just false fat, but also true fat. They create excess adipose tissue by disrupting the metabolism, by disturbing hormonal balance, and by creating intense food cravings. Millions of people have become obese because of these factors.

When my patients go on the False Fat Diet, most of them lose the false fat of bloating and swelling very quickly and then lose their extra adipose tissue gradually and steadily.

Over the years, I have seen patients try to lose weight with a number of other approaches, but no other weight control diet has been nearly as effective as my False Fat Diet. Other diets fail to keep weight off permanently because they ignore the terrible burden that food reactions place upon the body. When this burden is removed, most patients respond wonderfully well.

Clinical, controlled studies support my belief in the power of this diet. One important study is detailed on page 32. They irrefutably demonstrate that many people who have failed on other diets succeed with this approach.

Food reactions are not the only reason people gain weight. However, they are an extremely important reason – one that has gone largely unreported, except in medical literature. In actuality, an estimated 80 per cent to 90 per cent of all significantly overweight people suffer from these reactions and can lose weight if the condition is corrected.

Food reactions consist of **food allergies** and **food sensitivities**, which are similar to allergies. Some doctors refer to all food reactions as allergies, but most physicians feel that the term *reactions* is more accurate, because it's more inclusive. Strictly speaking, classic food allergies are relatively rare. Food sensitivities, however, are extremely common.

The incidence of food allergies and sensitivities has recently begun to increase dramatically for several reasons. The primary reason is that we eat too many staples, such as wheat, eggs, and milk, which exhaust our bodies' abilities to digest them. Also, we eat too many packaged, processed foods, which are loaded with reactive fillers and chemicals, such as corn syrup, wheat gluten, and MSG. Obesity and digestive problems, both very common health problems nowadays, also contribute to food reactions.

The increasing incidence of food reactions is mirrored by a recent sharp increase in obesity, which rose from 25 per cent of the American population in 1985 to 33 per cent today. If this rate continues, by the year 2030 most people in America will be obese. Childhood obesity has doubled since 1980. Even now 60 per cent of the population, while not obese, is overweight. Currently, obesity kills 300,000 Americans each year – more people than any other factor except smoking. Over-consumption also stresses digestive functions and leads to inefficient breakdown of foods and malabsorption of large molecules of food, which sets up food reactions.

Therefore, I believe that the important effect that food re-actions have upon weight control and digestive health must be brought to the attention of the American public and the world. At this point in the history of public health, few things are more vital.

Why This Diet Has Been Successful

The False Fat Diet has been successful because it corrects a serious biological flaw that has been proven to trigger weight gain.

Throughout the history of medical weight control, the most successful diets have been those that did not radically restrict calories, but instead corrected the metabolic problems that most often cause weight gain. For example, the *Sugar Busters* diet helped people by showing them how to correct the bio-logical flaw of insulin instability. Other successful approaches have included boosting the body's fat-burning thermogenesis and correcting deficiencies in the brain chemicals that make people feel satisfied after eating. Correcting biological flaws is a medically sound approach, because old-fashioned, caloric-restriction diets have been proven ineffective. They trigger the starvation response, which slows the metabolism and makes the body hoard its fat.

However, even the most successful diets have overlooked a critically important factor: most overweight people have in-dividualized food allergies and sensitivities that subvert the one-size-fits-all diets, in which all dieters eat the same foods. Therefore, some of the most popular diets have had high failure rates.

By correcting the common biological flaw of food reactions, though, the False Fat Diet achieves unprecedented rates of adherence and success.

How It Works: A Quick Overview

The False Fat Diet begins when you determine your own reactive foods, using either a blood test or an elimination diet, in which you eliminate foods, then reintroduce them gradually, to see which ones cause problems. I'll soon tell you about each method.

After you determine your reactive foods, you begin to avoid them during the first phase of the diet, the Cleansing Phase, which lasts about a week. During this initial phase, you may even experience withdrawal symptoms, such as food cravings, irritability, or headaches, as your body is cleansed of chemicals from reactive foods and as your metabolism begins to normalize. *These temporary symptoms are a sure sign that the diet is working.*

Then you quickly shift into the second phase of the diet, which is False Fat Week. During this 7- to 10-day period, you will lose your bloating and swelling and look 10 to 25 pounds thinner. Your energy, motivation, and well-being will begin to soar.

Then you progress to the third phase of the diet, the Balance Programme, which lasts as long as you want. In the Balance Programme, you can eat a varied, balanced assortment of non-reactive foods. During this phase, you will probably lose significant amounts of adipose tissue as your metabolic function improves and your food cravings vanish.

On the Balance Programme, you begin to rebuild your metabolic health, and overcome your food reactions. After 2 to 3 months, you can sometimes begin to eat even your most reactive foods, without incident. *Therefore, the Balance Programme becomes easier as time passes.*

During the Balance Programme phase, you'll also learn to balance your *lifestyle*, as well as your diet, by exercising and reducing stress. You'll discover that when you proactively follow a healthy, balanced lifestyle, your weight will naturally diminish and you'll begin to feel abundantly healthy.

Because the long-term Balance Programme is relatively easy and pleasant, adherence to the diet tends to be excellent. Another major reason dieters stick to the diet is because it often stops other common problems caused by food reactions, such as migraines, heartburn, insomnia, skin rashes, irritable bowel syndrome, nasal congestion, sinusitis, and recurrent infections. Becoming free from these common problems is extremely motivating.

During the Balance Programme, the maintenance phase, you are free to make your own food choices from a broad variety of non-reactive foods. In my medical practice and in this book, I provide several sample menu plans, with recipes, that serve as guidelines for dieters. The sample menu plans consist primarily of fresh, whole, unprocessed foods, such as vegetables, fruits, grains, fish, fowl, and legumes. The diet does not focus on caloric restriction, although most healthy, non-reactive foods do tend to be naturally low in calories. As a rule, it's much easier for dieters to stick to healthy foods on this diet than it is on other diets, because they are no longer driven by reactive food cravings.

The principle behind this diet is simple: when people stop eating their own particular reactive foods, their health almost always improves and their weight normalizes. This uncomplicated principle is powerful – and proven.

Five Innovations

Because this diet is a new, unique approach, it adds five important innovations to the battle against obesity. They are:

1. **This diet permanently rids the body of false fat.**
2. **This diet creates permanent loss of adipose tissue through avoidance of reactive foods.**
3. **This diet actually feels good.**
4. **This diet is notably proactive.**
5. **This diet is individualized.**

Now I'll explain these innovations in a little more detail.

Innovation 1. This diet permanently rids the body of false fat.
False fat is the unattractive bloating and swelling that makes
people look and feel *far more fat than they really are*.

No other diet ends the food allergies and sensitivities that
cause false fat. Often, people on other diets look overweight
even after their body-fat
ratio has significantly
improved because their
bodies still bulge with
reactive bloating and
swelling.

The human body is
composed of approxi-
mately 60 per cent to 70
per cent water by weight,
and the vast majority of
overweight people carry
at least 5 to 10 extra
pounds of water weight
at all times. This added
poundage is almost
always the result of
chronic swelling, or
edema, in the tissues,
caused by food reactions.

Unlike the temporary
loss of water weight that
occurs on some conven-
tional caloric restriction
diets, the loss of water
weight on the False Fat
Diet does not occur
because of the short-lived
effect of ketosis, the
urinary flushing of the fat
by-products called
ketones.

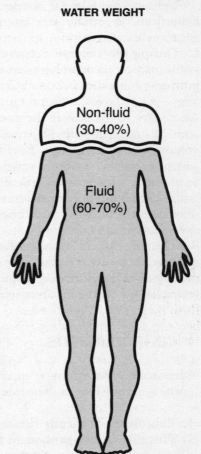

WATER WEIGHT

Non-fluid
(30-40%)

Fluid
(60-70%)

**The average person is
approximately 60–70 per cent water
by weight**

Instead, it occurs because of ongoing avoidance of the re-active foods that directly cause systemic edema. *A loss of at least 5 to 10 pounds happens almost immediately* and can endure for-ever. If the person is notably obese, the water weight loss is even greater. I have observed permanent decreases in tissue swelling in almost all of my weight-loss patients, with an accompanying loss of weight.

Although the false fat of edema is not adipose tissue, it is notably uncomfortable and unattractive, as every woman who gains water weight prior to menstruation already knows. In fact, people with allergic reactive edema frequently look even fatter than people who have more true fat, because edematous puffiness generally collects in the places that are most notice-able – in the face, the abdomen, the buttocks, the thighs, and the ankles. In the face, it often creates a plump, puffy appear-ance and a sagging double chin. In the thighs, it contributes greatly to the dimpling of cellulite; that's why temporary gimmicks, such as thigh wraps that squeeze water away, improve the appearance of cellulite for a short time.

Food allergies and sensitivities cause edema in much the same way that hay fever allergies cause the nasal tissues and eyes to become swollen and watery. When the digestive system is not able to break down foods, food molecules enter the system only partly digested. The immune system then targets these molecules as foreign invaders. It surrounds them with water, as part of the inflammatory response, in an attempt to flush them away. As more reactive foods are introduced, cells become congested with water, resulting in tissue swelling. Fortunately, hay fever season ends when pollen production stops. Food allergies and sensitivities, however, continue indefinitely; their season never ends – unless *we* end it.

The only way to overcome this phenomenon permanently is to avoid ingesting the reactive foods or to overcome your re-action to them. The False Fat Diet is the only diet that helps patients achieve both of these objectives.

As cellular swelling and tissue swelling subside, generally during the first week of the False Fat Diet, so does abdominal bloating. Abdominal bloating, which can add two to three inches to the waistline, is partly caused by the chronic retention of gas in the GI tract, particularly in the small intestine, which reactive foods 'stall'. Partially digested dairy products, for example, often ferment in the intestine for more than a day and cause considerable bloating. In addition, gut tissues themselves often swell with fluid and distend the abdomen. This abdominal distension caused by gas and fluid can create a 'pregnant' or a 'beer belly' look. Because the intestines are more than 20 feet in length, but are compressed into a small area, even moderate increases in gas and fluid retention greatly increase the gut's volume. When people on other diets fail to overcome this bloating, because they are still consuming reactive foods, they typically become discouraged.

On the False Fat Diet, my patients have found that this bloating was mostly resolved within three to five days. Many patients have quickly achieved flat stomachs, often after years of unproductive sit-ups and skipped meals. Bloating never returns, if the patient adheres to the diet and then overcomes his or her food reactions. In almost all cases, this quick success is very motivating.

As patients swiftly shed the false fat of edema and bloating, they often achieve the permanent appearance of a 15- to 25-pound weight loss. These fast, enduring results propel dieters into the Balance Programme, which is the most rewarding phase of all. In this phase, they cast off resistant pounds of true fat.

Innovation 2. This diet creates permanent loss of adipose tissue through avoidance of reactive foods.
As false fat dissolves, so does true fat. The same reactive false fat foods that cause swelling and bloating also trigger biological disasters that usually result in weight gain. The two primary disasters are **food cravings** and **metabolic disorders**.

Food Cravings
Food reactions are the single most common cause of the cravings that destroy diets. These cravings, which are far harder to resist than mere hunger, are similar to the physical urges experienced by alcoholics or cigarette smokers.

As long as a reactive food is in a person's system, it prevents discomfort, just as drinking alcohol prevents an alcoholic's discomfort. Food reactions can even cause the release of the body's own opiates, which is partly why you can become 'addicted' to certain foods. As reactive foods begin to leave the system, though, discomfort begins – just as anxiety and malaise occur when an alcoholic stops drinking. The withdrawal symptoms of food allergies and sensitivities are strongest for about two days, until the reactive foods are cleared from the body.

Conventional diets, unfortunately, usually allow people to eat reactive foods almost every day, and this perpetuates the allergic addiction of food reactions, just as ingesting alcohol or drugs every day would whet the self-destructive appetites of substance abusers.

For many years, it was presumed that most overweight people lacked willpower, but recent research on weight control indicates that overweight people have essentially the same level of emotional strength as thin people. A great many overweight people aren't weak – they're just trapped by the overpowering force of allergic addiction.

Many overweight people develop reactive cravings for junk food and sweets, but others crave 'healthy' foods. One patient of mine, for example, gradually developed a reactive craving for orange juice and grape juice, and ended up drinking about 1,000 calories' worth of these juices every day. She was convinced that juice was healthy for everyone. But she had never been informed that the tartaric acid in grapes and the citric acid in oranges can cause reactions in some people.

Metabolic Disorders

Food allergies and sensitivities contribute strongly to several catastrophic disorders of metabolism:

- They interfere with the hormonal balance of the endocrine system, including the thyroid and adrenal glands. This makes it harder for the body to burn stored fat.
- They disturb insulin levels, even in people who are able to

maintain normal function of the thyroid and adrenals. This signals the body to convert food energy into fat, and also contributes to hypoglycemia.

- They cause mood chemistry disruptions. Food reaction causes levels of the calming neurotransmitter serotonin to plummet, leading to depression, anxiety, and compulsive urges, all of which commonly trigger overeating. Serotonin instability also exacerbates many physical disorders, including migraines, premenstrual syndrome, fibromyalgia, and irritable bowel syndrome. These troublesome conditions often disrupt healthy eating patterns.
- They cause energy and immune dysfunction. Food allergies and sensitivities markedly decrease energy, contribute to insomnia, and dysregulate immunity (because food reactions are usually malfunctions of the immune response). All three of these problems interfere greatly with the ability to exercise. They also contribute markedly to the previously mentioned metabolic disorders.

In addition, food allergies and sensitivities indirectly contribute to the occurrence of candida yeast colonization in mucosal membranes, which causes symptoms similar to those of chronic fatigue syndrome and causes bloating. Unfortunately, yeast colonization then exacerbates food reactions.

The biological disasters that accompany chronic food reactivity occur in a self-perpetuating cycle, as you can see in the diagram on page 31.

Innovation 3. This diet actually feels good.
When I put patients on the False Fat Diet, I am helping cure them of a serious medical disorder – the medical condition of food reactions. Like patients who suffer other medical conditions, these patients, when cured of their allergies and sensitivities, *feel better*. They have notably *more energy*. They have better *cognitive function*. They have fewer *aches and pains*, in both joints and muscles. Their *moods* improve appreciably, and they experience significantly less depression, anxiety and compulsivity. They experience fewer *minor illnesses*. They *breathe* more freely. They have far fewer *PMS symptoms*.

THE FALSE FAT PHENOMENON:
The Fat-Creating Cycle of Food Reactions

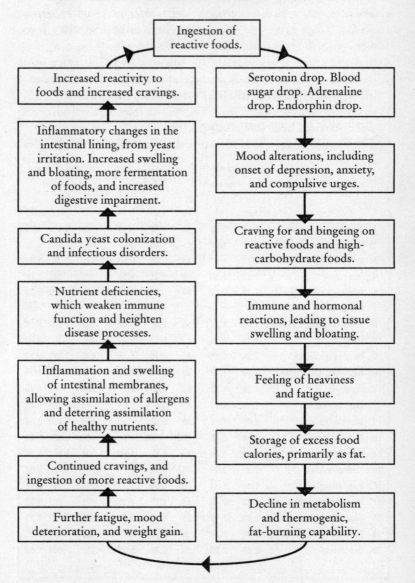

Ingestion of reactive foods.

Increased reactivity to foods and increased cravings.

Serotonin drop. Blood sugar drop. Adrenaline drop. Endorphin drop.

Inflammatory changes in the intestinal lining, from yeast irritation. Increased swelling and bloating, more fermentation of foods, and increased digestive impairment.

Mood alterations, including onset of depression, anxiety, and compulsive urges.

Candida yeast colonization and infectious disorders.

Craving for and bingeing on reactive foods and high-carbohydrate foods.

Nutrient deficiencies, which weaken immune function and heighten disease processes.

Immune and hormonal reactions, leading to tissue swelling and bloating.

Inflammation and swelling of intestinal membranes, allowing assimilation of allergens and deterring assimilation of healthy nutrients.

Feeling of heaviness and fatigue.

Continued cravings, and ingestion of more reactive foods.

Storage of excess food calories, primarily as fat.

Further fatigue, mood deterioration, and weight gain.

Decline in metabolism and thermogenic, fat-burning capability.

They have much less *heartburn* and gastroesophageal reflux. They have fewer migraine and tension *headaches*. They are far less likely to suffer from *irritable bowel syndrome, eczema, hives, recurrent urinary tract infections, or recurrent vaginitis*. They have less *insomnia*. And, of course, they have fewer *cravings for foods*.

I have seen this occur in hundreds of allergy and

COMPARISONS BETWEEN CHANGES IN SELF-REPORTS OF THE EXTENT TO WHICH DISEASE SYMPTOMS ARE BOTHERING THEM BETWEEN AN EXPERIMENTAL GROUP THAT FOLLOWED THE ALCAT FOR FOUR WEEKS AND A CONTROL GROUP THAT FOLLOWED A PROGRAMME OF THEIR OWN CHOOSING

	BASELINE SELF-REPORT Mean Scores			ENDING SELF-REPORT Mean Scores		P-VALUES* FOR CHANGE Mean Scores		
	[1] Exp	[2] Ctl	[3] p-Val	[4] Exp	[5] Ctl	[6] p-Val	[7] Exp	[8] Ctl
1. Migraine headaches	1.52	0.88	.06	0.71	0.56	.532	0.13	0.25
2 Irritable bowel syndrome	1.09	1.17	.81	0.33	1.02	.002	.005	0.59
3. Inflammatory arthritis	0.73	0.81	.78	0.48	0.63	.546	0.34	0.53
4. Gastroesophageal reflux	0.93	1.40	.19	0.21	1.26	<.001	.003	0.70
5. Recurrent sinusitis with infections	2.20	2.38	.64	1.05	2.02	.006	.002	0.33
6. Tension fatigue syndrome	1.59	1.76	.63	0.62	1.60	.001	.002	0.64
7. Eczema	0.36	0.36	.97	0.12	0.47	.023	0.12	0.55
8. Recurrent anxiety	1.34	1.50	.61	0.79	1.40	.042	.062	0.74
9. Recurrent depression	1.39	1.33	.87	0.55	1.23	.017	.003	0.76
10. Insomnia	1.36	1.31	.86	0.55	1.23	.004	.002	0.78
11. Low self-esteem	1.55	1.67	.72	0.64	1.35	.015	.003	0.32
12. Chronic tiredness	1.89	1.86	.93	0.93	1.86	.004	.003	0.99
13. Binge eating	2.34	2.36	.97	0.086	1.74	.004	<.001	0.09
14. Chronic tension	2.00	1.74	.41	0.60	1.58	.001	<.001	0.64
15. Lack of energy	2.34	2.17	.61	1.12	1.95	.011	<.001	0.52
16. Food allergies	1.14	1.29	.69	0.57	1.16	.049	.061	0.74
17. Feeling under stress	2.23	2.45	.48	1.17	2.33	<.001	.001	0.70
18. Cravings for sweets	2.80	3.19	.25	1.14	2.37	<.001	<.001	0.25
19. Cravings for other foods	2.41	2.79	.29	1.17	2.14	.003	<.001	0.07
20. Overeating	2.61	2.83	.56	0.74	0.74	<.001	<.001	.008

SOURCE: *The Bariatrician*, Spring 1996.   *P stands for probability

overweight patients. The table on page 32 presents the results of a study of improvements in the quality of life of patients on an allergy-free weight-loss diet. All of the patients in this study identified their food reactions by using the ALCAT cell-reaction testing system, which I'll describe later.

No other diet offers these improvements in quality of life.

Of course, many diets justifiably claim that when patients overcome obesity, they become less susceptible to heart disease, diabetes, and some forms of cancer. However, with most other diets, you've got to suffer to get there. With the False Fat Diet, getting there is half the fun.

The False Fat Diet feels good simply because people who engage in it are generally <u>cured of a medical disorder</u> and become healthier. **With the False Fat Diet, patients don't become healthy by becoming thin, they become thin by becoming healthy.**

Obviously, these quality-of-life *side benefits* are a tremendous motivating factor for patients. By far the biggest reason that people fail to achieve long-term success on most diets is because the diets are unpleasant. My patients, though, tend to have superior long-term adherence rates because they feel *good* on this diet.

Furthermore, they don't feel good when they go off the diet and eat their reactive foods, because their uncomfortable symptoms return. This negative reinforcement also makes adherence easier. It's similar to how easy it can be to avoid red wine after you've learned that it gives you migraines. You may miss the wine somewhat, but your main association with it is pain, not pleasure.

Innovation 4. This diet is notably proactive.
On most diets, it's not what you *do* that counts, it's what you *don't* do: you don't eat *much*. Often, the very best thing the dieter can do is to passively do nothing.

On the False Fat Diet, which focuses more on regaining health, fitness, and body shape than losing scale weight, patients participate in their own recovery from food reactions and obesity. They actively rebuild their health by following a systematic programme of rejuvenation.

The simplistic notion that weight control depends almost solely upon how much you eat and how many calories you burn through exercise is outdated. Even the most deadly diseases, such as cancer and cardiovascular disease, are caused by multiple factors and respond best to multidimensional healing approaches – and weight control is no different. Weight control is not as simple as 'You are what you eat.' Your weight is also influenced by what you breathe, what you do, what you drink, and even what you think. For example, toxins that congest the liver deter the liver from emulsifying fat. Therefore, the toxic additives in a synthetic non-fat food might cause a greater weight gain than ingestion of a similar full-fat, natural food. Toxin-induced weight gain is common because so many artificial flavours are added to foods, along with preservatives and fillers. (In fact, the average person eats about 5 pounds of these additives each year.)

By the same token, chronic exposure to stress impairs adrenal and thyroid activity, which can result in weight gain – even without overeating.

Therefore, my weight control patients engage in comprehensive, individualized health-building programmes. They practice various **detoxification** measures, such as short cleansing fasts, intestinal cleansing, saunas, dry skin brushing, and use of detoxifying herbs and nutrients. They take individualized **dietary supplements** to nurture their organs and glands of digestion and immunity, to increase energy, and to stimulate and support metabolism. They do aerobic and weight-training **exercise**, not just to burn calories, but also to eliminate toxins and improve metabolism. They practice various forms of **stress management**. They also work on curing **individual metabolic problems**, such as candidiasis.

All of these efforts help their bodies overcome allergies and sensitivities and regain health. In addition, these activities help shift people's focus away from scale weight to health and vitality. When my patients embrace the concept of becoming as healthy as possible, their food reactions invariably diminish, and their weight decreases *almost automatically*.

Furthermore, when my patients stay busy by proactively participating in a multifaceted programme, it often ends their emotional obsession with food. This obsession is relatively common among dieters, especially when they have fought allergic addictions during years of restrictive diets.

Innovation 5. This diet is individualized.
Conventional weight-loss diets recommend the same dietary programme for almost every person. Most diets do not even endorse the most rudimentary elements of individualization, such as adjusting portion sizes in relation to a person's weight and level of activity. For example, an obese 250-pound male construction worker would be advised to eat the same menu plan as a 130-pound female office worker.

The only recent diet that attempted to individualize its programme was one that based four diets on the four main blood types. My own clinical observation of this diet was that it did work well initially for some dieters – mostly those who significantly altered their food choices. In fact, other diets also work well initially, when people radically change the types of foods they eat. I believe that the reason this happens is because engaging in full-scale dietary change generally forces people to abandon the frequently eaten foods to which they've become reactive. If someone has been eating a low-fat, high-carbohydrate diet for years, they may lose weight when they switch to a higher-protein diet, since it will exclude many of their reactive foods. Therefore, rigid, extremist diets often work well in the early stages.

However, in the long term, people tend to develop new reactions to the foods they eat too frequently. This undoubtedly contributes to the eventual failure of many of the rigid diets.

On the False Fat Diet, though, patients comfortably participate for years at a time in the Balance Programme, in which they eat their own varied, balanced regimen of wholesome, non-reactive foods. This prevents new food allergies and sensitivities and provides the wide array of nutrients the body needs to heal.

Each patient's programme is somewhat different because each patient is different. On this diet you will not only learn your own reactive foods, but will also determine your own metabolic type. Your metabolic type largely governs the general kind of diet that you will thrive upon. For example, some dieters do best on an essentially vegetarian diet, while others do better on a diet that contains a moderate amount of meat and other animal protein. People with naturally efficient digestive metabolisms tend to do better on slowly oxidized foods, such as meat, while people with sluggish metabolisms generally fare better on quickly oxidized foods, such as fruits and vegetables. You will determine your own metabolic type by responding to the questionnaire in Chapter 9 on page 250.

You will probably discover that the False Fat Diet will be a pleasant return to the more balanced eating patterns you enjoyed before you began to engage in extremist, one-size-fits-all diets. Many of my patients have found that they can eat tempting foods that have long been denied to them, as long as they stay away from their reactive foods.

To recognize your reactive foods, however, you need the help of either a consulting physician or this book, because many reactive foods are hidden. For example, if your reactive food is corn, you need to become aware of all the foods in which corn products appear, including corn syrup, which is placed in hundreds of processed foods.

When patients first consult with me, they often presume that they have to give up all their favourite foods and suffer to be thin. But that's just not true. When my patients begin the False Fat Diet and start eating normal portions of a wide variety of foods, including foods that they had denied themselves for years, it can feel like a homecoming. Then when they quickly lose the swelling and bloating of false fat and begin to drop pound after pound of true fat, they sometimes are incredulous about the long melodrama of yo-yo dieting they had endured. They sometimes ask themselves, 'Is this really all there is to it? Why didn't someone mention this sooner?'

The Development of the Diet:
A Short History

The False Fat Diet was painstakingly developed through my large clinical practice over more than two decades. Most of the people who have been on the False Fat Diet have been my own patients or patients of my associates at the Preventive Medical Center of Marin, north of San Francisco. The first person to go on the diet, however, was not one of these patients – it was me.

In 1975, when I was just beginning my medical practice, I attended a lecture on the potential health benefits of short juice fasts. I decided to go on a lemonade fast myself for a few days, to see if it would produce any discernible improvements. I enjoyed it. It made me feel more energetic and clearheaded. Hoping to prolong my improved sense of vitality, I began to add foods back to my diet gradually, sticking to just healthy, whole foods, such as fresh fruits and vegetables. Then, during the first ten days of my new diet, a remarkable thing happened. I lost almost 15 pounds.

A great deal of the weight I lost – as much as 10 of the 15 pounds – seemed to be water weight, because it came off very quickly. Another sign that this loss was water weight was that it didn't come from just the fatty tissue in my midsection, but from throughout my entire body, including my hands, feet, ankles, and face.

My first thought was that this loss of water had come from the process of ketosis, which can happen during quick weight loss. But I didn't have any of the classic symptoms of ketosis, such as the characteristic odour in the breath. I began to think that the loss of water weight must have come from the correction of systemic edema.

Before my systemic tissue swelling had disappeared, I hadn't been particularly aware of it, although sometimes my hands had felt slightly swollen and occasionally my face had seemed rather puffy. But once the subtle swelling was gone, I could really feel the difference. Because the body is approximately two-thirds water by weight, I was carrying over 150 pounds of water, and any significant decrease in this water weight was very noticeable. Due to the loss of swelling in my face, I looked significantly slimmer to myself in the mirror, and my whole body felt more supple. To me, it looked as if I had lost even more than 15 pounds.

Another major reason I looked as if I'd lost more weight than I had was because my stomach was suddenly much flatter. My waist size decreased noticeably, even though I still carried almost as much adipose tissue around my midsection. My stomach had seemed to shrink, but this shrinkage was mostly just the absence of bloatedness. Prior to my new diet, my stomach had commonly expanded just after a meal into a tight, round balloon, and would stay that way for hours. Since I liked eating at night, I'd often go to bed bloated.

I'd never given much thought to this bloating and swelling, because I'd experienced them for as long as I could remember. As a boy growing up in Detroit at the height of the baby boom, I lived on the standard American fare of burgers, fries, sodas, and shakes. While I was still young, my father bought a neighbourhood shop with a long sweet counter, which I frequented, and I became somewhat pudgy, especially in my belly. I was active as a high school athlete, playing football, baseball, and tennis, but I was 30 to 40 pounds overweight.

At the University of Michigan's School of Medicine, I continued to eat carelessly and remained overweight. I often felt sluggish and suffered from allergies and chronic sinus congestion. Nothing in my med school curriculum, however, led me to believe that my lack of vitality was abnormal. By the medical standards of the time, I was considered quite healthy, because I didn't suffer from any overt diseases. In fact, among my fellow med students, feeling exhausted and depleted was a proud sign of diligence.

Nonetheless, the first seeds of the integrative medicine movement were beginning to bud during the late 1960s, and were particularly evident at the progressive University of Michigan in Ann Arbor, which was known as the 'Berkeley of the Midwest.' I was intellectually influenced by this movement but, true to the style of doctors of that day, didn't let it encroach upon my own lifestyle.

When I moved to the Bay Area for my early years of practice in the 1970s, though, I was further impressed with the
power of holistic ideas. The patients I saw who followed the
tenets of natural medicine were robustly healthy, but I wasn't
sure why. I remember one patient, a 64-year-old man, who still
ran marathons and looked about 40. His skin was smooth and
unwrinkled, and his eyes held a sharp spark of vitality. He'd
been on a nutritious whole foods diet, exercised, and taken
nutritional supplements since the 1950s, when many people
had teased him about being a 'health food nut.' At 64, though,
he was getting the last laugh. His health was truly extraordinary, but I didn't then understand the biochemical
complexities of how he'd done it.

Another patient, for whom I did some routine work, recovered from a supposedly incurable case of cancer while
following a strict diet and lifestyle programme. I was astonished by her recovery, and deeply puzzled.

I felt as if I had spent four years in medical school studying
diseases – many of them arcane diseases that no-one ever
seemed to have – but that I'd learned very little about health.
So I spent the next five years studying health and healing. I
learned about nutrition, herbology, mind-body medicine,
acupuncture, traditional Chinese medicine, and bodywork,
and I looked at how these techniques could be integrated into
modern medicine. I also began to apply these practices to my
own life, taking to heart the adage 'Physician, heal thyself.'

In the tradition of the Eastern healers, I adopted the
attitude that the highest aspiration for a doctor should be to
become a philosopher-physician who didn't play God with
patients, but simply taught them how to create and maintain
good health. I began a programme that charged patients a
yearly fee, and I would care for them without charge if they
became ill.

I soon decided to take my approach to a wider patient base
and moved into a large clinic with other doctors. Eventually I
became director of the clinic, having since expanded it twice
and added a branch. In accord with my role as a teacher, I also
began to write. My first book was *Staying Healthy with the
Seasons*, which has now had more than twenty printings. My

most prominent book is probably *Staying Healthy with Nutrition*, which is used in a number of college courses and nutrition certification programmes. My most popular book to date has been *The Detox Diet*, which helps readers overcome addictive habits.

It was still early in my career, though, when I went on my first brief fast, and then embarked upon the programme of dietary change that would become the False Fat Diet.

After my fast, as I added foods to my diet, I noted that several of them caused an immediate return of my former symptoms, including water weight gain, bloating, nasal congestion, and lethargy. I also found that eating some foods, such as wheat, could trigger withdrawal symptoms, including food cravings, which seemed similar to the cravings suffered by my substance abuse patients. The intensity of these food cravings surprised me.

I began to suspect that my reactions were symptoms of allergies. When I surveyed the medical literature, however, I found that most conventional allergists, almost all of whom focused their practices on airborne allergies, considered food allergy to be quite rare. They maintained that all food allergies occurred immediately upon eating, and were caused by reactions of an immune system substance called IgE (immunoglobulin E). The only effective way to test for food allergy, they said, was to scratch the skin slightly, insert a small amount of a suspected allergen, and note reactive changes. These skin changes were similar to symptoms experienced by people with classic food allergies: wheezing, hives, runny nose, and anaphylactic shock.

As I dug deeper, however, I found that there was a relatively small, progressive group of allergists who believed that a more subtle type of food reaction existed and was very common. Some of these allergists referred to this type of allergy as a food sensitivity, although others simply called it an allergy. This type of food reaction generally did not provoke *classic* allergic symptoms, such as a runny nose or wheezing. In addition, its symptoms frequently did not occur *immediately* (because of reactions of the IgE-releasing cells), but could occur as much as three days later, because of continuing reactions of an antibody called IgG (immuno-globulin G). Symptoms caused by these delayed food sensitivities, according to these allergists, covered a wide range, and could include headaches, joint pain, congestion, heartburn, fatigue, mood swings, immune dysfunction, recurrent infections – and tissue swelling and abdominal bloating. Furthermore, doctors who treated IgG-mediated delayed food sensitivities did not rely upon the orthodox scratch test, but instead used blood testing or elimination diets.

Many of the doctors I talked to felt that up to two-thirds of the general population had at least some minor food reactions. They also believed that this incidence was much higher among subpopulations of patients with certain problems, including migraines, asthma, hay fever, chronic nasal congestion – and obesity. Among these people, incidence of sensitivities was believed to be as high as 90 per cent.

By the time I had my own blood tested for food reactions, I had already figured out many of my own reactions by the simple trial-and-error method of the elimination diet, in which I limited my diet to just a few foods for a couple of days and then added foods one at a time, noting reactions. Because my metabolism had been severely stressed and overloaded for many years, I had at least minor reactions to many of the Sensitive Seven foods that most often cause allergies: wheat, sugar, dairy products, eggs, corn, soya, and peanuts.

Of course, it was somewhat difficult for me to avoid the foods I'd previously regarded as staples. I also had to start reading food labels more carefully and avoiding processed foods in order to avoid hidden foodstuffs, such as the more than 120 pounds of hidden sugars that the average person eats each year. But as my energy, mood, cognitive function, and general health began to rocket upward, it seemed a minor price to pay. As my cravings subsided, adherence became increasingly easy.

I continued to lose weight on the diet. In less than a year, I lost another 25 pounds, all of it in adipose tissue, or true fat. Combined with the 15 pounds I'd lost during the diet's first 10 days, I lost a total of 40 pounds. Of that 40 pounds, at least 10 to 15 pounds were from false fat water weight, which I lost permanently.

After I was sure the diet was safe and effective, I began recommending it to patients. The results they achieved were uniformly positive and sometimes spectacular. Patients consistently lost weight and were generally able to maintain their weight loss.

Most patients also recorded important secondary improvements, such as fewer headaches, a reduction in aches and pains, less frequent colds and infections, and more energy. As a rule, these secondary gains synergistically supported weight loss. One patient, for example, who lost about 25 pounds, told me that she could never have stuck with the diet just to lose weight, but she stayed with it because it made her irritable bowel syndrome and migraines go away. Because the diet improved her whole life so much, she said, it was 'practically addictive'.

Many of my weight control patients were not obese, but were mildly to moderately overweight, as is approximately 60 per cent of the public. As a rule, these people responded even better than obese patients. In general, the less weight people have to lose, the easier it is for them to reach their goals. After going on the diet, my mildly overweight patients – many of whom didn't carry much extra adipose tissue, but were primarily just bloated and swollen from allergies – often looked and felt great. One of my patients, Chloe, 29, lost only about 5 pounds of adipose tissue on the diet, according to a body-fat ratio test, but looked remarkably slimmer. She had lost a great deal of false fat and reported that most of her friends thought she'd lost at least 20 pounds.

A great many patients also succeeded, however, even when they were clinically obese, which is defined as being 20 per

---

THE SENSITIVE SEVEN:
MOST COMMONLY REACTIVE FOODS

1. Dairy products	5. Soya
2. Wheat	6. Eggs
3. Corn	7. Peanuts
4. Sugar	

cent over your ideal weight. I clearly recall the success of one of my early patients on the diet, Meaghan, who was 40 pounds overweight. Meaghan, who was 35 at the time, was really unhappy when I first consulted with her. Besides her obesity, she was clinically depressed and suffered from chronic nasal congestion, which often led to sinus infections. At first she was reluctant to try any kind of diet, because she had gone hungry on many diets in the past and had always regained more weight than she'd lost. This is a common phenomenon, because of the destruction that severe caloric restriction wreaks upon the metabolism.

Also, she told me, three other doctors who had placed her on diets had, as she put it, 'given up on me,' after their diets had failed. All three of them had implied that she was weak-willed. I ultimately convinced Meaghan that my diet was different from any other she'd ever tried.

We used a standard elimination diet to determine Meaghan's food reactions. For several days she ate only a few different fruits and vegetables, and occasionally grilled chicken. She ate more than enough to keep from being hungry, but at first she still craved bread, cheese, and yogurt, which she had previously been eating excessively. Her prior dependence upon these foods and her craving of them were both strong indicators that these were her reactive false fat foods. Usually, as part of a vicious cycle, people become re-active to the foods they eat most often and then begin to overeat the foods to which they've become reactive. This is very common and extremely destructive. A small part of the craving is psychological, but it's mostly a biochemical reaction.

After Meaghan had avoided dairy products and wheat for a little less than a week, however, most of the biochemical traces of them had left her body, and her craving for them decreased greatly. I also helped her manage these cravings with nutritional supplements, which you'll learn about later on.

As her cravings vanished, Meaghan began to feel much better, physically and emotionally. Her nasal stuffiness cleared up, and she told me it was 'like taking a clothespeg off my nose – I could *breathe* again.' She felt more energetic, and her depression lifted.

After approximately one week, Meaghan 'challenged' her system by eating a pot of yogurt. It was a high quality organic plain yogurt, which she had always considered a very healthy food. But for her, it was practically poison. The same hour she ate it, her nasal passages clamped shut, she got heartburn, and her energy level plummeted. I wasn't surprised at the intensity of her reaction, because people who have eliminated reactive foods from their systems often respond dramatically when that food is reintroduced.

During the uncomfortable period after her symptoms returned, Meaghan felt an almost overpowering urge to eat more yogurt. She had the intuitive feeling – which was quite correct – that if she ate more yogurt, it would make her symptoms go away, at least temporarily. Caught in the web of allergic addiction, she was terribly tempted by yogurt, just as an alcoholic is tempted to keep drinking after he's fallen off the wagon and taken his fateful first drink. She wasn't just hungry for yogurt – she *craved* it.

Meaghan told me that her craving was an odd sensation. 'My stomach was full, but I was *dying* for more yogurt. It tasted fabulous – sweet and creamy – and I just started spooning it into my mouth, almost hypnotically.' She ate three more containers of yogurt.

It was obvious that we'd discovered one of her primary reactive foods.

Meaghan wasn't just hungry.
She had reactive food cravings.
There's a big difference.

Meaghan stopped eating dairy products again, and the first couple of days were difficult. She was puffy and bloated, and felt irritable, but I helped her get through her withdrawal phase with several powerful techniques – all of which I'll tell you about later – and soon she was feeling great again.

Next, she challenged her system with wheat. Similar results: disaster! This time, though, she knew what to expect, and didn't give in to the urge to binge. Her symptoms settled down much more quickly, and her well-being returned.

After those two experiences, she didn't feel very tempted by wheat or dairy products. She associated them more with pain than pleasure. She kept adding foods back to her diet, but some of them significantly provoked her symptoms. She had mild reactions to shrimp, broccoli, and oranges, but everything else seemed to 'agree' with her.

Meaghan quickly found substitutes for wheat and milk. This was much easier than she thought it would be, because almost all supermarkets now stock a rich variety of non-dairy and non-wheat substitutes for their allergic customers.

Almost every day, Meaghan's health and vitality reached new levels. She became very enthusiastic about her new eating strategy, because it made her feel and look so much better. Right away she lost about 10 pounds, mostly by overcoming her reactive cellular swelling. Her lactose intolerance had also caused considerable bloating, since dairy products are the most common cause of chronic gas, bloating, and diarrhoea. In addition, she had far more energy, because her adrenal glands no longer had to pump out adrenal hormones, day and night, just to combat her allergic symptoms. Her increased adrenal efficiency also improved her mood.

Within three months, she lost nearly 40 pounds. She also improved her life in other ways. She ended an unsatisfying relationship and even got a better job. She became much more active and content and, to my knowledge, has never regained an excessive amount of weight.

Meaghan's success, early in the development of this diet, was very heartening to me. It showed me that most weight-control patients – even those that other doctors had discarded – really weren't weak or self-destructive. They just had a simple physical problem: food reactions.

Most people, including overweight people, are *strong*. They work hard all their lives and make the best of every bad situation. They endure low energy, food cravings, and even the scorn of other people. *But they don't quit.* They try one approach after another, even when each new approach fails.

Too often, though, when a medical approach fails these

people, it's not because the patients failed to follow their doctor's orders — it's because the *doctors failed their patients*. They didn't give the patients the right kind of information to solve the problem.

When people know the right action to take, they'll usually take it. Nobody's perfect, but *perfection isn't necessary* for health and fitness. All that's necessary is good information, hard work, and the faith that fuels motivation.

In Chapter 2, I will give you all the information you'll need to melt off false fat. By this time next week, you can be rid of the bloating and swelling that make you feel fat.

In Chapter 3, I'll tell you how to burn away the true fat that's hurting your health and holding you back.

I know you can do it!

Let's get started!

2

WHY YOU WILL LOSE FALSE FAT

DONNA DIDN'T LOOK FAT, AT LEAST NOT IN THE LEGGINGS and long sweater she was wearing as she entered my office. Her legs looked slender and fit, and her sweater hid the rest. But she *felt* fat.

'I've got a guy's type of weight problem,' she said as she sat down. She was animated and energetic, but obviously frustrated. 'Women are supposed to collect fat in their hips and thighs – aren't they? – but mine sticks right here.' She patted her stomach. When she was sitting, I could see that it bulged, even under the thick sweater. 'I hardly ever overeat,' she said, 'but since I've hit 40, I get *no forgiveness* from my body. It's like my metabolism took early retirement. I take *two bites* and I can feel the fat cells around my waist start to expand. *Literally.* I pinch my love handles, and they're *thicker* before I even get up from the table.' She looked at me expectantly, as if I might not believe her. 'My last doctor,' she said with a sour look, 'told me there's no way that food could make me fat that *fast*. But I can *feel* it happening.' Again, she searched my face for reassurance. She had an upbeat personality, but she was almost ready to give up. She ate carefully, exercised hard, and still carried 20 extra pounds.

'It's not your imagination,' I said. 'That feeling of instant weight gain happens to a lot of people. But it's not fat you're gaining. It's fluid retention and bloating, and you're probably getting it from food reactions. A lot of the swelling and bloating from food reactions occurs directly in and around the gut.

That's why you feel it in your midsection right away.'

'If it's not fat,' she said, 'why doesn't it leave as fast as it comes? I look like this almost all the time.'

'Your biochemistry won't allow it to go away, because your body is trying to *protect* you. When you eat reactive foods, your body sees them as foreign substances, almost as poisons, and it goes all out to protect you. It can take two to three days to stop reacting to some foods.'

'But it's not like I eat *junk*. I'm an old-time you-are-what-you-eat type. I was eating granola before they even had a name for it.' She smiled, but I could see she felt cheated. For many years, she'd followed all the rules – but the rules had been wrong.

'People can become reactive to *healthy* foods,' I said, 'even granola, if you eat it all the time. Do you eat a lot of non-fat and artificially sweetened foods?'

'Now that my metabolism has slowed down, I've *got* to.'

'I hate to say it, but some of those "lite" foods may be doing you more harm than good. If you're reactive to a food, it can be virtually calorie-free and still make you gain weight. Even diet soda can cause bloating and swelling.' She looked surprised. Most people these days are so accustomed to counting calories and fat grams – the *quantity* of their food – that they forget about the importance of *quality*.

'I don't think you're eating too many calories,' I said. 'And I don't think your age is the real problem. Your metabolism is slowing down just 5 per cent every decade, and that's not enough to cause what you're experiencing. I think you've just developed some food reactions over a long period of time. When you resolve them, you'll lost your weight.'

'But I was tested for allergies and they didn't find any.'

'Did they explain that not all food reactions are allergies?' I asked.

'No.'

I wasn't surprised. Most doctors don't really understand food reactions. They usually have an all-or-nothing attitude; they think that you either have a classic food allergy, with hives and wheezing, or you have nothing at all.

I gave Donna a brief rundown on how food reactions work

and how they cause bloating and swelling. I explained it out of respect for her. Some doctors think it's acceptable to tell patients what to do, without telling them why, but I object to that approach. If patients are willing to change their lives by taking my advice, they deserve to know exactly *why* these changes will help.

As I gave all the details to Donna, she listened attentively and took notes. Over the next few weeks, she eliminated her false fat foods – one of which was oats, a primary ingredient in most granola – and dropped about 15 pounds.

Now I'll give *you* the details on how food reactions get started. Then we'll look at how they cause bloating and swelling.

If you're going to make changes in your life, you deserve to know exactly what's going on.

I'm sure some of this information will hit home. Often, when I tell patients about food reactions, they say, 'That's *me* you're describing.'

For years, Donna
followed all the rules.
But the rules were wrong.

The Risk Factors That Cause Food Reactions

The primary cause of most food reactions is incomplete digestion. At almost every meal, we eat foods that we don't completely digest. The results are disastrous. When we eat foods we can't digest, we almost always have some type of reaction.

Food that isn't completely digested can enter our systems in large food macromolecules that cause a great deal of trouble. The body perceives these macromolecules of partly digested food as foreign invaders, similar to bacteria, viruses, or parasites. Then the body attacks them with the full force of the immune system.

This immune inflammatory attack creates the symptoms that you hate: fatigue, weakness, heartburn, aching joints and muscles, nasal stuffiness – and false fat.

There are several factors that most often cause incomplete digestion. To get started on the False Fat Diet, you've got to understand these factors and avoid them. In order of importance, here they are.

Risk Factor 1. We eat too narrow a range of foods.

It's estimated that the average person gets about 75 per cent of his or her calories from just ten different foods. Most of us have our favourite foods, such as wheat and dairy products, and we rely on them far too much. When we overeat any one food, we exhaust our body's ability to fully digest it.

Risk Factor 2. We eat too many fake foods.

We eat synthetic foods, such as fake fat and artificial sugar, that are manufactured in factories. No wonder we can't digest this stuff! Furthermore, most of our packaged foods have been crammed with chemicals that human bodies cannot adequately metabolize. Often, a synthetic food has a long shelf life precisely because it *can't* be broken down by nature.

Risk Factor 3. We have digestive enzyme deficiencies.

Many people are dangerously low in the enzymes that digest food. Even when these people eat healthy foods, they don't have enough pancreatic enzymes to break the foods down properly.

Millions of people haven't been genetically endowed with the right digestive enzymes to thrive on a modern, industrialized diet. For example, African Americans are ten times more likely than Caucasians to lack the enzyme that breaks down milk. Because a lack of enzymes is a common problem, the False Fat Diet generally includes supplementation with specific enzymes.

Another cause of enzyme insufficiency is our failure to ingest the natural enzymes that exist in foods. Many whole, unprocessed foods automatically come with the enzymes that are needed to help digest them, but before we eat these foods, we often *kill* the enzymes by cooking, processing, irradiation, and storage.

Because it's important to eat foods with live enzymes still in them, patients on the False Fat Diet tend to eat a lot of fresh, whole, raw foods.

Another critically important digestive substance that millions of people lack is stomach acid, or hydrochloric acid. Unfortunately, production of this acid decreases as we age, which is why indigestion is more common among older people. Many people mistakenly think they have *too much* stomach acid, because they often get heartburn – but the opposite can be true. Heartburn can also be a sign of *low* acid. When you don't have enough existing stomach acid from day to day, your stomach secretes *too much* when you eat to make up for the deficiency. Later on, I'll tell you how to fix this deficiency.

Risk Factor 4. We eat food that is too refined.
Too much of our food is stripped of fibre and then shredded, pulverized, powdered – and finally stuck back together again with gluey fillers. By the time we eat it, it's not much more than a predigested mush of starch and sugar. Unfortunately, this excessive processing often allows the food to rush into the bloodstream before it undergoes the complete digestive process. If this 'predigested' food still had its fibre, it would stay in the gut long enough to be fully digested, or it would be carried all the way through the system by the fibre and eliminated. Because of this factor, I urge people to avoid overly refined foods.

Risk Factor 5. We create our own intestinal problems.
One of the most common and harmful of these problems is a condition that allows undigested food macromolecules to slip through the intestinal wall. This condition is called 'leaky gut syndrome,' and doctors have only recently realized how hazardous it is. A leaky gut's wall is more permeable than it should be.

This permeability can be caused by eating chemical additives and also by drinking coffee or alcohol with meals. If you've noticed that you most frequently have food reactions when you have a cocktail with dinner or coffee with breakfast, you may have leaky gut syndrome.

Another primary cause of leaky gut syndrome is overgrowth of the natural yeast *Candida albicans*. Candida is usually present in the body and is mostly found in the mucous membranes – especially those in the intestines. It normally stays in balance with other healthy bacteria, but it can get out of control and increase gut wall permeability. It proliferates if you:

- Take antibiotics, which kill all bacteria.
- Take birth control pills.
- Take steroid drugs.
- Eat foods, such as sugar, that cause yeast to multiply.
- Eat things that contain lots of yeast, such as bread and beer.
- Have impaired immunity.

Candida is a major cause of bloating and often causes a 'beer belly' look. In fact, I think that many heavy beer drinkers with beer bellies aren't nearly as far as they look, but are just swollen with candida, reactive gas, and fluids. I had one patient who lost his beer belly in a matter of days on the False Fat Diet. He was thrilled with his quick response, and it motivated him to stay with the diet.

Risk Factor 6. We eat too much at once.
Overeating causes food reactions by overwhelming the digestive system. Unfortunately, *reactions* also cause *overeating* by creating food cravings, and this destructive cycle ruins many lives. The problem gets even worse when people eat the exact foods that cause them to experience reactions. This often happens, however, because of the cravings caused by allergic addiction.

Overeating also disrupts the immune response, which further heightens food reactions.

Risk Factor 7. We're under too much stress.
Stress hurts digestion. When you're under stress, your stress

hormones – such as adrenaline and cortisol – take blood away from your organs of digestion and shift it to the fight-or-flight organs and systems, such as the muscles, eyes, and heart. Sometimes, when you're nervous, you feel this loss of circulation in your digestive system as butterflies in the stomach.

Proper digestion is most likely to occur when we take time to eat our meals in a relaxed atmosphere. However, the average worker sits down for lunch for only eleven minutes, and many for only five minutes, or eats a sandwich unconsciously while working.

Risk Factor 8. We don't chew our foods completely.
This interferes significantly with digestion. Foods that remain in excessively large pieces can't be broken down properly, even when enough digestive juices are available.

Risk Factor 9. We drink too many liquids with our meals.
This dilutes digestive juices and stomach acid, keeping them from fully digesting our foods.

Risk Factor 10. We combine too many of these risk factors.
If we regularly made just *one* of these mistakes, we might not have a problem. Most people, though, combine several of these risk factors, and soon they experience the straw that breaks the camel's back. Doctors call this reaching the allergic threshold.

All of these risk factors can cause your digestive system to dump large, unwieldy macromolecules of food into your bloodstream. When this happens, it generally triggers your immune response.

If your immune system is *already* impaired, your immune reaction to these macromolecules of food will be even worse. You'll get reactions to a wider variety of foods, and your symptoms will be more severe and more frequent. Many forces can impair immunity: poor nutrition, exposure to toxins, stress, and lack of sleep.

Therefore, to avoid food reactions, you should not only minimize your risk factors, but should also try to optimize your immune strength, with a healthy lifestyle, ingestion of specific nutrients, and avoidance of toxins. I'll soon tell you how to do this.

In addition, a number of *non-food factors* can make food reactions worse by contributing to the allergic threshold. The body doesn't care if an allergen is a food-borne allergen or an airborne allergen, such as pollen. To the body, an allergen is an allergen. Food reactions are worse in people who inhale airborne allergens, are exposed to toxic chemicals, or are under stress.

Therefore, *you are not just what you eat.*

Food reactions — and therefore fat — can be caused by many factors, and food is just the most obvious one.

I know that this is a new, strange concept for many people. But I have tested this concept clinically and have seen it work wonders.

Here's an example: a patient of mine worked in a paint shop and regularly inhaled airborne toxins. This man was bloated, puffy, and red-eyed most of the time, and reacted strongly to a number of foods. He also got sick a lot because the toxins he breathed were stressing his immune system. When he switched jobs and escaped the constant assault of airborne pollutants, his sensitivity to foods decreased dramatically. His progress on the False Fat Diet accelerated tremendously when he quit his job, and he soon lost almost all of his false fat and most of his true fat. Simultaneously, he stopped having frequent minor illnesses.

If any of these risk factors apply to you, you are vulnerable to food reactions.

You are not just *what you eat.*
Fat can be caused by many factors.
Food is just the most obvious one.

Now I'll tell you how food reactions develop within your body, after you engage in these risk factors. Once you understand how food reactions work, you'll be better able to stop them — forever.

How Food Reactions Work

When large food macromolecules enter the system, they wreak havoc. They create the two different types of food reactions, **allergies** and **sensitivities**.

IS THIS YOU?

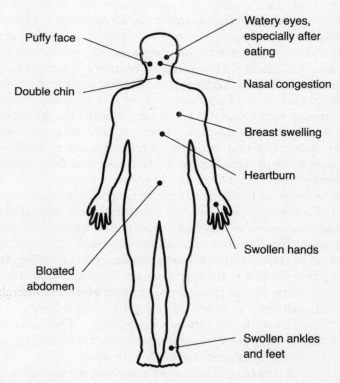

Puffy face

Watery eyes, especially after eating

Double chin

Nasal congestion

Breast swelling

Heartburn

Swollen hands

Bloated abdomen

Swollen ankles and feet

Food allergies are more immediate and usually more severe than sensitivities, and are harder to cure, but they aren't at all common. Sensitivities are usually more subtle, but unfortunately, they're extremely common. Both of these conditions can make you fat. Let's take a look at them so that you'll know how to get over the problems they cause.

Food Allergies

Allergy has been recognized for centuries. Even the ancient Egyptians knew that certain substances, such as cat hair, pollen, and shellfish, 'didn't agree' with some people. But they didn't know why.

The first person to categorize food allergy as a medical condition was Hippocrates, the father of modern medicine, who noted that some people reacted negatively to cheese while others didn't. But Hippocrates couldn't figure out why this happened.

In the 1920s, doctors finally began to understand the biochemistry of allergy. They found a substance in itchy, allergic skin that wasn't in healthy skin. It wasn't until the 1960s, though, that researchers realized that this substance was an immune system substance known as an antibody. Antibodies are sent out by the immune system to kill foreign invaders, such as bacteria and parasites. Antibodies are essential for keeping us healthy and are powerful enough to kill worms in the intestines.

The name of the antibody that is found in allergic skin is IgE, or immunoglobulin E. IgE antibodies are most abundant in the mucous membranes of the digestive tract, lungs, eyes, and nose – the very places allergic symptoms are strongest. IgE antibodies not only attack foreign substances themselves, but also signal the rest of the immune system to launch an all-out attack. When this happens, the immune system inaugurates the inflammatory response, flooding the affected areas with extra fluid to wash away the foreign invaders. This can result in swollen, itchy eyes, a congested nose, and swelling and bloating in the abdomen.

These protective inflammatory reactions often involve the release of several chemicals, one of which is well known: histamine. Histamine dilates capillaries and makes them release fluid into tissues, causing swelling. You've probably taken antihistamines when you wanted to dry up cold symptoms, which are partly caused by histamines attacking viruses.

Other protective chemicals are also released, including kinins and leukotrienes, both of which pull water out of the blood and force it into tissues. They can help make your eyes puffy and can make your abdomen swell with false fat.

Once an IgE antibody has recognized a macromolecule of food as a foreign invader, it has an indelible 'memory' of this food. Each antibody is marked for a specific substance and attacks only that substance. After the first encounter, the antibody is programmed to attack the food *every time it enters the system*.

Antibodies live in white blood cells, which can have as many as 100,000 available areas, or receptor sites, for IgE antibodies. A person with *no* allergies will have white blood cells that are almost *empty* of IgE antibodies, but people who have allergies will often have *every one* of these 100,000 sites filled — on billions of white blood cells.

Therefore, once you've developed an allergy, your body is primed to make a powerful response every time the allergen enters your system.

Allergies can begin at any time, but seem to be somewhat more common in youth, and in midlife and beyond. At their most severe, classic allergies can cause the response known as anaphylactic shock, which results in wheezing, dizziness, and even death from airway swelling. More than one hundred people die each year from food allergies, making food allergies a more common cause of death than bee stings.

In the event of anaphylactic shock, the best treatment is immediate injection with the stimulating hormone adrenaline. Adrenaline counteracts many of the effects of allergy, such as the constriction of the lungs. In fact, people with severe allergies often carry around a hypodermic needle filled with adrenaline, in case they mistakenly eat allergenic food.

This strong need for adrenaline reveals the demand that *milder* food reactions constantly place on the adrenal glands. If you're consistently experiencing subtle food reactions, you're draining your natural supply of adrenaline. When this happens, it can rob you of your energy, good mood, and motivation.

One good thing about classic food allergies is that they're rare, striking only about 2 per cent of the population. Therefore, you probably don't have a classic allergy. That's the good news.

The bad news: you probably *do* have at least one food sensitivity, because most people do. They're extremely widespread. Unfortunately, sensitivities are very similar to allergies. They often *feel* almost exactly like allergies.

Let's take a look at them, because they're probably the primary cause of your false fat.

Food Sensitivities

There are three major types of food sensitivities: (1) **delayed reactions**; (2) **direct cellular reactions**; and (3) **immune complex reactions**.

These three types of food reactions are, in all probability, the culprits behind your false fat. They are, in effect, the usual suspects.

FOOD SENSITIVITY 1:
Delayed Reactions
These are the single most common cause of false fat.

Arguably, delayed food reactions cause as many health problems as some of the most horrific of life's various risk factors, such as smoking or stress. The effects are often subtle and accumulate slowly, but the harm is undeniable. Without a doubt, delayed food reactions cause weight gain. Because 300,000 people die each year from obesity-related problems, anything that exacerbates weight gain is a serious issue.

Therefore, the average person's ignorance about delayed food reactions is a serious public health problem. Don't let yourself be a victim of this lack of knowledge!

Delayed food reactions are very similar to classic allergies. The biggest difference is that when you have sensitivities, you often don't notice symptoms right after you eat. Sometimes it can take as long as three days for symptoms to appear. The reason for the delay is that this type of food reaction is caused by a different antibody than the one that causes classic food allergies, and it takes longer for allergens to come in contact with this antibody. This antibody, IgG (or immunoglobulin G), is found only in the bloodstream, so food molecules need to reach the bloodstream for problems to occur. As long as food macromolecules stay in the digestive tract, no symptoms may appear. Sometimes food molecules move out of the digestive tract almost immediately, but sometimes they don't.

When reactive food macromolecules do eventually meet up with IgG antibodies, the antibodies wage the same basic type of battle fought by IgE antibodies, which cause classic allergies. The IgG antibodies call the immune system into the fight, and histamines and other chemicals are released, causing swelling and other symptoms.

The IgG antibodies are by far the most common antibodies in the body. They're three times more common than the IgE antibodies that cause classic allergies; that's one reason delayed food reactions are more common than classic allergies.

Because IgG reactions are delayed, people are often unaware of their real cause. If you feel a symptom on Monday morning, it may be hard to link it to something you ate Friday night.

Another reason people are often unaware of their IgG reactions is that these reactions often don't occur in obvious places, such as the skin, as do classic IgE allergies.

Even though an IgG reaction may not be obvious, it can still be very harmful. For example, if you're allergic to bee stings and get an IgE reaction on your skin from a sting, you'll be sure to notice and treat it. However, an internal IgG reaction to a food may ultimately cause you much more generalized, systemic swelling than a bee sting; it's like getting a bee sting to the whole body. But because your reaction is spread over your whole body, you may not be very aware of it. All you'll notice is that you don't feel good and have more bloating and swelling. After you've read this book, though, and learned what to look for, I guarantee that you *will* notice how drastically food reactions affect your body.

Another antibody that can cause delayed reactions is IgA. IgA fights at the front lines — at the mucous membrane sites and in the digestive tract itself — trying to stop allergens from being absorbed by the body in the first place. To do this, it stimulates secretion of mucus, which blocks absorption.

Studies show, though, that almost half of all Americans

don't secrete enough IgA. Non-reactive people secrete 3,000 to 5,000 mg of IgA every day, but some reactive people don't secrete much at all. If you're low on IgA, sooner or later a re-active food molecule will work its way through your intestinal wall and cause a reaction. The more reactive foods you eat, the more likely you'll be to use up your supply of IgA and lose your front-line force against food reactions.

Therefore, if you do 'cheat' and eat an allergenic food, it's smart not to eat too *much* of the food. One jam doughnut might get blocked by IgA, but three doughnuts may over-whelm your forces and push you past your allergic threshold.

Another factor that depletes IgA is use of certain medic-ations, including antibiotics, antacids, ulcer drugs, cortisone and aspirin. Again, as you can see, it's *not just what you eat* that can hurt your metabolism and make you fat.

FOOD SENSITIVITY 2:
Direct Cellular Reactions

In a very real sense, *everybody* has direct reactions to foods. Direct reactions are reactions caused directly to cells by chemicals in foods. Among the most obvious direct reactions are those caused by alcohol. If you drink alcohol, you are almost certain to experience sedative effects, due to the direct effect of alcohol on your brain cells.

Often, people with Asian heritage react quite negatively to alcohol, and the common belief is that they're allergic to it. Technically, though, they don't have an allergy; they have a sensitivity – because this is a *direct* reaction, which doesn't involve the immune system. I believe that it's clearer and more sensible to say simply that Asians often have a food *reaction* to alcohol, since food reactions include both allergies and sensitivities.

Direct reactions, however, can eventually involve the immune system, because sooner or later the immune system is called in to repair the mess that direct food reactions cause. Therefore, the symptoms of direct reactions can *feel* much like allergies. Because of this, direct food reactions are sometimes called false food allergies.

Alcohol has obvious direct actions, but most direct food

reactions are more subtle. Often, direct reactions occur when chemicals in foods bind with the cells that produce histamine; these cells are called mast cells. When this happens, it can cause the release of histamine. The food chemicals that are most likely to do this are lectins, which are most often found in wheat, peanuts, and beans. Another cause can be certain partial proteins, or peptides, that are found in tomatoes, strawberries, shellfish, pork, chocolate, and eggs.

Other foods that often seem to cause direct food reactions are mustard, pineapple, papaya, buckwheat, and sunflower seeds. Ironically, one patient of mine had terrible digestive symptoms, including severe heartburn, and took large amounts of digestive enzymes to help the problem. However, his enzymes were full of papaya, which he later found he was reactive to. When he stopped taking the digestive aids, his digestion improved immeasurably. Moral of the story: don't trust common knowledge about what's healthy – *trust your own experiences*. Everyone is different.

Other foods that sometimes cause direct reactions are those that contain high levels of natural histamines. Histamines are formed in foods that are allowed to age and ferment. Therefore, histamines are often found in aged cheese, sausage, and salami.

Other foods that can cause direct reactions are those that contain the partial proteins tyramine, phenylethylamine, and octopamine. These chemicals, like histamines, can cause blood vessels to expand and contract, which causes tissue swelling. In the head, blood vessel constriction and expansion can cause migraine headaches. That's why people who get migraines often shun the foods that are high in these partial proteins, such as wine, aged cheese, citrus fruit and yeast.

Another common foodstuff that often causes direct reactions is the artificial sweetener aspartame. Aspartame is mostly composed of the partial protein, or amino acid, called phenylalanine. In some people, it acts directly on brain cells, causing symptoms such as agitation and depression. In other people, it causes blood vessels to contract and expand, triggering migraines. In most people, though, it causes no reaction at all.

Many people also react to MSG, or monosodium glutamate, with headaches, nausea, dizziness, heart palpitations, and confusion. Others react to various additives, including nitrates, sulphites, and artificial food colours.

Another name for direct food reactions is pharmacologic reactions. That's a good description, because it implies an important point: *foods, like drugs, are chemicals*. Not all drugs are good for you – and not all foods are, either.

Now let's look at the last type of food reaction: immune complex reactions. This type of reaction is not well known. But it should be. It can be a killer.

Foods, like drugs, are chemicals.
Not all drugs are good for you,
and not all foods are, either.

FOOD SENSITIVITY 3:
Immune Complex Reactions

These occur when antibodies attack allergens but don't manage to kill them. The result is an allergen (called an antigen) with an antibody stuck to it. This creates a whole new animal (an antigen-antibody complex) that the body doesn't recognize. When this happens, the 'new animal' starts circulating around the body, and this circulatory immune complex, or CIC, can eventually lodge in tissue.

CICs create many of the same reactions as classic allergies. When they circulate through or lodge in tissues, such as those of the kidneys, lungs, liver, or joints, they can cause terrible problems by starting immune and inflammatory responses. They can cause joint problems similar to arthritis, and they can cause organs to malfunction. They often interfere with the body's filtering mechanisms, such as the lymphatic system and kidneys. Some researchers believe they contribute to many types of kidney disease, some of which are eventually fatal.

Sometimes, people with serious CIC problems experience widespread conditions – such as migraines, kidney problems, and joint pain – and never realize that all of these problems have a single cause.

Frequently, patients come to me hoping only to lose weight, but when they resolve problems such as excessive CIC production, they also overcome other serious health conditions. One recent patient, for example, not only lost 22 pounds but also recovered from chronic joint pain, migraines, and gallbladder inflammation. This patient was happy to lose her weight, but was *overjoyed* to solve the other problems. Of course she had to make a serious commitment to her health and change her lifestyle. But she *enjoyed* the whole process, because she felt *so much better* every step of the way.

This reinforced my belief in the adage, '*If you just strive for thin, you'll never win. Strive for health, and thin will follow.*'

Now you know about the risk factors that make you vulnerable to food reactions, and you know how food reactions work. Good for you! You now have more knowledge about this subject than many doctors do.

Now that you have a good foundation of knowledge, you'll be able to understand why food reactions cause bloating and swelling. Once you understand this, you need never again be a victim of false fat.

How Food Reactions Cause Bloating and Swelling

Bloating and swelling are *false* fat. But bloating and swelling look so much like true fat that most people can't tell the difference. I once had a patient who developed a significant false fat problem after taking a long course of steroid-type drugs, which are notorious for causing swelling and bloating. After his course of medication ended, he told me he wanted to 'get some of this fat off.'

I told him that his abdominal distension wasn't really fat. But he was dubious. He said, 'Hey, *fat is fat.*'

He was dead wrong. *Adipose tissue* is fat. Bloating and swelling are *fluid and gas*. There's a big difference.

Fluid is the biggest component of false fat. For the most part, this fluid is simply water, mixed with other secretions.

Because your body is 60 per cent to 70 per cent water, even *minor* changes in the volume of your water can make a huge difference in your weight. There are 10 pounds of water in your blood alone. Even your bones, which you may think of as 'bone dry,' are 30 per cent water. Muscles can be up to 75 per cent water; that's partly why athletes are careful not to become dehydrated – it weakens their muscles.

Your body is constantly using all of this water in your metabolic processes. You filter about a litre of blood through your kidneys *every minute*, and every one of these litres carries as much as an ounce and a half of soluble waste. Water is, in fact, your primary medium of waste disposal. When your body finds toxins or any type of foreign invader, it flushes the site of the toxin with water to flood it away. Even the carbon dioxide that you exhale needs water for elimination. Water moistens every part of your respiratory system and keeps it functioning. Every day you lose about a half a litre of water just from breathing. If you're under a lot of stress and your breath is quick and shallow much of the day, you can lose one to two litres of water.

You lose even more water when you sweat. When you're working hard in the heat, you can sweat up to one litre per hour. A high fever can make you lose 10–15 litres a day.

We replenish most of our water supply by drinking, but we also consume a lot of water in food. Fruits and vegetables are often about 90 per cent water, and meat is usually about 60 per cent water. Even supposedly dry foods, such as bread, can be as much as 25 per cent water. That's why dried-out bread is so different in texture from fresh bread.

About two-thirds of your water is inside your cells. The rest is in your blood, in various bodily fluids, and in the tissue spaces between your cells. The water inside your cells and outside your cells is all affected by food reactions.

Food reactions make you retain water. And when you retain water, *you gain false fat*.

In fact, one of the first symptoms of food reactions is thirst. Thirst often occurs when we begin to store water. If you feel unusually thirsty after eating a suspected reactive food, chances are good that you're experiencing a food reaction.

Here's why food reactions make you *gain false fat*:

1. Food reactions cause fluid to surround invading food particles. When food macromolecules are identified as foreign invaders, your body launches the inflammatory response, which includes flooding an area that's under attack. Your body will hold onto this water as long as reactive food substances remain in your tissues. This water dilutes these substances and reduces their effects, but at the same time the cells and tissues swell with water. This often accounts for swelling under the eyes and chin, in the hands, feet, ankles, and midsection.

2. Food reactions release hormones that cause fluid retention. To offset the effects of the allergic inflammatory response, the body produces hormones, such as adrenaline. But these hormones cause water retention. The adrenal hormones cortisol and aldosterone increase sodium uptake, and sodium attracts water to cells and tissues.

This action also triggers other hormonal changes, apparently through effects of the pituitary gland, which orchestrates your body's 'hormonal symphony.' These other hormonal changes may include excessive secretion of anti-diuretic hormone, which causes fluid retention. Anti-diuretic hormone is also often secreted in response to stress, and is commonly released by women as part of premenstrual syndrome. The female hormone estrogen, which can be affected by food reactions, also increases water retention. Furthermore, growth hormone, which helps boost the metabolism, can be *depressed* by food reactions.

Besides these hormones, which circulate throughout the body, food reactions also have strong effects on certain gut hormones (including cholecystokinin and somatostatin), which can cause water retention and swelling *directly in the gut tissues*. Sometimes, when people experience immediate abdominal swelling after eating, it is due to the influence of gut hormones.

Because women tend to have more problematic hormonal profiles than men, the hormonal elements of false fat tend to be worse for them. For example, when some menopausal women are given extra hormones, their bloating and swelling increase.

When people stop eating their false fat foods, however, these hormonal problems usually stabilize quickly.

3. Food reactions make intestinal membranes swell. There is often pronounced swelling of intestinal membranes, in response to irritation by allergens and in response to hormonal imbalances. This can account for the 'pregnant' look that often characterizes false fat. The result of this type of swelling is a feeling of heaviness and congestion in the abdomen, particularly in the small intestine.

4. Food reactions disrupt cell chemistry, causing fluid storage. Food reactions cause a condition called cellular acidosis, which harms cell chemistry and results in fluid retention. Here's how it works. The inflammatory response, caused by food reactions, causes calcium and sodium to enter cells, and this attracts water. It not only causes swelling, but also depresses the function of the cells' energy centres, or mitochondria. When the mitochondria are disturbed, it saps your energy.

This action also causes even *more* release of the stress hormones cortisol and aldosterone, which try to correct the chemical imbalance. But this in turn just causes more fluid retention.

Furthermore, as the food reactions subside, the cells release all of these acidic chemicals into the tissues. This can cause a new round of inflammation and the release of even more protective fluids. Over a long period of time, this tissue acidity can contribute to the onset of degenerative diseases, including arthritis.

5. Food reactions cause capillaries to leak fluids. As you may recall, many food reactions release chemicals, such as histamine, that make blood vessels expand and contract, in the process leaking fluids into tissues. This leakage of fluids causes further inflammatory reactions, with accompanying swelling. Sometimes this swelling can impinge upon nerves and cause aches and pains. It can also cause hives, due to the swelling of capillaries near the surface of the skin.

Often, when this fluid leaks out of capillaries, it carries

protein with it. This protein in turn attracts sodium, which causes even more fluid retention. The combination of sodium and fluid outside the cells can 'smother' cells by making it harder for oxygen to reach them. This contributes to further cell malfunction, and even to the death of cells.

When cells die, even more water is drawn to the area to flush away the dead cells.

6. Food reactions cause gas production. Food reactions allow the proliferation of abnormal bacteria and yeasts, and these factors lead to fermentation of food. Fermentation, primarily of carbohydrates, forms wind or gas, including methane.

Secondarily, it creates by-products of alcohol metabolism, such as the chemical acetaldehyde, and alcohol itself. Both of these substances can impair mood and cognitive function when absorbed by the body.

Food reactions also tend to slow the natural squeezing of food through the digestive tract by the bowel-muscle process of peristalsis. When food transit through the bowel is slowed, more gas and fermentation products are produced. Also, this 'constipation effect' causes more irritation of the bowel lining. This can create even more gas and can also contribute further to leaky gut syndrome, allowing reactive macromolecules to slip through the intestinal wall.

Bacterial overgrowth in the small intestine also causes fermentation and gas. This causes pressure and discomfort in the small intestine, because the small intestine is relatively narrow and doesn't have much room for expansion. Another major contributor to gas buildup in the small intestine is lack of the digestive substance hydrochloric acid, which is abnormally low in approximately 70 per cent of all people over 60. Hydrochloric acid, or stomach acid, also tends to be chronically low in people who are under stress, in people who eat lots of processed foods, and in people with food reactions.

Gas formation is also increased by use of anti-inflammatory drugs, such as aspirin, which irritate gut mucosa. It can also be exacerbated by antacids.

In addition, poor digestion also causes increased excretion of the amino acid taurine, which lowers cellular magnesium

---

HOW FOOD REACTIONS CAUSE FALSE FAT

1. Food reactions cause fluid to surround invading food particles.
2. Food reactions release hormones that cause fluid retention.
3. Food reactions make intestinal membranes swell.
4. Food reactions disrupt cell chemistry, causing fluid storage.
5. Food reactions cause capillaries to leak fluids.
6. Food reactions cause gas production.

---

and slows peristalsis, resulting in *more* intestinal gas.

Lastly, women's menstrual cycles upset hormonal balances, and this also impairs peristalsis.

All of these factors are insidious. They feed off one another and contribute to bloating and swelling. The result of this entire range of forces is a swollen, distended belly and puffy, spongy flesh all over your body. Until now, you may have thought that this was fat. Now you know it's not. It's false fat – and you can get rid of it in a week or less if you make the necessary effort.

I'm sure you can do it! Every day that you make the effort, you're going to feel a little better. You'll look better, too.

Now, let's look at your *real* fat fight: your war against the true fat that's dragging down your health. You can lose that, too. And you can lose it exactly the same way you lose false fat – by overcoming your food reactions.

Let's start now!

3

WHY YOU WILL LOSE TRUE FAT

MARILYN WAS ASHAMED OF HERSELF. SHE WAS ASHAMED OF how she looked. And she was ashamed of how she ate. She looked very overweight, and she ate compulsively.

When she first consulted with me, in 1995, she was desperate to lose weight. She told me that if she could just suddenly wake up thin one morning, it would change her life. When she said that, she had a distant look in her eyes, as if she could see the future.

But I strongly disagreed with her. I thought that suddenly being thin wouldn't change her life at all. Many patients have come to me who had become suddenly thin – through liposuction, crash dieting, or pills – but it had *never* really changed their lives. Most of them still *felt* fat. In their minds, they still carried a mythical image of a perfect body – an image that had never been gradually modified by the day-to-day challenge of life in the real world – and they still hadn't achieved that image. When they looked in the mirror, they didn't see that perfect body; they just saw a starved-down version of their own imperfect body – and it *wasn't good enough*.

Even worse, most of these people were *hungry*, and felt like ticking time bombs, ready to blow up the first time they binged.

Worst of all, even when they *had* starved themselves into slimness, they still had not achieved the Big Prize that their various diet gurus had promised: self-respect.

Self-respect doesn't come from being thin. Being thin comes from self-respect.

The only thing any of these people had really achieved was to become a thinner version of their same old self. And because they were their same old selves, their slimness never lasted. It was invariably subverted by old habits, by pent-up hunger, and by the metabolic damage done by dieting.

I explained all this to Marilyn. 'Don't try to get thin so that your life will change,' I urged her. '*Change your life* – and then you'll get thin.'

Marilyn, a very bright 30-year-old systems analyst, seemed to instantly understand my point. She saw the logic in it.

Still, she was pessimistic about her ability to change her lifestyle. She had tried many times to alter her stormy relationship with food, to no avail. When she got hungry, she said, the feeling wasn't at all like the simple desire to eat that she had experienced as a child. Instead, it was a gnawing, unsettling feeling in her stomach that made her weak, irritable, and shaky. It was an overpowering sensation, much like a symptom of an illness. Her ravenous hunger sometimes focused on a few beloved foods – frozen yoghurt, peanut butter and jam sandwiches, and breakfast cereal. Other times, she was hungry for *anything* and stuffed down whatever was in the refrigerator. But no matter how much she ate, she never felt fully satisfied. She told me that she sometimes ate five or six bowls of cereal over a couple of hours, and still felt hungry.

Many times, she said, she had forced herself to go on tortuous diets, but she had rarely lost much weight. She told me that her metabolism was 'stuck in reverse,' and that every bite she ate seemed to convert to fat. Since college, Marilyn said, her eating habits had got progressively worse, and by 1995 she was about 55 pounds over her college weight.

As she spoke, though, I became increasingly convinced I could help her, because I believed that she had a classic case of *reactive food addiction*. Her food reactions had created intense food cravings, and these cravings were almost as powerful as a drug addiction.

In addition, her food reactions had badly harmed her metabolism and had made her terribly vulnerable to weight gain – *even when she managed to eat moderately*.

Marilyn, sad to say, was a relatively typical weight-loss

patient. Because she was so overweight that it was hurting her health, she was classified as morbidly obese, a category that had increased 370 per cent in America since 1970. Also, like an estimated 95 per cent of all women, she perceived herself as being even more overweight than she really was. She told me she wanted to lose 70 pounds, but that would have been *too much*. Like one-half of all American women, she was a frequent dieter, and like most overweight American girls and women, she was obsessed with her weight; on average, overweight American women say they would sacrifice five years off their life span to be thin.

Despite Marilyn's fervent desire to lose weight, though, her approach to weight loss had been all wrong – as is the approach of most dieters today. She still thought that people got fat mainly because they lacked willpower. This perspective on obesity is very common, even among doctors, but it's outdated. In fact, the American Heart Association recently called for a conceptual housecleaning in medicine's approach to obesity, away from the simplistic concept that almost all overweight people just eat more calories than they burn with exercise. The new approach to obesity, the association said, should be to view obesity as a chronic disease, like hypertension or diabetes, caused by specific physiological factors. I strongly endorse this new perspective.

The most important single physiological factor in the disease of obesity, I am convinced, is food reactivity. The disease of obesity can almost never be cured until food reactions are overcome.

Marilyn took my advice to heart and put the full force of her personality to work on overcoming her food reactions. She quickly ascertained her reactive foods – dairy products, sugar, wheat, corn and peanuts – and soon overcame her cravings for them. Being free of these cravings, she told me, was 'like getting out of a prison.' Suddenly she stopped experiencing the painful, exaggerated feeling that she had learned to identify as hunger. After she resolved her food reactions, hunger once again became merely the desire to eat. If she had to wait an hour or two to eat, it wasn't a big problem. With her new power over food, she became far more discriminating in her food choices and ate a smart, wholesome diet, free of the foods that had battered her metabolism.

In her first week on the False Fat Diet, Marilyn lost about ten pounds of false fat, and this strengthened her resolve even more.

When she realized she wasn't just a weak-willed glutton, it made a remarkable difference in her ability to change her life. She engaged in the Balance Programme enthusiastically, making sure she also balanced work with play, rest with exercise, and relaxation with activity.

For many years, Marilyn told me, she had been waiting to start her life as soon as her fat was gone. But with her new-found confidence about eating, she had the courage to *start her life anyway*, while she was still overweight. Before she'd even lost much weight, she took the emotional risk of reaching out to a man she liked and beginning a relationship. She remarked to me that this 'was the smartest thing I ever did, because it made me realize I could be loved for *me*, and not just for being thin.'

After the quick loss of Marilyn's false fat, the rest of her weight came off at the rate of about three-quarters of a pound per week. Once her metabolism was free from the assault of food reactions, it normalized and began consistently to burn adipose tissue.

Marilyn's slow, measured progress was ideal; it didn't trigger the starvation response, nor did it impair her health or energy in any way. In fact, she felt stronger and healthier with each passing week. As she began to approach her ideal weight, she even lost interest in weighing herself, which is very healthy. I want my patients to be concerned with their fitness, energy, health, and mood – not their scale weight. Scale weight is an artificial measure of body composition that frequently fluctuates, and doesn't even differentiate between fat and muscle.

Actually, when Marilyn got all the way down to the weight at which she thought she looked best, she didn't feel quite as energetic, so I urged her to put a couple of pounds back on. Most people, including me, don't feel their best at what they believe to be their ultimate 'skinny' weight. I feel best when

I'm about 5–10 pounds over my lowest weight. In winter, when my body tends to require more stored energy, I sometimes gain up to 10 pounds. Lots of people, of course, spend their lives trying to be as thin as movie stars, but that's foolish. Movie stars usually have to suffer to look the way they do, and even then their appearance is only temporary. Most stars diet down for movies and often starve themselves for certain revealing scenes. They may look momentarily perfect, but it rarely lasts.

Perfection is not just a burden – it's an illusion.

Marilyn gradually realized she didn't have to look *perfect* to look *beautiful*, and that realization was her saving grace. She was quite happy just knowing that she was no longer a food addict.

Food cravings aren't just hunger.
They are an intense, painful,
'need-to-feed' reaction.

Food addiction, caused by intense food cravings, is very common, and it's terribly destructive. Allergic addiction is most insidious, though, when you don't realize that *your food reactions are causing your craving*s. If you're not aware of this, you may think that you're just neurotic, indulgent, or weak. You're not! You have a medical condition – food reactions – and now it's time to get rid of this condition.

Let's look at how food reactions *cause the cravings that make you overeat*, and also *cause your metabolism to gain weight easily*. When you understand these two things, you'll have a tremendous advantage. You'll be well on your way to gaining power over food.

First, let's see if you actually have food cravings. Try the checklist on the next page.

If you answered yes to only one or two of these questions, you may not have any food cravings. If you answered yes to three to five questions, you probably have moderate food cravings. If you answered yes to six or more, you almost

DO YOU HAVE FOOD CRAVINGS?

YES	NO	
☐	☐	Do you frequently eat until your stomach is uncomfortably full?
☐	☐	When you get hungry, does it make you feel tense, weak, or irritable?
☐	☐	When you get hungry, do you sometimes focus on one or two specific foods?
☐	☐	Do you snack often, usually eating the same snacks?
☐	☐	Have you ever had other addictive habits, such as smoking or drinking too much alcohol or overconsuming caffeine?
☐	☐	Are you often hungry after a meal and stay that way until you've eaten one of your favourite foods?
☐	☐	Do you usually need dessert after dinner to feel satisfied?
☐	☐	Do you tend to eat a relatively narrow range of foods?
☐	☐	When you eat your favourite foods, do you often intend to eat only a moderate amount, but end up eating a larger amount?
☐	☐	Do you sometimes feel as if you lack control over what you eat?
☐	☐	If you snack on foods other than your favourite foods, do you tend to feel unsatisfied?
☐	☐	Do you binge on food more than once per week?
☐	☐	Even if you know a food doesn't agree with you, do you eat it anyway?
☐	☐	When you eat your favourite foods, do you frequently drift into an almost trancelike state of relaxation?
☐	☐	When you eat one of your favourite foods, does it generally improve your mood?

certainly have pronounced food cravings, caused by food reactions.

If you answered yes to six or more questions, you are probably overweight. If you're not, you must have a tremendous degree of willpower or an exceptional metabolism.

To understand these cravings and to understand yourself better, let's briefly examine why these cravings occur. When you understand this, you'll be better prepared to overcome the cravings and stop eating compulsively.

When this happens, you will *stop eating as much as you now eat*, and your *metabolism will heal*. You will then begin to lose adipose tissue gradually, painlessly – and permanently.

How Food Reactions
Cause Cravings

When healthy people eat wholesome, non-reactive foods, their bodies automatically shut off hunger and convert this food to energy. As these people eat, hormones and nerve pathways in their stomachs and guts send signals to the part of their brains that controls hunger, the hypothalamus. When the hypothalamus gets the message that the stomach is full and that the body has a new supply of blood sugar, it releases various brain chemicals that evoke satisfaction and contentment.

These 'contentment chemicals' include hormones and brain messengers, or neurotransmitters. One of the key hormones in the process of satiety is insulin, which helps carry blood sugar into your cells to give you energy. Thyroid hormones also give you a boost. The primary neurotransmitter that gets released is the 'feel-good' neurotransmitter serotonin.

The combination of these calming chemicals, with the surge of blood sugar, shuts off your appetite and makes you feel energetic and fulfilled.

However, when *food reactions* enter the picture, this whole wonderfully orchestrated symphony of satisfaction *breaks down*. As you probably remember, when you eat reactive foods, they enter your system as macromolecules that your body doesn't recognize. This triggers the inflammatory response, which causes water to rush into afflicted cells and be held in tissues, which results in swelling and bloating. As this rescue mechanism takes place, your body, thinking that it's under attack from a foreign invader, goes into a condition of distress.

When this happens, you *do not* experience the release of contentment chemicals, along with extra blood sugar. Instead, you experience a nasty bout of metabolic upset, which will soon leave you hungry, weak, and miserable.

In response to the distress triggered by food reactions, you begin to pump out your own natural opiates, called endorphins, which are almost always secreted in response to trauma. When these opiates hit your system, they give you a feeling of relief. You feel physically and mentally fulfilled. If the distress is significant and causes abundant release of endorphins, you even feel an opiate 'high.'

This is the pleasant phase of allergic addition – the *only* pleasant phase. For at least a few minutes, and quite possibly for several hours, any negative feelings you may have had are masked by this release of these natural opiates.

Soon, though, this endorphin high wears off and leaves you with a depleted supply of endorphins. When this happens, your natural instinct is to eat the same food that produced the pleasurable feelings in the first place. After years of gaining pleasure from this food, you probably have a strong association between this food and feeling good.

This endorphin fluctuation alone can make you feel virtually addicted to certain foods. But this is only the beginning of the process of allergic addiction. It gets worse.

As you crash from your opiate high, *other* chemical reactions occur that are equally disastrous. These other chemical reactions strongly reinforce your powerful desire to again eat your false fat food – as fast as possible. When these reactions begin, only an iron will can stop you from eating.

One of the most disruptive of these other chemical reactions is the release of adrenal hormones. You may remember that when your body is under allergic assault, it counters the effects of this assault with adrenal hormones, such as adrenaline, norepinephrine, and cortisol. When these stimulating hormones first hit your bloodstream, you feel good. They boost your energy level and mood. They directly stimulate your glands and organs and help convert stored blood sugar into energy.

As these adrenal hormones course through your system, your heart beats faster. In fact, one of the tests for food reactions is to take your pulse after you eat. If it's elevated, it means that you probably ate a reactive food. Unfortunately, though, your adrenal rush fades as fast as your endorphin high. When it's gone, you drop into a slump of fatigue, irritability, and mental lethargy. This makes you want to eat more of your false fat foods, but when you do eat more, you tend to have an even stronger reaction to them, because you no longer have enough adrenal hormones to protect you from your food reactions.

The third major chemical reaction that's caused by eating false fat foods is a drastic *decrease* in the blood sugar entering your cells. This reaction is devastating, because blood sugar is the very 'food' that feeds each one of your cells. When you don't get enough blood sugar into your cells, you quickly run out of physical and mental energy. You feel weak and have an overpowering desire for food. This desire for food may feel like hunger, but it's really your body's cry for help. Your body feels as if it's starving to death.

This drop in blood sugar is caused by hormonal disturbances that destabilize your levels of insulin, the hormone that moves blood sugar into cells. When blood sugar levels, adrenal hormone levels, and endorphin levels all drop, you're in big trouble. You're not just hungry – you have a *need-to-feed* reaction.

But then things get even *worse*. The fourth and final cause of food cravings is probably the most painful of all: a decrease in your levels of the neurotransmitter serotonin.

Serotonin is a veritable elixir of contentment. It helps us feel happy, healthy, and well-fed. As you probably know, drugs that boost serotonin levels, such as Prozac, are tremendously popular, because they help people feel calm and content. Many diet medications are designed to increase serotonin levels, because serotonin helps shut off hunger.

Obese people often have low levels of serotonin. This serotonin deficit makes them very vulnerable to hunger. When they develop food reactions, though, their serotonin levels plunge even *lower*, because food reactions destabilize serotonin.

Someone who has *normal* serotonin levels can eventually develop the same low serotonin levels as an obese person by constantly suffering from food reactions. Serotonin levels are decreased by food reactions because serotonin is mostly carried by white blood cells – the very same cells that the immune system uses to fight the invasion of reactive food molecules. When these cells are busy fighting reactive foods, they are less able to deliver adequate serotonin.

WHY FOOD REACTIONS
CAUSE FOOD CRAVINGS

1. Endorphin drop	Discomfort
	+
2. Adrenaline drop	Fatigue
	+
3. Blood sugar drop	Hunger
	+
4. Serotonin drop	Anxiety
Together =	Food Cravings

One of the most harmful aspects of this serotonin drop is that it creates specific cravings for *high-carbohydrate foods*, such as sugar and starch. Carbohydrates help move serotonin into the brain, and when the brain is low on serotonin, it creates an overpowering urge to eat high-carbohydrate, sweet, and starchy foods.

Because of this effect, millions of people crave sweet and starchy foods. *Of all food cravings, carbohydrate craving is the most common.* My weight control patients crave carbohydrates more than any other type of food. In fact, Fuller Royal, M.D., one of the modern pioneers in the field of food reactions, coined the term 'carboholic' to describe people who seek a serotonin boost by cramming down carbohydrates.

As you can see, it can be almost impossible to withstand the force of these four factors: (1) endorphin drop, (2) adrenal drop, (3) blood sugar drop, and (4) serotonin drop. These noxious factors create a need-to-feed reaction that very few people can consistently resist.

Unfortunately, this need-to-feed reaction can often be satisfied only by eating the specific false fat foods that created the problem in the first place. But when you eat these foods, it just perpetuates the problem. Millions of people get trapped in this destructive cycle and have to endure not only the pain of their cravings but also the pain of low self-esteem, brought on by their continual failure to control what they eat. As if this isn't bad enough, they also endure the scorn of society and even their own families, who often regard them as weak and indulgent.

But their misery doesn't end here. Their cravings are only *half* of the problem. The other half of the problem is that food reactions *badly damage the metabolism*.

Once you see the damage you're doing to your metabolism with food reactions, you'll be even more motivated to pull yourself out of this trap and enjoy a life of power over food.

---

*Food reactions decrease the
'contentment chemicals'
that turn off hunger.*

How Food Reactions Hurt Your Metabolism

Food reactions, I believe, *harm the metabolism more than any other single dietary factor*. Even if you never, ever gave in to your food cravings and never ate too much, your food reactions would still make it very hard for you to be thin. That's because food reactions make it easy to gain weight and hard to lose it.

Food reactions create five metabolic roadblocks to weight loss:

1. **They slow the metabolic rate.**
2. **They increase the hormones that cause weight gain.**
3. **They create hypoglycemia.**
4. **They depress energy.**
5. **They contribute to illness** (which makes regular exercise much more difficult).

This is a powerful array of forces. Any one of these forces can make you fat. The combination of all five is almost certain to make you feel as if your own metabolism is your worst enemy.

Food reactions **slow the metabolic rate** partly by blocking the absorption of essential fatty acids, which rev up your metabolism, just like oxygen revs up a fire. Some common false fat foods, including several of the Sensitive Seven most commonly reactive foods, prevent full absorption of the essential fatty acids. Among the foods that do this are eggs, wheat, dairy products, and sugar.

Food reactions also slow your metabolism by gradually depleting your supply of adrenaline. When this happens, your metabolism can become sluggish and more prone to storing fat.

Another way food reactions can slow your metabolism is by interfering with the hormonal balance of your thyroid gland, which is directly involved with metabolic rate and the burning of fat. You'll know your thryroid may be malfunctioning if you are especially sensitive to cold; if you're depressed, lethargic, or prone to easy weight gain; or if you have dry skin or are losing hair.

Food reactions also hurt your metabolism by **increasing hormones that cause weight gain**. Several hormones are involved, and they're all very important.

Insulin is probably the most obvious hormone that can make you gain weight. If you produce too much of it, it moves excessive amounts of blood sugar into your cells and makes you fat. If you produce too little of it, your cells become 'hungry' and you tend to overeat to satisfy this hunger. Food reactions can trigger both overproduction and underproduction, depending upon the types of reactive foods you eat.

Food reactions can even contribute to a condition called insulin resistance, in which the *quality* of insulin declines and insulin has a hard time moving blood sugar into cells. An estimated 20–25 per cent of the population has at least a moderate degree of insulin resistance, brought on in part by overconsumption of carbohydrates. This condition is more common now than it used to be, partly because a common dietary approach of the 1990s was a high-carbohydrate diet, based mostly around grain products.

Another hormone that can impair fat burning is the adrenal hormone cortisol, which is increased by food reactions. Cortisol reduces the activity of a natural fat-burning enzyme called *delta-6-desaturase*. A shortage of this enzyme makes it much harder to lose weight.

Cortisol is increased by eating too much refined starch and sugar. It is also drastically increased by stress. Therefore, stress can indirectly contribute to weight gain – even when it doesn't cause you to overeat.

Other important hormones that are affected by food reactions are the eicosanoids. In his groundbreaking book *The Zone*, Barry Sears showed that certain eicosanoids could make people fat by inhibiting the burning of adipose tissue. The eicosanoid most responsible for slowing down fat burning is called PGE-2 (prostaglandin E-2). PGE-2 is produced during the inflammatory response that occurs during food reactions.

Besides disturbing the levels of hormones, food reactions also make you gain weight more easily **by causing hypoglycemia**. As your probably remember, hypoglycemia, or low blood sugar, is also a major factor in food cravings. In fact, *cravings* and *metabolic problems* are closely related.

Food reactions cause hypoglycemia mostly by interfering with the hormones that help control blood sugar levels, such as insulin and adrenaline.

Food reactions also *indirectly* contribute to hypoglycemia by prompting you to eat foods that trigger hypoglycemia, such as refined starches and sugar. When you have hypoglycemia, you have an overwhelming urge to eat in order to raise your blood sugar levels. You feel weak, tired, mentally foggy, and irritable. Hypoglycemia appears to be more common now than ever before, due mostly to our society's heavy intake of refined grains, sugar, and processed foods.

Ironically, many people who have tried hard to eat wisely have become hypoglycemic, because they ate too many carbohydrates and not enough protein. People who live on carbohydrates – mostly fruits, grains, and starchy vegetables – become hypoglycemic more easily than people who have a more balanced diet, with higher amounts of protein.

Interestingly, hypoglycemia can be directly caused not only by food reactions, but also by allergies and sensitivities to non-food substances, such as toxic inhalants, and even cigarette smoke. Again, as you can see, it's not just food that can make you fat.

The final way that food reactions make you gain fat is by making you **feel sick and fatigued**. When you feel like this, it's almost impossible to lose weight. You don't feel like exercising, and you may feel so discouraged that you go off your healthy diet.

Food reactions also help cause many serious medical conditions, including migraines, irritable bowel syndrome, insomnia, chronic pain, arthritis, skin rashes, sinus problems, and chronic fatigue syndrome. Any one of these conditions can destroy your quality of life and make you turn away from exercise and prudent eating.

Even when they don't make you sick, food reactions still sap your energy. When the energy loss becomes severe, you can feel almost as tired as if you had a bad cold. The energy-draining immune response caused by food reactions can feel similar to the fatiguing immune response caused by a virus. Even when this energy loss is not severe, though, it can still be very troublesome. You might feel weak, lethargic, and un-motivated, but not know why.

Food reactions increase your cravings,
and disrupt your metabolism.
The result: weight gain.

When you feel like this, you may not have the energy or the motivation to do the things you need to do to be thin.

By now, you should know that you're not weak. You just have a *medical condition* that's making you fat: food reactions. The medical condition of food reactions causes your *food cravings*, and it also causes your *metabolic dysfunction*. These two problems make people fat. Correcting these two problems will over time have a tremendous impact upon your body's adipose tissue. *You will lose fat.*

Unfortunately, if you're a woman, these two elements may be even more severe than they are for men. Women, because of their special metabolic profiles, are particularly vulnerable to these forces. In Chapter 4, I'll tell you why this is and what you can do about it.

Once you understand your food reactions, you'll understand your own body much better. And with this understanding will come power over food.

4
WHAT WOMEN NEED TO KNOW

WOMEN NEED TO KNOW THAT THERE IS A CRUEL crossover effect between food reactions and premenstrual syndrome. Symptoms of both conditions are *very similar* and *cross over* from one condition to the other.

- Each of the two conditions makes the other worse.
- Both cause weight gain in very similar ways.

When both conditions are present at the same time, the effects can be devastating. This isn't fair, but it's a fact of life.

Food reactions and female hormones *both* cause: **(1) food cravings, (2) mood disturbance, (3) metabolic disorders (including low thyroid function, hypoglycemia, and insulin instability), (4) swelling and bloating, and (5) energy and immune dysfunction**. Considering the power of these two combined forces, it's a wonder that *any* woman is thin. It's a testament to the willpower of women that so many of them can resist these two potent biological factors.

Furthermore, even though it's much harder for women to stay slim than it is for men, women are expected by society and by themselves to be *thinner* than men. Ironically, this expectation makes many of them even more overweight, by tempting them to use harmful weight-loss gimmicks, such as crash diets, which often cause rebound weight gain.

But I have excellent news! Women can end this cruel crossover effect by controlling their food reactions. When they do this, the crossover effect disappears and life becomes much more fair. Many of my female patients have escaped this double-trouble crossover effect. For some of them, it was the best thing they ever did for their physical health and their emotional well-being.

The crossover effect is most apparent in women who suffer from *severe* premenstrual syndrome. For these women, the added burden of food reactions makes PMS into a virtual nightmare of pain, bloating, swelling, irritability, and food cravings. In addition, not only do their food reactions make their PMS worse, but their PMS also makes their food reactions worse. They tend to have terribly exaggerated responses to reactive foods. When they eat a false fat food during a bad bout of PMS, it often makes them feel much more sick, irritable and moody.

Because of this insidious crossover effect, most of my weight-loss patients are women. Many of them are aware that their PMS is part of their weight-control problem, but they don't know how to end their PMS. Many have already tried to reduce their PMS symptoms with herbs, exercise, a balanced diet, and medication, but this approach generally fails if they are still having food reactions. When food reactions are controlled, however, PMS symptoms invariably subside.

When food reactions and PMS simultaneously decline, women almost always lose weight. They quickly lose a great deal of false fat as bloating and swelling disappear. Then they gradually lose adipose tissue as their food cravings vanish and their metabolic functions heal.

For many women, the combination of PMS and food reactions is the most severe chronic health problem they face. This was true, for example, for a patient of mine named Rita, who was 34. Before I met with her, she had been to four doctors for her PMS, but none of them had really helped her. She told me at her first consultation that, at least ten days each month, her life was, as she put it, 'a living hell – or more like a *dying* hell.' I still remember that phrase, mostly because of how she looked when she said it. She didn't look just sad or frustrated. She looked frightened. She genuinely feared the inevitable return of her symptoms. She'd been so depleted by

PMS so many times that she'd come to see it as a force that she could not combat.

When I saw her four weeks later, though, after she'd begun the False Fat Diet, she seemed to *exude* power. The first thing I asked her was how her last premenstrual period had gone.

'It was bad,' she said with a shrug.

I was confused. Her words didn't fit the way she looked. 'I'm sorry to hear that,' I said.

'Oh, no,' she replied. 'Bad is *good*. It wasn't horrible like it usually is. It was just . . . bad.' She was smiling.

A month after that, her PMS was even better, and a month later, it was well within the range of normal. She still had some cramping and breast tenderness, but she no longer suffered from the physical and emotional battering that her PMS had previously inflicted. Furthermore, she had lost about 10 pounds of false fat, and nearly 15 pounds of true fat.

For Rita, though, the weight loss was just the icing on the cake.

If you're a woman, it's critically important for you to understand how your own unique hormonal make-up affects your weight and your life. Female hormones have an almost magical ability to create and nurture new life. They also seem to help promote positive traits that are often associated with women, such as empathy, expressiveness, and closeness to the elemental forces of nature. In fact, studies show that when female hormones reach their monthly peak, women tend to have a heightened ability for communication and word recall. Anecdotal evidence suggests that they are also more intuitive at this time.

But the delicate balance of female hormones is easily upset. When this happens, PMS occurs. Contrary to conventional wisdom, painful, difficult PMS symptoms are not normal. They're *common*, but that doesn't mean you should accept them as normal.

Even when female hormones are in perfect balance, however, they *still* predispose women to easy weight gain.

THE DOUBLE-TROUBLE CROSSOVER EFFECT

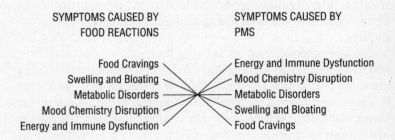

SYMPTOMS CAUSED BY
FOOD REACTIONS

SYMPTOMS CAUSED BY
PMS

Food Cravings
Swelling and Bloating
Metabolic Disorders
Mood Chemistry Disruption
Energy and Immune Dysfunction

Energy and Immune Dysfunction
Mood Chemistry Disruption
Metabolic Disorders
Swelling and Bloating
Food Cravings

Why Women Gain Weight Easily

Human beings are genetically programmed for survival, and part of human survival depends upon women gaining weight easily. Why? In a single, simple phrase: *fat equals fertility*.

When a woman's body-fat ratio drops from the average of 29 per cent to below 20 per cent, her fertility decreases markedly. This happens in part because *fat helps to produce estrogen*. When a woman's body-fat ratio falls between 12–15 per cent, as if often does among female athletes, fertility can cease entirely, along with the cessation of menstruation. In fact, even sexual desire can begin to decrease when a woman's body-fat ratio dips significantly.

In addition, a woman's monthly gain of water weight, shortly after ovulation, is a biological preparation for pregnancy, which requires extra fluids for fetal development. During pregnancy, the body also requires approximately 10 extra pounds of fat, to protect the health and energy of mother and child.

When a mother nurses, she also requires extra body fat, because nursing requires the expenditure of an extra 500–1,000 calories per day.

To ensure the availability of the extra fat that women need for fertility, women store fat differently than men. Female hormones dictate the storage of extra fat in an area of the body where it burns relatively slowly: the hips, thighs and buttocks. Fat in the hips, thighs, and buttocks accounts for only 8 per cent of all the fat in men, but about 20 per cent of the fat in women. Men tend to store most of their extra fat in their abdomens, where fat is more easily burned by exercise and dieting.

Most people think of fat as being biologically inert and lifeless, but fat is always changing. The triglycerides that form fat are constantly being broken down and rebuilt, and this happens much more readily in abdominal fat than it does in lower-body fat. Lower-body fat, which is sometimes called 'quiet fat,' tends to process insulin less efficiently than abdominal fat does.

Because women need more fat for fertility, they're born with more and gain even more during puberty. Female infants have an average of 10–15 per cent more fat tissue than male infants, and during puberty, their body fat increases by approximately 50 per cent as their estrogen levels rise. By contrast, when boys hit puberty, their increased testosterone helps them to burn fat more efficiently and build more muscle. This extra muscle allows them to burn even *more* fat, since muscle burns more calories than fat. Men tend to burn 10 per cent to 20 per cent more calories at rest than women, because of their extra muscle and their male hormones.

By age 20, the average amount of body fat among women – approximately 29 per cent – is much higher than a man's 18 per cent to 20 per cent. The average female body-fat ratio by midlife is an average of 38 per cent.

Estrogen, the primary female hormone, appears to have a generally negative effect upon natural fat burning, or thermogenesis. In fact, a common practice among farmers has been to feed female hormones to cattle to fatten them up.

Unfortunately, not only does estrogen increase fat production, but *fat also increases estrogen production*. This creates a vicious cycle. Due to this natural, biological proclivity that women have for adding extra fat, it's much harder for women to lose weight and easier for them to gain it. In an analysis of a number of studies conducted between 1976 and 1980, approximately 25 per cent more women were overweight than men.

Even women who have a very healthy balance of hormones, with no evidence of premenstrual syndrome, tend to have more body fat than men. However, 85 per cent of pre-menopausal women have at least mild PMS, which makes them *far* more vulnerable to weight gain.

Most doctors have long believed that women gain weight more easily than men solely because of their female hormones and because of the imbalances that often disrupt these hormones. While I was in medical school, that's what I thought, too. I now believe, however, that this is a simplistic, limited perspective.

The *real* reason that women are far more prone than men to weight gain, it now appears, is not just female hormones, but also the crossover effect between PMS and food reactions.

Let's look at the specific effects that PMS has on weight control. You'll see that it causes the same five problems that food reactions cause: (1) food cravings, (2) metabolic disorders, (3) mood swings, (4) energy and immune dysfunction, and (5) swelling and bloating.

PMS and Food Cravings

Almost all of my female patients who have moderate to severe PMS report food cravings. Most of these patients also suffer from food reactions. These patients most commonly crave sweet foods – especially chocolate. One patient of mine, for example, craved chocolate so much that sometimes, just before her period, she ate an entire batch of brownies in a single evening, with chocolate milk.

Once, she told me, she was walking through town just before her period was due and was overwhelmed by the smell of chocolate wafting from a nearby factory. Smell is the only one of our five senses that goes straight to the brain's cortex without first being filtered through the hypothalamus, and it's therefore especially powerful at triggering memories, emotions, and endocrine secretions. The smell of chocolate was so overpowering for this woman that it made her literally feel faint. She rushed to the nearest shop and ate four chocolate bars, one after the other.

Soon she suffered a severe food reaction and craved even more chocolate. She went on a two-day binge. It took more than a week for her metabolism to return to normal.

She believed that this episode would never have happened if she hadn't been suffering from PMS at the time, and she was probably correct. One of the primary effects of PMS – and also of food reactions – is to lower the levels of the brain's primary contentment chemical, serotonin. That's mostly why women feel depressed and anxious during PMS. Chocolate, however, is the richest dietary source of a substance called phenyl-ethylamine that gives the brain a big emotional lift. Some people are more sensitive to this substance, which is somewhat similar to amphetamine, or speed, than others, and women appear to get a far more profound boost from it than men. Thus, it's very common for women to crave chocolate when they have PMS. In fact, in a study of PMS and food cravings, chocolate was the food most craved. Furthermore, the women with the worst PMS symptoms were those who craved chocolate the most.

The other type of food that is very commonly craved is *any* kind of sweet, starchy dessert. This is understandable, because eating sweet, starchy foods is the best dietary way to directly increase serotonin. Sweet foods also quickly reverse low blood sugar, which commonly occurs during PMS due to metabolic disturbances of several endocrine glands.

The food cravings that PMS cause are almost exactly like the cravings that food reactions cause. In both situations, serotonin and blood sugar are driven down. The cravings that result are not at all like mere hunger; they are a need-to-feed reaction that feels intense and urgent.

The need-to-feed response caused by either PMS or food reactions *alone* can be painful, but when these two powerful forces are combined, the cravings can become virtually irresistible. These cravings cause many women to eat voraciously for several days each month, and these several days of overeating destroy many diets.

Recently, pharmaceutical researchers developed several weight control medications, such as fenfluramine, that increase serotonin, but I almost never prescribe these drugs. I prefer to get to the root of the problem by preventing serotonin slumps before they begin. The best way to do this is to eliminate food reactions. It's also quite helpful to decrease PMS symptoms using the natural therapies that I'll describe in the last section of this chapter. For the most part, many of the same procedures and practices that eliminate food reactions also help correct PMS.

When PMS is corrected, menstruation can become a positive experience, according to my female patients who have achieved hormonal balance and overcome their food reactions. These women have learned to approach menstruation as a time of cleansing and renewal, during which they further purify their diets and cast off the metabolic impurities in their systems.

PMS and Mood Disturbance

As I mentioned, PMS lowers levels of the important feel-good neurotransmitter serotonin. This not only causes food cravings but also disturbs overall mood. A low level of serotonin is by far the most common cause of mood disorders in our society today. Almost all antidepressant medications, including Prozac, are designed to increase serotonin.

Women, unfortunately, are vastly more vulnerable to serotonin slumps than men. Many researchers now believe that the female hormone estrogen has a powerful direct effect upon serotonin, often lowering its levels.

The worst problems with serotonin occur when estrogen levels fluctuate. This almost always lowers serotonin levels and causes mood problems. There is some evidence, however, that even when estrogen levels are normal and stable, estrogen still has a negative effect upon serotonin levels. Several animal experiments have indicated that estrogen *destabilizes* serotonin, while the male hormone testosterone *stabilizes* serotonin. This, however, has not been conclusively proven.

It has been proven, though, that some of the abrupt swings in female hormones that can accompany menstrual cycles are antagonistic to the serotonin system. Researchers have charted serotonin levels on a monthly basis in women, and have found that as hormonal levels fluctuate, serotonin levels decline. These dips in serotonin are almost certainly the cause of the monthly bouts of insomnia, depression, anxiety, vulnerability to pain, and food cravings that characterize PMS.

One biochemical reason for this drop in serotonin is that estrogen changes the way women metabolize the nutritional building block that produces serotonin, the amino acid tryptophan. When tryptophan metabolism is impaired, the body is unable to produce sufficient supplies of serotonin.

Again, this isn't fair, but it's a fact of life.

Because of this, women are prone not only to PMS but also to a number of other disorders that are caused by low serotonin. Some of these disorders are quite obvious, such as depression and anxiety. Women suffer from clinical depression almost three times more often than men.

Other disorders have a less obvious link to low serotonin, but this link is still very real. For example, most doctors now think that low serotonin levels are the primary cause of migraines, because serotonin keeps the blood vessels in the brain from expanding uncontrollably, as they do during migraines. Migraines strike women three times more often than men. Another serotonin-related malady is chronic pain, because serotonin is a natural painkiller. Chronic pain is also about three times more common among women than men. Women also suffer almost ten times as much fibromyalgia, the painful muscle condition that appears to be related to low serotonin.

Many researchers have tried to figure out exactly why female hormones cause serotonin to decline so that they could fix the problem. For the most part, they've tended to see estrogen as the culprit, and the female hormone progesterone as the possible 'cure.' But just giving women more progesterone doesn't seem to work, because hormone interactions are very complex. The fundamental problems appear to be *imbalance* of female hormones and fluctuation. It's quite difficult, however, to control imbalance and fluctuation, because they're influenced by so many factors.

I occasionally prescribe hormonal replacement therapy to women, primarily during menopause, but my fundamental approach is to help women find their own most healthy lifestyles and nutritional habits, and allow the innate wisdom of the body to balance the hormones naturally.

Lately, I've begun to theorize that two other weight-related conditions that mostly strike women may also be related to low serotonin.

The first is the body image problem called body dysmorphic disorder, or BDD. People with BDD, which is far more common among women than men, think they look much fatter than they really do. Many of the people who have this problem are quite normal in appearance, but feel obese. If they eat a biscuit or piece of chocolate, they feel even fatter.

Some of this irrational perception is caused by societal expectation. Women in particular, are bombarded by contrived images of slimness, and they often feel they must conform. This factor certainly contributes to BDD. However, I think that for most women with severe BDD, the problem isn't primarily psychological, but biochemical. I believe that the most important causative factor in BDD is a lack of serotonin. Serotonin helps us to feel good about *every* aspect of our lives, including our finances, our families, our jobs – and our bodies. Often, the women I treat who have BDD are dissatisfied with almost *every* aspect of their lives. They don't yearn for just a slimmer body, but also for more money, a better job, and a happier marriage. When they go on the False Fat Diet, however, their hormones generally stabilize, their PMS tends to subside, and they often begin to see things differently. They accept themselves. They accept their lives. Often, of course, they'd still like to be a little thinner, but they're no longer obsessed with slimness and no longer have a distorted body image.

Many doctors have achieved success by treating BDD with Prozac-type drugs, which boost serotonin. I prefer to increase serotonin with a more natural approach, but do sometimes prescribe antidepressants.

* * *

The second condition that I think is linked to low serotonin is the presence of eating disorders, particularly bulimia and anorexia. Eating disorders are a largely female phenomenon; women and girls account for 90 per cent to 95 per cent of all cases. Eating disorders are very common among women who have body dysmorphic disorder. When women perceive their bodies irrationally, they often eat irrationally. Virtually all anorectics have BDD.

Recently several studies have shown that both bulimics and anorectics have low levels of serotonin. Some researchers think that eating disorders *cause* low levels of serotonin by restricting nutrients, but I think it's the other way around. I believe the problem *starts* with low serotonin (which generally occurs for reasons that are obscure or unknown). Then, after an eating disorder is established, it may indeed drive serotonin levels even lower, as part of a vicious cycle. One indication that low serotonin starts the problem came from a study in which bulimic women and non-bulimic women were given a diet that was normal in every way, except for a deficiency of the amino acid that creates serotonin (tryptophan). The bulimic women became very depressed and had increased urges to engage in bulimic behaviour. The non-bulimic women weren't particularly affected. The researchers concluded that bulimic women are much more sensitive to low serotonin levels than non-bulimic women.

Another indication that low serotonin causes bulimia is the fact that bulimic women tend to have *other* personality traits that are associated with low serotonin. Among the traits are obsession, compulsion, heightened stress response, impulse control difficulty, and a proneness to addictive disorders, including alcoholism. One patient of mine, for example, was not only bulimic but also a compulsive shopper and a chain smoker. She had a rather brittle, sensitive personality and didn't handle stress well, particularly when she was suffering from PMS. After she eliminated her food reactions, however, her PMS subsided dramatically, and her hormonal mood swings became much less pronounced. Over a period of about six months, she became much calmer and stopped shopping every time she felt tense. She hasn't been able to stop smoking, but she's no longer chain-smoking and is trying to quit.

Recent studies have also linked low serotonin to anorexia, which strikes about 1 per cent of all women – mostly adolescents, at the height of their hormonal turmoil. Anorexia causes greater damage to the metabolism than any other eating disorder, due to its severe caloric restriction, and this makes the condition very difficult to treat. Anorexia grossly distorts endocrine function and greatly exacerbates existing disorders of the serotonin system. Anorectic women tend to be rigid and perfectionistic, which are also traits associated with low serotonin.

I haven't treated enough anorectic patients to draw any conclusions, but a number of other physicians have achieved some success by treating anorexia with serotonin-boosting medications. Currently, Prozac-type drugs are the treatment of choice for this complex physical and emotional disorder.

As you can see, hormonal instability wreaks havoc upon mood chemistry, mostly by lowering the levels of serotonin. When the mood chemistry disruption caused by PMS is combined with the mood problems caused by food reactions, women can suffer terribly. Twenty years ago, most doctors blamed these mood problems solely on psychological factors, such as unhappy childhood memories. This made millions of women see themselves as neurotic and hysterical. This was unfair and unenlightened. Nonetheless, many doctors still cling to this old-fashioned view.

PMS and Metabolic Disorders

Hormonal instability causes two metabolic disturbances that pile on the pounds; low thyroid function, or hypothyroidism, and low blood sugar, or hypoglycemia. As you may recall food reactions *also* cause both of these problems. When food reactions and PMS are both contributing to these two serious problems, weight control can become almost impossible.

Low thyroid function is more common than most people

realize. Doctors almost always detect hypothyroidism when it becomes severe, but often overlook the problem when it is mild. Nonetheless, this mild, sub-clinical hypothyroidism can cause significant problems, including weight gain, a feeling of coldness, constipation, fatigue, and depression. It can also trigger hypoglycemia.

Hypothyroidism often occurs in women whose estrogen levels are much higher than their levels of progesterone. In general, estrogen decreases thyroid function, and progesterone increases it. Because estrogen can lower thyroid function, hypothyroidism is five to ten times more common among women than men. It is often triggered by puberty, menopause, and pregnancy; an estimated 30 per cent of all women experience sub-clinical hypothyroidism after pregnancy.

The thyroid, a large endocrine gland located in the neck, secretes hormones that help provide energy and growth, and help the body to adjust to heat and cold. Symptoms of poor thyroid function include not only lethargy but also sensitivity to cold. Abnormal hunger is also sometimes caused by hypothyroidism.

Low thyroid function also contributes to *hypoglycemia*, because thyroid hormones help signal the pancreas to produce insulin. When the thyroid isn't functioning well, it can trigger low blood sugar. It's very common for women to experience hypoglycemia as part of their PMS symptoms. When hypoglycemia hits, people can literally feel as if they're starving. People with hypoglycemia generally feel tired, irritable, weak, confused, and hungry. To compensate for this lack of blood sugar, the body secretes extra adrenaline, which often adds to the feeling of agitation. When this adrenaline wears off, hunger and fatigue become even worse.

The brain is especially hard hit by hypoglycemia, because brain cells, unlike other cells in the body, have no capacity to store extra blood sugar. That's why one of the first signs of hypoglycemia is inability to concentrate, often accompanied by depression or anxiety. When hypoglycemia strikes, it's almost impossible to refrain from eating. In fact, it's not even smart to refrain from eating, because a depleted source of blood sugar can actually damage and kill brain cells. Some brain researchers believe that hypoglycemia can kill almost as many brain cells as other well-known biological insults to the brain, such as drinking too much alcohol.

To temporarily stop the uncomfortable effects of hypoglycemia, many people use mild stimulants, such as caffeine and nicotine, which can replenish blood sugar for a short time. These substances stress the adrenal glands, though, and have many other harmful effects.

The only truly effective way to deal with hypoglycemia is to prevent it. The best ways to do this are to avoid reactive foods, avoid foods that are metabolized too quickly (such as sugar and starch), and to eat more frequently (without adding extra daily calories).

PMS and Swelling and Bloating

Swelling and bloating appear to be increasingly common as a symptom of PMS, perhaps because of the increasing incidence of food reactions in our society. In a major study done in 1953, swelling and bloating were reported to occur in only about 6 per cent of women with PMS. In a more recent survey of studies conducted by the FDA, however, swelling and bloating were reported by 31 per cent of women with PMS.

Among my female patients with food reactions, swelling and bloating are commonly a significant symptom of PMS.

Most of my female food reaction patients have swelling and bloating even before their monthly premenstrual symptoms begin. Then, when PMS occurs, their swelling and bloating become even worse. The crossover effect between food reactions and PMS often transforms tissue swelling into a significant medical condition characterized by pain, blockage of sinus drainage, proneness to migraine, and dizziness (due to inner ear disturbance).

It appears as if tissue swelling during PMS is caused by the imbalance between estrogen and progesterone. Low progesterone seems to be the primary causative factor, possibly because it increases levels of anti-diuretic hormone. As you'll recall, storing extra water is a natural preparation-for-pregnancy phenomenon, which supports the health of a developing fetus. The average water weight gain during PMS is 4 to 7 pounds, although gains of up to 14 pounds have been reported. At the end of this water-storage period, a woman may urinate an extra four to five litres of urine per day, for several days.

Water weight often collects in fat cells, but can also be stored in most of the cells in your body. It is also often stored in the spaces between cells. Fluids commonly make your extremities swell. Your hands, feet, ankles, and breasts may become swollen. These changes may be uncomfortable and may cause shoes, rings and even bras to no longer fit.

More serious problems occur, however, when water is stored in areas that do not allow for the stretching of tissues. This occurs in the labyrinth of the inner ear (causing dizziness), the sinuses (causing congestion and headaches), the spinal discs (causing backache), and the joints (causing stiff, achy joints). Some researchers believe that minor swelling of the brain can also occur, resulting in cognitive and emotional problems, but this has not been proven. In the lungs, PMS-related swelling, or cyclical idiopathic edema, can aggravate asthma, and can also create a heavy, congested feeling. In the eyes, it can cause pressure similar to that of glaucoma.

Water retention is most likely to occur in cells that are already inflamed due to injury, infection, or food reactions. Therefore, water may tend to migrate to areas such as the abdomen, where tissues are already swollen from food reactions.

The orthodox therapy for water retention is use of diuretics, but I rarely employ this approach. Some diuretics cause depletion of potassium, which increases fatigue and weakness. Furthermore, diuretics have a notoriously short-lived effect. Water is replaced almost as quickly as it is excreted.

The only sound approach, in my opinion, is to prevent water retention before it becomes significant by ameliorating premenstrual syndrome and by avoiding food reactions.

PMS and Energy and Immune Dysfunction

Similarly to food reactions, PMS drives down energy, contributes to insomnia, interferes with normal immune function, and exacerbates yeast colonization, which can produce flu-like symptoms. When the crossover effect is in force, these characteristics are doubly disabling.

Lethargy is a common symptom of PMS. Sometimes it is directly caused by a deficit of progesterone, which generally has an energizing effect. At other times, it's indirectly caused by other PMS factors, including depression, insomnia, hypoglycemia, hypothyroidism, and a shortage of adrenaline. As you'll recall, food reactions can also cause depression, insomnia, hypoglycemia, hypothyroidism, and adrenal deficit, with a secondary effect of lethargy.

Frequently, I see women who have several of these disorders, caused by both PMS and food reactions, and these women often suffer from a profound sense of fatigue. They feel exhausted and describe their fatigue vividly, using terms such as 'bone tired,' 'half dead,' and 'asleep on my feet.'

However, when the symptoms related to their crossover effect begin to lift, they often experience an intense resurgence of energy. One young woman described her recovery by saying, 'It was like someone lifted the proverbial bell jar off me' – making a reference to Sylvia Plath's book *The Bell Jar*. It was an interesting analogy, because Sylvia Plath is well known among readers for her sensitive portrayal of gloom, but is well known among endocrinologists as a famous victim of premenstrual depression. Unfortunately, Plath, who committed suicide during one of her periodic bouts of depression, lived in an era when virtually all depression was thought to be of psychological origin, rather than biochemical, and never received adequate medical treatment.

Besides sapping energy, PMS also has a moderately negative effect on immune strength. One way PMS hurts immunity is by increasing the secretion of the stress hormone cortisol. Cortisol is similar to adrenaline, but has a stronger effect and stays in the system longer. When too much cortisol is in your system, it sends extra energy to your fight-or-flight organs and systems, such as your muscles and heart. Unfortunately, this robs energy from your immune system's gland and organs, such as your thymus or liver. In one interesting experiment, during a flu epidemic, researchers discovered that 90 per cent of the people who had high levels of anxiety and depression caught the flu. These people didn't recover for an average of three weeks, compared to just five days for people who weren't depressed or anxious.

Another way PMS hurts immunity is by harming the function of the thyroid, which plays a secondary role in immunity. Thyroid hormones stimulate the liver to produce the white blood cells, called phagocytes, that kill bacteria and viruses.

PMS and Candida

One of the most debilitating effects of PMS is to increase proliferation of common yeast, or *Candida albicans*, in the body's mucous membranes, especially in the intestinal and genitourinary tracts. Candida overgrowth, which is also exacerbated by food reactions, is extremely common and can be a serious health problem. Candida overgrowth in the gut causes fermentation of foods and inflammatory thickening of the gut wall, which can cause severe abdominal bloating. It is therefore a significant cause of false fat.

The most obvious yeast infections are vaginal. Most women get them from time to time. But yeast overgrowth occurs just as often in the intestines, and frequently goes unnoticed. When this happens, the results can be quite problematic. The overgrowth itself often makes people feel sick. It also contributes to food reactions; this happens when tiny yeast 'roots' bore into the wall of the intestine and dig microscopic holes. This creates the condition called *leaky gut syndrome*, in which undigested food macromolecules slip through the holes and enter the body's tissues and fluids. When this happens, they often cause food reactions by triggering the immune response.

Yeast infections are not only exacerbated by hormonal imbalance but also *cause* hormonal imbalance. This is another one of the vicious cycles that are so common when the metabolism gets out of balance.

Yeast is almost always present in the intestines, but is generally controlled by the probiotic friendly flora of other helpful, food-digesting bacteria (such as *Lactobacillus acidophilus* and bifidobacteria, the healthy bacteria in yogurt). However, a number of factors cause candida to proliferate. Some of these factors increase candida by killing friendly bacteria, while others increase candida by feeding the yeast itself. Among the factors that cause yeast overgrowth are: use of antibiotics; eating foods that contain yeast, such as baked goods and beer; stress; birth control pills; impaired immunity; eating foods that cause yeast to multiply, such as sugar; use of cortisone-type drugs; exposure to airborne moulds (which is more common in wet weather); and sexual contact with a person who carries candida microorganisms.

Some of the symptoms of candida overgrowth are obvious, but others are frequently mistaken for other problems. The most obvious symptom is itching and discomfort from a vaginal yeast infection. However, yeast can grow in any mucous membrane – including those of the throat, nose, and sinus – and yeast overgrowth in those areas is often mistaken for a virus or for allergies. In the intestines, yeast overgrowth is sometimes mistaken for flu symptoms or for food reaction symptoms. Often, yeast overgrowth in the intestines – which causes significant abdominal bloating – is mistaken for fat. This frequently happens among people who are heavy beer drinkers. They think the beer they drink is just making them gain adipose tissue, but it's also often making them bloated from yeast overgrowth and fermentation. This seems to be somewhat more common lately, due to the increased popularity of yeasty micro-brewed beer.

The main reason candida overgrowth causes bloating is because it ferments foods in the digestive tract. It especially ferments sweet, sugary foods, as well as foods that tend to be naturally hard to digest, such as diary products. The most obvious sign of this fermentation is abdominal distension, and the next most obvious sign is presence of gas and excessive flatulence.

Candida overgrowth is much more common among women, but it also frequently occurs among men. Men often overlook the condition, however, because many of them incorrectly assume that a man cannot get a yeast infection. In men, candida overgrowth is most likely to occur in the intestinal tract. However, men can also develop redness and itching on their penis, scrotum, or groin area from a yeast infection, and it may also aggravate the prostate. Sometimes this occurs after they have sex with a woman who has a yeast infection. It's not uncommon for a man and woman to pass a yeast infection back and forth, through sexual activity.

When people have chronic candida overgrowth, they often feel weak, depressed, irritable, and tired. Periodically they may experience a mass die-off of yeast organisms, and this may make them feel even worse, as the necrotic material is dumped into the body's tissues and fluids. The symptoms of chronic candida overgrowth, therefore, are quite similar to those of chronic fatigue syndrome. I've had several patients who were certain they had chronic fatigue syndrome, but who actually had candida overgrowth.

Fortunately, yeast overgrowth is relatively easy to control. This can be done with nutritional therapy medication, and herbs. *Nutritional therapy* consists of avoiding yeasty and sugary foods, as well as yeast-increasing foods such as mushrooms, cheese, pickled vegetables, vinegar, dried fruit, fruit juices, baked goods, alcohol, and bread. You should also, of course, avoid reactive foods.

It's also very important to ingest nutrients called probiotics: *Lactobacillus acidophilus* and bifidobacteria. Both of these probiotics are present in some cultured yogurts and are also available as nutritional supplements. Many people who are reactive to dairy products take their probiotics in dairy-free supplement form. Other people who are not reactive to dairy products still take their probiotics in supplement form, because supplements usually contain more organisms than yogurt. An appropriate dosage provides about 4 to 10 billion acidophilus micro-organisms daily.

Other helpful nutrients and herbs, taken on a daily basis, include: caprylic acid; grapefruit seed extract; coenzyme Q_{10}; GLA, or gamma linolenic acid; betaine hydrochloride; goldenseal; pau d'arco; echinacea; and garlic extract. In addition, you should take a multivitamin/mineral supplement that includes vitamins C, A, E, K, beta-carotene, and the B-complex, along with calcium, chromium, copper, selenium, iodine, and iron (for dosages, see the chart on page 104). Most of these are included in a multivitamin/mineral.

If you are not accustomed to nutritional therapy, this may seem excessive, but it is not. It takes a strong regimen of nutrients to pack the power that is needed to overcome potentially serious medical conditions, such as candida over-growth. Another nutritional therapy approach is to take a nutritional formulation designed to fight candida. If you do this, make sure you buy a powerful formula. Seeing a prac-titioner experienced in treating candida may be necessary.

When the condition is cleared, you will be almost certain to feel the effects and can then scale down your nutritional therapy accordingly. To prevent recurrence, it's important to ingest some healthy, probiotic bacteria virtually every day. This will also help your general digestion and should help prevent food reactions.

The most commonly used systemic medication for yeast infection is fluconazole, which is sold under the brand name Diflucan. Doctors generally prescribe only a single pill of Diflucan for vaginal yeast infection. However, for intestinal yeast overgrowth, I often administer the medication for a week or more to kill the many thick layers of yeast that can reside in the gut and other tissues. Other frequently used medications are nystatin, ketoconazole (Nizoral), which is less expensive than fluconazole, and itraconazole (Sporanox). These drugs are sometimes irritating to the liver, but this side effect is relatively rare. My patients seem to tolerate them well.

Now let's look at natural therapy for premenstrual syndrome. If you employ this therapy, it will greatly improve

CANDIDA THERAPY

Dietary and Metabolic Factors
- Avoid foods that stimulate yeast growth, such as sugars, sweets, bread, baked goods, alcohol, vinegar, cheese, fruit juice, and dried fruits.
- Eat vegetables, proteins, nuts, seeds, and legumes, and limit fruit to 2 per day (avoiding sugary melons).
- Exercise, reduce stress, and keep the bowels active.

Supplements (Nutrients and Herbs)

GENERAL SUPPORT NUTRIENTS
- Multivitamin/mineral: 1–6 daily, as directed on the bottle, in evenly divided dosages after meals
- B-complex: 25–50 mg; with 300–500 mcg of biotin, once or twice daily
- Vitamin C: 500–1,000 mg, twice daily
- Vitamin E: 400 IU, once or twice daily
- Selenium: 100–200 mcg (take with vitamin E)
- Beta-carotene: 15,000–30,000 IU (or mixed carotenoids)

SPECIFIC ANTI-YEAST NUTRIENTS
- Acidophilus or other probiotics, with at least 5 to 10 billion live organisms per dosage (other probiotics include rhamanosa and bifidobacteria)
- Garlic capsules, odourless or oil: 2–3 capsules, twice daily, before or after meals
- Caprylic acid: 500–1,000 mg, 2 or 3 times daily
- Grapefruit seed extract: 1–3 capsules, twice daily (also available as a liquid extract)
- Pau d'arco: 1–2 capsules, once or twice daily (also available as a liquid extract)

OTHER HELPFUL NUTRIENTS
- Echinacea: 1–2 droppers of liquid extract, or 1–2 capsules, twice daily, between meals, for no more than 3 consecutive weeks (to avoid 'antibiotic' side effects)
- Goldenseal: 1–2 droppers of liquid extract, or 1–2 capsules, twice daily, between meals (for two consecutive weeks only)

- Hydrochloric acid (or betaine hydrochloride): 1–2 capsules just before eating meals containing fat or protein
- GLA oils (from evening primrose or starflower seed): 1–2 capsules, 2 to 3 times daily, after meals
- Coenzyme Q$_{10}$: 30–50 mg, twice daily

Pharmaceutical Medications

Take these as directed by your physician.
- **Fluconazole** (Diflucan)
- **Ketoconazole** (Nizoral)
- **Itraconazole** (Sporanox)
- **Nystatin**
- **Lamisil**

---

your chances of ending the cruel crossover effect between food reactions and PMS.

PMS Therapy

The best way to overcome PMS is with nutritional therapy and exercise. There is no reliable medication that will solve the root problem of PMS.

Your diet should be relatively low in fat, high in fibre, nutrient dense, wholesome, and free of reactive foods. Soya can be especially helpful, because it contains isoflavones that help to naturally balance female hormones. In fact, women in Asia tend to have far less PMS than women in the West, theoretically because they eat more soya products. It may also be because they eat less fat, which stresses the liver and deters it from adequately balancing hormones.

Because the liver is important in hormonal balance, it's also essential to avoid other foods stressful to the liver, such as sugar, fried foods, and foods contaminated with pesticides, herbicides, and additives. It's also helpful to avoid beef and chicken from animals that were fed hormones; to do this, buy organic, hormone-free meats.

Among the specific nutrients that are most important are vitamin B_6 and magnesium. B_6 supports the liver and is especially helpful for preventing the false fat of water retention. Magnesium is a powerful antioxidant that exerts a notable calming effect and also increases cell wall permeability. It's important, though, to take the full spectrum of B-complex vitamins, because each supports the functions of the others. (For dosages on all suggested nutrients, see the chart on page 107.)

Other special nutrients for PMS, which should be taken on a daily basis, include evening primrose oil, omega-3 fatty acids, multiple vitamins and minerals, vitamin E, vitamin C, calcium, phenylalanine, and 5-HTP.

Herbs can be extremely helpful. Among the best is dong quai, which has been used for centuries to balance female hormones. Others are vitex (chasteberry), ginger, parsley, and juniper berry, all of which help reduce water retention. A number of good PMS herbal formulations are available at health food shops and pharmacies, and many of my patients have benefited from them.

It's also important to exercise. A number of studies indicate that PMS symptoms decline in direct relation to exercise, in part because exercise increases the output of endorphins and also increases the stimulating neurotransmitter norepinephrine. Exercise is also a powerful detoxifier.

It may also help to use bright light therapy in the dark winter months. Many women with elevated PMS suffer from the depressive condition of seasonal affective disorder, which is caused by a lack of sunlight. Sunlight or artificial full-spectrum lights naturally increase output of norepinephrine, which is crucial for avoiding depression. When women simply turn on bright full-spectrum lights for about an hour in the morning, it often stops their premenstrual depressive symptoms.

If you're a woman, you owe it to yourself to overcome the cruel crossover effects between PMS and food reactions. When you do overcome them, your strength and your peace of mind will increase every day, and you will feel better than you have in years. I know you can do this! Others have. Now it's your turn.

PREMENSTRUAL SYNDROME THERAPY

Dietary and Metabolic Factors

- Avoid sugar and sweets, wheat, refined flours, and reactive foods. Eat a variety of wholesome foods and soya protein (for helpful isoflavones and hormonal support).
- Exercise, and sweat, to eliminate toxins and support the metabolism.
- Express your feelings and emotions to family and friends.

Supplements

- Multivitamin/mineral: 1–2 capsules, twice daily, as directed on bottle
- Vitamin E: 400 IU, once or twice daily
- Vitamin C: with bioflavonoids, 500–1,000 mg, twice daily
- Calcium: 400–600 mg (taken with magnesium in the evening to promote sleep and decrease cramps)
- Magnesium: 300–500 mg (taken with calcium in the evening to promote sleep and decrease cramps), plus 250–500 mg, twice daily, during the day
- Vitamin B_6: 50–100 mg, 2 to 3 times daily
- Evening primrose oil: 2 capsules, 2 to 3 times daily
- Omega-3 fatty acids: 1–2 capsules, twice daily after meals
- 5-HTP: 50–100 mg, at night, to promote sleep, if needed
- Phenylalanine: 250–500 mg, twice daily
- Dong quai: 1–2 capsules, once or twice daily

This natural programme is often very helpful for relieving PMS within two months. Other helpful herbs, individually or in combination, may include ginger, ginseng, juniper berries, and vitex, or chasteberry.

There are many good commercial formulations, containing multiple nutrients and herbs, for PMS. They are available from health food shops and mail-order supplement companies. Take as directed. Also, natural progesterone can be used medically during the second half of the cycle to reduce PMS symptoms that often result from a low progesterone-to-estrogen ratio. Consult with your doctor or health practitioner about this therapy.

We now have only one more chapter before we get into the details of starting the False Fat Diet. It's an amazing chapter that covers *twenty-one different medical conditions* that are caused or aggravated by food reactions. You probably have one of these conditions, because they're very common.

You can get rid of it – and lose weight at the same time!

5

THE EXTRAORDINARY SIDE BENEFITS

PATIENTS OFTEN BEGIN THE FALSE FAT DIET HOPING JUST to lose weight — but soon *extraordinary, unexpected things begin to happen*. Their depression, migraines, insomnia, and muscle pains often disappear. Frequently their joint pain, asthma, or eczema also improves significantly. They sometimes even recover from disorders that are generally considered incurable, such as irritable bowel syndrome.

These recoveries are astonishing to my patients and very rewarding for me. I love to see people achieve full, robust health and break free from the countless destructive conditions that plague modern life. I also love helping them break free from the lifestyle habits that often contribute to these conditions. For me, that's what being a doctor of integrative medicine is all about — the great 'side benefits' that patients experience when they treat one problem with improved habits and natural therapies. This, to me, is real *health* care. Too often, doctors settle for just suppressing negative symptoms, instead of trying to evoke healing and vibrant health. When they do this, *they fail their patients*. Suppressing negative symptoms is, in my opinion, just a glorified version of first aid.

In contrast, when I place patients on the False Fat Diet, it often helps them reach their full physical and mental potential. The diet does this by reversing many of the terrible conditions caused by food reactions.

Look at this long list of problems that are often caused by, or exacerbated by, food reactions.

- Arthritis
- Asthma
- Candidiasis (yeast overgrowth)
- Cardiovascular disease
- Chronic ear infections
- Chronic fatigue syndrome
- Chronic pain
- Cognitive disorders (including memory and concentration impairment)
- Diabetes
- Digestive disorders (including heartburn, indigestion, and ulcers)
- Eating disorders (including bulimia, bingeing, and anorexia nervosa)
- Eczema, acne and hives
- Fibromyalgia
- Hay fever and airborne allergies
- Headaches (especially migraines)
- Hyperactivity and attention deficit disorder
- Hypoglycemia
- Insomnia
- Irritable bowel syndrome
- Mood disorders (including depression and anxiety)
- Sinusitis

When food reactions are eliminated, these problems are frequently cured or controlled. *No other weight-loss diet can make this claim.* That's because the False Fat Diet is much *more* than just a weight-loss diet – it's a *health recovery diet*, which also results in normalized weight.

When my food reaction patients first consult with me, most of them are not only overweight but also suffer from at least one of the conditions on this list. This occurs so often because food reactions have such pervasive, far-reaching effects. They are a systemic disorder and cause problems throughout the body.

Most patients, however, aren't even aware that several of their problems have the same cause. They don't see how a number of very different conditions – such as arthritis, insomnia, and heartburn – could possibly be connected. Too often, their doctors also miss this connection. Most doctors, unfortunately, tend to focus on just one problem at a time. This happens for several reasons. One reason is that patients usually come in with just one complaint at a time. Also, doctors are trained to deductively isolate problems, and this sometimes makes them miss the big picture. Furthermore, many doctors are specialists, treating just one disorder or one part of the body.

Therefore, doctors and patients often overlook the *single, root cause* of a host of related problems. This frequently happens for many years – and sometimes for a patient's entire life.

It happened to my patient Walter, who went most of his life without an accurate diagnosis of his primary, pervasive problem – food reactions. Walter, 38, was about 30 pounds overweight. He had a high-stress technological job at a company based near my centre. Walt blamed job stress for his insomnia and chronic anxiety, and felt it was also related to his severe heartburn, occasional migraines, and the eating binges that aggravated his weight problem.

When I first met Walt, his doctors had him on an anti-depressant, two medications to reduce the level of his stomach acid, migraine medicine, and an appetite suppressant. However, these medications were only exerting temporary effects on his symptoms and didn't help with his insomnia at all.

He was miserable. He hated his job but couldn't afford to quit. He felt trapped.

However, when he went on the False Fat Diet, and eliminated eggs, corn, oranges, and soya, it had a wonderful effect upon him. He lost all of the weight he wanted to, which made him look good and feel good. Even more exciting, though, were his *side benefits*.

The first symptom that went away was his severe heartburn, or acid reflux disease. Severe heartburn is extremely common these days, partly because of food reactions. Some people get heartburn from reactive foods, simply because they can't readily digest these foods. Often, digestive disorders, including heartburn and excess gas, are the first symptoms that improve for people on the False Fat Diet.

Walt loved being free from his heartburn, because it had caused him a great deal of discomfort. When it had been bad, he told me, 'it felt like somebody was scratching the inside of my stomach with a wire brush.' Previously, he'd often had to gulp Maalox all day, just to feel normal.

The next symptom to clear was Walt's anxiety. This was extremely gratifying for him, because it was his most troubling symptom. When his food reactions were eliminated, his levels of the key neurotransmitters serotonin and norepinephrine seemed to stabilize, and he just didn't, as he put it, 'worry every little thing to death anymore.'

His mood remained calm and upbeat even after he discontinued use of his antidepressant, a Prozac-type drug called Serzone.

His reduction of anxiety tracked closely with a reduction of his insomnia, leading me to believe that the same neurotransmitter problems were largely responsible for both conditions.

As his other symptoms declined, so did his migraines. His migraines, like his insomnia and anxiety, were probably also related to his serotonin deficit. In recent years, researchers have concluded that a lack of serotonin causes most migraines, because serotonin keeps blood vessels in the brain from expanding uncontrollably.

After Walt began to feel better, he made a fascinating discovery: his job wasn't as inherently stressful as he'd thought. When his mind and body were no longer deviled by anxiety, insomnia, heartburn, and headaches, he was able to perceive his job stressors quite differently. He began to see them as challenges, instead of threats. In a matter of months, Walt turned his whole life around.

After Walt overcame his food reactions, he found his job wasn't as stressful as he'd thought.

After about twelve weeks on the diet, Walt told me that I

was 'a genius' for solving all his problems. But I couldn't take the credit. I had only solved *one* of his problems – food reactions. His own body, with its innate healing wisdom, had solved the rest.

There is wisdom in your body, too. You just have to learn to pay attention to it. And you have to know the signs and symptoms to look for.

Let's now take a closer look at the list of conditions that may be caused by food reactions. If you have one or more of these conditions, you may soon be able to end it. If you do, you'll have even more motivation to stick with your False Fat Diet – and change your life.

Arthritis

The most common type of arthritis, osteoarthritis, is caused by the gradual deterioration of the spongy cartilage that cushions the bones in joints. Cartilage keeps them from rubbing together and causing pain. Food reactions can contribute to this deterioration, because the inflammation they cause can gradually break down cartilage.

However, food reactions also have a much more *immediate* effect. Long before they actually destroy cartilage, food reactions can *mimic the effects of arthritis* by causing swelling and inflammation in joints. I believe this mostly happens because of immune response to circulating immune (antigen-antibody) complex food reactions. It can happen to anyone, including young people with healthy cartilage. When it happens, it can be almost as painful and restrictive as classic arthritis.

This pseudo-arthritis of joint swelling and inflammation is quite similar to the second most common type of arthritis, rheumatoid arthritis. Rheumatoid arthritis frequently strikes young people, and is characterized by swelling and inflammation in the joints, similar to that caused by food reactions. In fact, many arthritis experts believe that food reactions are a major cause of classic, immune-related rheumatoid arthritis.

The pseudo-arthritis caused by food reactions often strikes

people who also have actual, classic arthritis caused by cartilage deterioration or by rheumatic factors. When this happens, it can make their symptoms much worse and can make them think that their arthritic condition is far more advanced than it really is.

Unfortunately, when these two conditions gang up, patients often begin to take large amounts of aspirin, and this can make things even worse. Aspirin can actually aggravate cartilage deterioration. In addition, it can also make food reactions more frequent and more severe by irritating the stomach and gastrointestinal tract lining.

I recently had a patient who suffered from the pseudo-arthritis of joint inflammation caused by food reactions and overall toxicity. She was a 37-year-old nurse-practitioner whose hands were becoming crippled by joint pain. Her primary care physician had prescribed Motrin, but it wasn't very effective, and she feared its long-term side effects.

She went on the False Fat Diet, beginning with the detox phase, where she eliminated wheat, milk, sugar, and corn. She became free of arthritis-like symptoms in her hands *in one week*. Her doctor thought that this was a remarkable recovery from arthritis, but she didn't really *have* arthritis.

Over the next six months, she also lost about 12 pounds, overcame her insomnia, cleared up her chronic nasal congestion, began to feel much more energetic, and was still pain-free and more flexible in her hands.

It is, of course, quite common for patients to break free from a constellation of associated symptoms on the False Fat Diet. False fat does not occur in a vacuum – it's just one symptom of a systemic disorder.

According to conventional wisdom, the foods that seem to cause pseudo-arthritis most frequently are the nightshade family of plant foods, including tomatoes, peppers, potatoes and aubergines. These foods contain the chemical solanine, which can interfere with enzymes in muscles and aggravate pain. However, I believe that *any* food that a person reacts to can cause joint pain.

It's also important for people with joint pain to avoid heavy consumption of most animal fats and hydrogenated oils.

However, the omega-3 and omega-6 oils, the essential fatty acids, are generally quite helpful for the joints. They act, in effect, as lubricants.

Another food family that often contributes to joint pain is the rue family, which includes citrus fruits, such as oranges, grapefruits, lemons, and limes.

If you're beginning to suffer from joint pain – especially if you're under 50 – you should eliminate your food reactions. If you do, you may well find that your 'arthritis' isn't arthritis at all. If you're over 50, you may find that your arthritis isn't nearly as bad as you thought. If you do have classic osteo-arthritis, you may gain some relief from glucosamine sulphate and chondroitin, taken as directed by your physician.

Asthma

Food reactions appear to play an important secondary role in asthma, the condition of respiratory symptoms that include wheezing, shortness of breath, coughing, and increased mucus production in the lungs.

When an asthma attack strikes, muscles constrict in the small breathing tubes of the lungs. No one is certain why these muscles go into spasm. At the same time this happens, the lungs produce too much mucus. Researchers aren't sure why asthmatics produce more bronchial mucus, but we do know that food reactions often create overproduction of mucus.

Asthma is often triggered by airborne allergens – chiefly dust, pollen, mould, feathers, animal dander, cigarette smoke, and chemical pollutants. As I've mentioned, sensitivity to airborne allergens is usually heightened by food reactions. Food reactions often tip the scale and push people past their allergic thresholds. For example, many people aren't very reactive to pollen unless they also eat reactive foods.

Another potent trigger of asthma is eating foods that contain the food additive tartrazine, which is in yellow food dye #5, a common additive in yellow confectionery and snacks, margarine, cheese, coloured cereals, pickle relish, and some flavours of ice cream, pudding, and yogurt.

Preservatives are another frequent food trigger of asthma. The worst are the sulphites, which may be used by restaurants and are common in dried fruits.

Aspirin and ibuprofen also can trigger asthma attacks.

If you have asthma, eliminate your food reactions, and your allergic attacks may subside substantially. This has happened with several of my patients, including one 10-year-old boy, who was reactive to wheat and sulphites. When he eliminated them, his attacks decreased significantly.

Candidiasis

Candidiasis is often connected to food reactions; each makes the other worse. It is an insidious problem that creates symptoms similar to those of chronic fatigue syndrome. This condition tends to be overlooked by many physicians and often causes intermittent suffering for years at a time. Candidiasis was discussed at length in Chapter 4.

Cardiovascular Disease

Food reactions contribute to cardiovascular disease in several direct and indirect ways. Because cardiovascular disease is such a terrible problem in the United States, killing almost half of all Americans, anything that can decrease it is valuable. There is evidence that eliminating food reactions can help prevent certain cardiovascular diseases.

An important indirect way that food reactions contribute to cardiovascular disease is by causing food cravings, which provoke us to make poor food choices. Food cravings often make us eat unhealthy foods, and this can: (1) make us overweight; (2) thicken our blood; (3) clog and harden our arteries; and (4) raise our blood pressure and cholesterol. Each of these risk factors contributes significantly to cardiovascular disease.

Food reactions also directly damage the walls of blood vessels when circulating immune complexes enter the circulatory system. For more information on circulating immune complexes, see Chapter 2.

Food reactions also contribute to cardiovascular disease by stressing the liver, the only organ that breaks down cholesterol. As you probably know, high LDL cholesterol is a major risk factor in heart disease.

Food reactions also interfere with blood vessel flexibility by lowering the levels of serotonin. Serotonin helps blood vessels readily expand and contract and stay supple. Without enough serotonin, vessels can become stuck in a state of constriction or expansion.

If you have any of the risk factors for cardiovascular disease, such as high cholesterol or high blood pressure, I urge you to eliminate your food reactions. This will help you to stay on a healthy diet, containing only moderate amounts of fats and calories, and will help your blood vessels stay healthy. It will also make you feel better and may help save your life.

Cognitive Disorders

One of the most common side benefits that occurs when people eliminate food reactions is improved cognitive function – better concentration, mental focus, and memory. Dozens of my food reaction patients have told me that when they eat their false fat foods, they feel spacy and fuzzy-headed.

This happens for several reasons. One reason is that food reactions interfere with the assimilation of brain nutrients, including the nutritional building blocks that are used to manufacture neurotransmitters. For example, to manufacture the neurotransmitter acetylcholine – the primary carrier of thought and memory – your body needs the nutrients choline, vitamin B_5, and vitamin C. Food reactions can disturb the assimilation and absorption of these nutrients and decrease the manufacture of acetylcholine. This can interfere immediately with thought and memory.

In addition, among reactive people, certain chemicals in foods can have a direct pharmacologic effect, as I explained in Chapter 2. This pharmacologic effect often occurs in the brain. An obvious example of this happens when alcohol hits the brain and disrupts the normal function of brain cells. In much the same way, a macromolecule of a partially broken-down foodstuff can also alter normal brain function. One of my patients once told me that eating wheat made him feel light-headed and forgetful, as if he'd taken a neurologically active drug. The effect was even more pronounced when he ate wheat and corn together.

Food reactions also affect hormonal balance, and this too can trigger cognitive problems. Hormones are primarily associated with mood, but also affect cognitive functions, such as concentration and memory. For example, the adrenal hormone cortisol, which is often increased by food reactions, can significantly interfere with the neurotransmitters that support thought and memory. This neurotransmitter interference may have happened to you during a period of stress, when you were overstimulated by excessive cortisol and were unable to operate at your peak mental level. This is known colloquially as the stress-induced 'bonehead effect.'

Food reactions also hurt brain function by causing hypoglycemia. Brain cells do not store blood sugar as efficiently as other cells do, so they are very vulnerable to drops in blood sugar. When brain cells are low on blood sugar, cognitive function is grossly impaired. When this happens to people, they often grab a cup of coffee or a high-carbohydrate snack to quickly boost blood sugar levels. But this quick fix soon backfires by disturbing insulin levels. Soon blood sugar falls again, lower than before.

To prevent hypoglycemia, you should eliminate food reactions and cut down on sugary and starchy foods. Eat a diet rich in protein, with moderate amounts of fat. If you eat grains, also eat some protein with them. For example, an appropriate daily regimen for someone prone to hypoglycemia might include sautéed tofu and vegetables for breakfast, a chicken breast for lunch, and fish for dinner. Add vegetables to each meal. These high-protein meals should be accompanied by healthy snacks between meals, such as high-protein nuts and seeds. You should also take the mineral chromium, because it helps to stabilize blood sugar levels.

Chronic Ear Infections

This problem can occur in adults who have food reactions, but is much more common among reactive children, because their ear canals and eustachian tubes are smaller and more vulnerable to swelling, blockage, and subsequent congestion.

When people eat reactive foods, they often experience swelling, minor inflammation, and increased mucus production in many parts of their bodies, including their nasal passages, ear canals, and eustachian tubes. When the ear tissues swell, the ear doesn't adequately drain fluid through the eustachian tube, and this causes fluid to build up in the ear. The fluid buildup can cause pressure and pain and can lead to infection.

Frequently, babies who are reactive to cow's milk suffer from this problem. Cow's milk, however, is not the only food that causes ear infections and congestion in babies. Babies can also become reactive to low-allergy soya formula and even to breast milk — especially if their mothers are eating foods that the babies can't tolerate.

For example, one infant patient, Adrianna, suffered from this problem because of a reaction to a low-allergy soya formula. When Adrianna was first born, she'd had a bad reaction to cow's milk and had suffered severe colic, with pain, bloating, and diarrhoea. Because of this, her pediatrician had placed her on soya formula.

After five months on the soya formula, though, she began to react negatively to it, just as she had previously reacted to cow's milk. Her ears became congested, and she developed an infection. Her pediatrician prescribed an antibiotic.

The pediatrician advised her parents to leave her on the soya formula, on the theory that soya was less allergenic than cow's milk for most babies. The problem with that theory, of course, was that Adrianna was not most babies. She wasn't even the same baby that she'd been five months earlier. People change, and so do their food reactions.

I recommended that Adrianna be taken off the soya formula. I thought that five months of eating nothing but soya formula had probably caused her to become reactive to it.

This is, of course, a common phenomenon among people with food reactions.

My basic approach is: if one food isn't working, try something else. Experiment. Be flexible.

Adrianna's parents put her back on cow's milk, and she responded terrifically. Her digestive problems disappeared, and so did the congestion in her ears. Her ear infection healed up and didn't return.

One child was first allergic to cow's milk, then soya milk. People change – and so do their food reactions.

Some parents ignore the role that food reactions play in the development of their children's ear 'infections', and I think this is a terrible mistake. Food reactions aren't the only cause of ear infections, or otitis media, but they are a very common cause.

The standard therapy for ear infections – antibiotics – can sometimes cause disastrous problems. Antibiotics are an excellent short-term treatment for many kinds of infections, including ear infections, but they have serious limitations. They kill many of the bacteria in the body, including the helpful bacteria in the gut, and this can harm digestion terribly. Even a single course of antibiotics can kill enough intestinal flora to dramatically increase food reactions. Repeated courses of antibiotics are even more disruptive.

Antibiotics are also the most common cause of candidiasis, or yeast overgrowth, because they kill the helpful bacteria that keeps yeast in check. For more on yeast overgrowth, see Chapter 4.

In addition, repeated courses of antibiotics can interfere with natural immunity. Therefore, antibiotics often perpetuate a repeating cycle of various infections including ear infections.

It's much wiser to eradicate the root causes of ear infections, such as food reactions, exposure to airborne allergens, and impaired immune function. Immune function in children can be bolstered with prudent dosages of children's and infants' vitamins. Also, immune-boosting herbal and homeopathic medications are now formulated especially for children. For example, children past infancy may take chewable echinacea tablets, and infants can safely be given many homeopathic medications.

Some infant homeopathic medications, such as those for colic and teething pain, can be exceptionally helpful. Colic and ear infections can be extremely painful, and I feel that parents owe it to their children to treat this pain aggressively with safe, natural medications. Ask your doctor to oversee the treatment.

Infant ear infections and congestion can also be helped with natural herbal ear drops, which powerfully inhibit infection. These ear drops contain natural anti-bacterial agents, such as garlic and mullein. They're known to be safe and effective, and also help decrease pain.

If you do give your child antibiotics – which is often advisable for virulent infections – you should also give him or her *Lactobacillus acidophilus* and bifidobacteria, in dosages appropriate for children. This will replenish the healthy bacteria in the gut and help break the cycle of repeated infection.

Chronic Fatigue Syndrome

This condition is called a syndrome, instead of a disease, because no one is sure what causes it. It is a collection of symptoms and probably has many different contributing factors among different people. I believe that the most common cause of CFS is a virus – probably one or more of the family of herpes viruses. However, some people seem to develop CFS symptoms from other causes – exposure to toxins, allergies, infections, and food reactions.

Most CFS symptoms appear to be the result of a hyper-vigilant immune system, which is responding to real or perceived attacks from foreign invaders. These symptoms include fever, fatigue, poor concentration, sore throat, swollen lymph nodes, exhaustion after exercise, and night sweats. A hyper-vigilant immune system can be triggered by viruses. It can also be triggered by food reactions.

As you'll recall, food reactions are essentially a malfunction of the immune system. For example, the most obvious CFS symptom – ongoing, severe fatigue – often appears to be the result of an overproduction of the immune substance called cytokines. Cytokines are produced by the immune system to help kill foreign invaders, such as viruses. But they are also produced when reactive foods are mistaken by the immune system for foreign invaders. Regardless of what causes their release, though, cytokines almost always make people feel tired and weak.

I have treated many patients who suffered from chronic fatigue syndrome, and food reactions are usually part of their problem, and are sometimes the *entire* problem. Often, patients have combinations of *several* disorders – including viruses, food reactions, candidiasis, and PMS – all of which have similar, CFS-type symptoms. It's common, for example, for CFS patients to have high levels of the herpes virus – mostly Human Herpes Virus, type 6 (HHV-6) – along with food reactions, candidiasis, and premenstrual symptoms. Not only do these conditions have similar symptoms, but they also exacerbate one another. When people have this kind of multi-condition medical problem, solving just one problem is never enough. *All* of the problems have to be solved in order for them to feel fully well again.

Fortunately, many of the same forces create these similar problems, and addressing these few forces often solves several problems at once. For example, eliminating reactive foods not only stops food reactions but also helps wipe out the symptoms of PMS and candidiasis, when used as part of a complete programme.

People with CFS, like people with ear infections, should be careful not to rely too heavily on antibiotics. Sometimes a secondary bacterial infection is a component of CFS, but it's almost never the cause. Antibiotics sometimes make people with CFS feel better temporarily, but they can ultimately depress immunity.

Besides eliminating food reactions, people with CFS should

take the amino acid lysine, which inhibits herpes virus repro-
duction. Very high dosages of lysine may be advisable for some
people – up to 10 or even 20 grams daily, depending upon the
severity of symptoms. Results are often noticeable in less than
a day. In some people, this high amount may provoke mild
intestinal upset, such as loose stools. If this is uncomfortable,
the dosage may be reduced. Lysine is also extremely valuable
for preventing recurrence of symptoms, once they've been
controlled. For prevention, dosages of 500 mg to 5 grams daily
may be appropriate.

Lysine may be purchased inexpensively as an individual
amino acid. It may also be purchased as one component of an
immune-boosting formulation, which might also include
echinacea, vitamin C, goldenseal, propolis, or elderberry.

Presence of a cold sore generally indicates a herpes infection, usually herpes type 1 virus. Herpes 2 causes genital
herpes more commonly and this responds less well to lysine.

People with CFS should also overcome possible candidiasis
(see the information on candidiasis in Chapter 4). They should
also eliminate any possible intestinal parasites, which can contribute to chronic fatigue symptoms. Many anti-parasite
nutritional formulations are available at health food shops and
from mail-order supplement companies. These products may
include grapefruit seed extract, artemesia herbs, and
berberine, a goldenseal extract.

In addition, people with CFS symptoms should take
energy-enhancing nutrients, including CoQ_{10}, ginseng, and
carnitine. They should avoid regular use of protein powder or
high amounts of the amino acid arginine, which negates the
virus-inhibiting power of lysine.

Even if CFS patients control the viral and bacterial compo-
nents of their problem, though, they still must eliminate food
reactions. If they don't do this, they may never feel much better.

Chronic Pain

My co-author, Cameron Stauth, noted in his book *The Pain
Cure*, written with Dharma Singh Khalsa, M.D., that eating

reactive foods is one of the worst possible mistakes for people with chronic pain. Food reactions increase pain by triggering widespread inflammation. When existing inflammation is amplified by food reactions, the results can be disastrous. It can turn moderate, manageable discomfort into severe, deep-seated pain.

Food reactions also increase pain by lowering the levels of the body's primary natural painkiller, serotonin. Many people think that endorphins are our most dependable natural analgesic, but it's really serotonin that most effectively mutes pain.

Another way food reactions increase pain is by decreasing the brain's energy. You've probably noticed that pain is almost always worse when you're tired. This is mostly because the nervous system loses much of its ability to screen out pain if it's exhausted. If your brain and nervous system are being irritated by food reactions, you'll be far less able to mentally block pain. You'll react to pain you would usually ignore.

Furthermore, food reactions directly contribute to several of the conditions that cause chronic pain, such as arthritis, migraines, and irritable bowel syndrome.

To overcome chronic pain, you should avoid reactive foods and eat plenty of the omega-3 oils, because they have a natural anti-inflammatory effect. It's also helpful to exercise, because physical activity naturally increases resistance to pain. In addition, you should try to manage your stress well, because both anxiety and depression physically amplify pain by interfering with various functions of the brain.

Diabetes

Food reactions are one of the predisposing factors that lead to adult-onset diabetes. Other factors include obesity, stress, a diet high in sugars and other carbohydrates, and lack of exercise.

Food reactions contribute to the onset of diabetes mostly by interfering with the body's steady supply of insulin. Food reactions have an effect on insulin that is similar to the effect caused by eating too much sugar. When someone suffers from food reactions for many years or overeats sweets for many years, it can eventually exhaust the organs and glands that produce insulin or help metabolize sugar. These include the pancreas, thyroid, and adrenals.

Food reactions also cause overproduction of the inflammatory hormones called prostaglandins. Excessive prostaglandin production can also harm the pancreas.

There is, in addition, some evidence that food reactions can make *existing* diabetes worse by destabilizing insulin and blood sugar levels. There is even evidence that food reactions can contribute to *juvenile onset* diabetes. In a 1992 article in *The New England Journal of Medicine*, the authors concluded that milk allergies had caused diabetes in some children, in whom food reactions had destroyed insulin-producing cells in the pancreas.

If you are at risk for diabetes, you should eliminate your reactive foods. If you are obese, you should also lose weight and eat a low-carbohydrate diet. Try to avoid alcohol and caffeine. In addition, it may be helpful to take supplements that help stabilize blood sugar levels and increase energy production within cells. These daily supplements include chromium (200–400 mcg), omega-3 fish oils (500–1,000 mg), magnesium (200–400 mg), carnitine (500–1,000 mg), and CoQ_{10} (50–100 mg). Dosages should be divided evenly into two portions and taken after breakfast and dinner.

Digestive Disorders

Most food reactions *are* digestive disorders. They are an inability of the digestive system to thoroughly break down foods. Often this causes acute, immediate symptoms of digestive distress, including heartburn, gas, flatulence, and bloating. If food reactions occur regularly, they can contribute to gastrointestinal inflammation and ulcers.

When you eat foods that you can't readily digest, your stomach tends to produce excess acid to help break down these foods. When excess stomach acid is squeezed out of the stomach by internal pressure or by physical movement, it rises into the esophagus and causes heartburn. If this condition is pronounced or persistent, it is called acid reflux disease. If the esophagus has already been irritated by previous acid reflux, the condition can be quite painful.

Heartburn is becoming increasingly common in our society, mostly because we eat too many reactive foods and too many fatty, chemicalized foods that are hard to digest. Most people treat heartburn with antacids, and this is a good temporary solution. However, it's much wiser to *prevent* heartburn. Many people prevent it with medications that decrease stomach acid secretion. This is a reasonable approach, but it is far from ideal. One problem with it is that many people oversecrete stomach acid when they eat simply because they don't have *enough* of it in their stomachs *before* they begin to eat. If you're chronically low on stomach acid – as many people are, especially older people – you should take 1 to 2 capsules of betaine hydrochloride (also known as hydrochloric acid) just before you eat. This natural supplement, available at almost all health food shops, will supply you with enough digestive acid to keep you from overproducing it when you eat.

Another way to keep from overproducing stomach acid is to take digestive enzymes with your food. Enzymes help break down foods, which helps prevent the release of excess acid. Because betaine hydrochloride and digestive enzymes help digest foods, they not only help stop heartburn but also *help stop food reactions*. Therefore, most of my food reaction patients take digestive enzymes, betain hydrochloride and pepsin (which helps digest protein).

Interestingly, the condition of a hyper-acid stomach appears to be related to tissue swelling throughout the body in some people. One of my patients told me that when he takes antacid tablets for heartburn, he immediately feels less nasal congestion and can breathe more freely. This apparently happens because of a reduction of swelling in the tissues of the nasal passages.

In addition, many doctors of integrative medicine believe that healing in general occurs optimally in a relatively alkaline body environment, rather than in an acidic one. They believe that alkalinity favours the activity of the body's calming parasympathetic branch of the nervous system, rather than the stimulating sympathetic branch of the nervous system, and that the parasympathetic branch is more conducive to immune strength. The parasympathetic branch shifts energy away from the fight-or-flight organs and glands and sends it to organs and glands that confer immunity, such as the thymus and liver. This is part of the reason that stress can make us sick and can slow healing.

Unfortunately, many people take digestive disorders for granted or believe that they are just a minor nuisance. This is a potentially dangerous attitude, because digestion is the well-spring of all of the salubrious effects of nutrition. Running your body with poor digestion is as risky as running your car with a bad fuel system. If you do it, your entire physical organism will suffer.

Furthermore, your digestive system may soon break down entirely and develop a debilitating digestive disorder, such as duodenal ulcers, irritable bowel syndrome, Crohn's disease, or ulcerative colitis.

In addition, acid reflux disease can make a person as much as forty times more likely to contract esophageal cancer, according to recent research.

For good digestion, eat good foods, not reactive foods. Take betaine hydrochloride and digestive enzymes. If you already have stomach problems, you may also want occasionally to drink a diluted solution of aloe vera juice, because it can help heal irritated digestive system membranes. Taking probiotics, such as *Lactobacillus acidophilus*, can also help.

Eating Disorders

The most common eating disorder is bingeing on foods. And the most common cause of bingeing is food cravings, created by food reactions.

The next most common eating disorders are bulimia and anorexia. As I mentioned in Chapter 4, it appears as if the serotonin deficit caused by food reactions is a primary trigger of both bulimia and anorexia.

For more information on eating disorders, see Chapter 4.

Eczema, Acne, and Hives

It is well documented that food reactions commonly cause skin problems. I've seen this happen in dozens of patients.

One reason food reactions cause skin problems is because they stimulate the skin's mast cells to release histamines and other chemicals. When these chemicals are released, they cause the capillaries around them to become relatively more permeable, often allowing fluids from the blood to leak into the skin. This can interfere with the normal function of the skin and may ult-imately result in hives, eczema, or other skin reactions, such as acne.

When the normal activities of the skin are disturbed by food reactions, it excites the nerves in the skin and makes them sensitive and irritated. I have one patient who can tell if he's having a food reaction by how his skin feels. If it feels touchy and irritated, he knows he's eaten something he shouldn't have. He told me that before he figured out the problem, he almost always wore extremely soft clothing, such as cotton or cashmere, to avoid frequent discomfort.

I've treated several patients with acne who improved considerably on the False Fat Diet. The mechanism of action isn't exactly clear, but food reactions probably contribute to acne by increasing sebaceous secretions, heightening inflammation and toxicity, and reducing immune strength.

As you may remember, for many years it was widely believed that chocolate and fried foods triggered acne outbreaks. Then, about ten years ago, researchers announced that only a small percentage of people in a study got acne from chocolate. The researchers concluded that chocolate didn't cause acne. I disagree with that conclusion. I believe this study shows that chocolate *can* cause acne, but only in people who react to chocolate. *Everyone is different.*

This same principle holds true for other foods. Acne can be caused by animal fat, sugar, spices, shellfish, and many other foods, but only among people who react to these foods. Intestinal candidiasis also contributes to acne by causing food fermentation toxins, which irritate the skin.

A number of studies prove that people with skin problems

can recover when they eliminate food reactions. In one study, 100 per cent of patients with hives were able to control their symptoms when they eliminated food reactions. In another study, 66 per cent of patients with eczema improved on a diet free of reactive foods, while a control group of eczema patients on diets of their own choosing became significantly worse.

Another study showed that 67 per cent of people who had no skin pathologies still achieved smoother, softer, healthier-looking skin when they eliminated food reactions.

---

*Food reactions are a major cause
of unhealthy skin.*

If you have skin problems, one of the best things you can do is to take supplements of omega-3 or omega-6, found in fish or flaxseed oils. Some patients with eczema find these essential fatty acids to be a veritable wonder drug. Interestingly, I had one 11-year-old male patient who took omega-3 oils and noted improvement in all three of his problem areas: eczema, weight control, and impulse control. These are three supposedly unrelated disorders, but in this boy, they were all helped by a single dietary change. This indicates the pervasive, far-reaching impact of nutrition: it's the fuel that runs your entire body.

Other important nutrients for healing the skin and maintaining its health are vitamin A (10,000–30,000 IU daily), vitamin E (200–400 IU daily), vitamin C (2–4 g daily), and zinc (50–100 mg daily), in divided dosages. It also helps to drink 6 to 8 glasses of water per day.

Fibromyalgia

Fibromyalgia – widespread, chronic muscle pain, with tender trigger points – has been an enigma for many years, but now many researchers believe it's a disorder of the metabolism, caused primarily by low levels of serotonin. Serotonin indirectly helps heal muscle pain.

Interestingly, fibromyalgia is closely associated with other low-serotonin conditions that are often caused by food reactions. Among them are insomnia, headaches, irritable bowel syndrome, painful menstruation, swelling in the extremities, anxiety and depression, and cognitive impairment. Most people with fibromyalgia have one or more of these conditions. Because these conditions are sometimes related to food reactions, it's reasonable to assume that food reactions may contribute to fibromyalgia causation in some people.

Low serotonin indirectly contributes to the muscle pain of fibromyalgia by depriving people of deep, delta-wave sleep. Without enough serotonin it's hard to drift into delta sleep. Delta sleep is crucially important for muscle health, because only during delta sleep does the body secrete the hormone that repairs muscle strains: human growth hormone. Without this nightly repair, minor muscle aches and pains accumulate and become worse.

Fibromyalgia is very common, afflicting an estimated 7 to 10 million Americans, or about 3 per cent to 4 per cent of the population. About 20 per cent of all fibromyalgia patients are disabled by it, and 30 per cent have to find different jobs. Fibromyalgia is ten times more common among women than men. This may be due to the fact that female hormonal fluctuations often drive down serotonin levels.

One of the best nutritional therapies for fibromyalgia is ingestion of the supplement 5-HTP (5-hydroxy-tryptophan), which is available at health food shops and pharmacies. This supplement is a form of tryptophan, the amino acid that is the nutritional precursor of serotonin. In a study reported in the *Journal of Internal Medicine Research*, 50 fibromyalgia patients who received 300 mg of 5-HTP daily (in 2 to 3 divided doses) showed significant improvement.

Tryptophan can also be purchased, but requires a hospital prescription. Because 5-HTP is so similar to tryptophan but does not require a prescription, I generally recommend it instead of tryptophan. If you do take tryptophan, follow your doctor's recommendations on dosages. A common dosage of 5-HTP is 50–100 mg three times daily, including one administration at bedtime, to promote sleep.

Other nutrients that help manufacture serotonin are vitamin B_6 and pycnogenol, a derivative of pine bark used for centuries as a folk remedy for rheumatism.

It's also important for fibromyalgia patients to take 300–500 mg of magnesium daily, because magnesium helps keep muscles flexible and reduces muscle spasms. Other nutrients that are good for muscle tissue are magnesium malate or malic acid (in dosages of 1,200–2,400 mg daily), and CoQ_{10} (in dosages of 100–200 mg daily). The amino acid creatine also helps repair muscles. A dosage of approximately 1–2 grams daily of creatine may be appropriate for most people, but people with fibromyalgia or people who exercise extremely hard may need more – up to 5–10 grams daily, in three divided dosages. In healthy people, it is usually taken before exercise to improve workout capacity.

Hay Fever and Airborne Allergies

Many patients of mine find that when their food reactions are eliminated, their hay fever goes away. This happens because food reactions push patients past their allergic thresholds and leave them more reactive to airborne allergens. When they then come into contact with pollen, dust, ragweed, or animal dander, their mast cells are already sensitized, and they often react. But when my patients eliminate food reactions, they frequently don't react as much to airborne allergens.

---

*When food reactions are eliminated,
hay fever often goes away.*

Many studies confirm this phenomenon. In one study, 42 per cent of people with hay fever recovered from the condition when they eliminated food reactions. In another study, 67 per cent of patients found that their hay fever was badly exacerbated by food reactions.

If you have hay fever, you should definitely avoid reactive foods. It may also be helpful to take 2–3 grams of vitamin C daily, because this seems to reduce direct-contact allergies, such as those that occur when pollen contacts the nasal membranes. Vitamin C helps strengthen cell walls and may prevent some allergens from entering cells. Also, the bioflavonoid quercetin, in dosages of 200–300 mg three times daily, reduces the histamine response, and decreases allergies.

Headaches

Food reactions are a major cause of migraines. They contribute to migraines in two primary ways: (1) by lowering serotonin levels and (2) by triggering blood vessel constriction.

Migraines were once considered a mystery, but in the past few years many researchers have concluded that they are probably the result of blood vessel *constriction* in the brain, followed quickly by an overreaction of blood vessel *dilation*. When blood vessels become overly dilated, they leak blood and irritate nerves. Pain also comes from constriction of swollen blood vessels. The main reason that blood vessels get 'stuck' in a state of overdilation is because of a lack of serotonin. Serotonin helps keep blood vessels flexible and prevents them from getting stuck in an overdilated condition.

Food reactions also cause migraines by directly causing blood vessel constriction (which is followed by dilation). Among the worst blood vessel constrictors are foods that contain high amounts of the amino acid tyramine. The foods richest in tyramine are red wine and aged cheese. Other blood vessel constrictors are foods that contain nitrates and nitrites, such as hot dogs, bologna, bacon, and other cured meats. MSG, or monosodium glutamate, also constricts blood vessels, as does the amino acid phenylalanine, the primary ingredient in the artificial sweetener aspartame. Another constrictor is caffeine.

In one study, 93 per cent of young migraine patients stopped having headaches after they eliminated all of their individualized reactive foods.

Nutrients that help *prevent* migraines include magnesium, which helps keep blood vessels relaxed. In one study of migraine patients, 40 per cent had a magnesium deficiency. Another nutrient that may help is vitamin B_2, or riboflavin, which helps support the brain's energy-producing mitochondria. The supplement 5-HTP can also help, by building up levels of serotonin (see the entry on fibromyalgia). To help prevent migraines, take daily dosages of 25–50 mg of B_2 (riboflavin) (once or twice daily); 400–800 mg of magnesium (in 2 doses, 1 during the day and the other at night); and 50–100 mg of 5-HTP (at bedtime).

Migraines are relatively common among my food reaction patients. When my patients go on the False Fat Diet, though, their headaches tend to significantly subside. A number of patients stopped having migraines entirely after they stopped eating their false fat foods.

Common tension headaches, caused by spasm of the muscles of the neck and shoulder, also seem to decrease among patients on the False Fat Diet. I believe that this happens primarily because these patients feel generally stronger and calmer and are less reactive to stressors. Also, they are less prone to inflammation and tend to have less muscle tightness.

Hyperactivity and Attention Deficit Disorder

These two problems are often considered as a single disorder – attention deficit hyperactive disorder, or ADHD – because they frequently occur in tandem. No-one is certain what causes ADHD, but there is widespread agreement that this is a physical disorder, rather than a psychological problem. For many years, it's been theorized that ADHD is caused by food reactions. This concept was first proposed by Benjamin Feingold, M.D., who noted improvement in children who avoided foods containing preservatives, salicylates, artificial flavouring, and food dyes. Later researchers also implicated commonly reactive foods, such as sugar, milk, eggs, and soya.

As a result of this research, it became conventional wisdom that virtually all children who ate foods high in sugar would react with a sugar high and become hyperactive. I believe this is a gross oversimplification. Some children do react badly to sugar, but others seem to tolerate it. A more realistic perspective, I believe, is that children can become hyperactive from any food that they're reactive to, just as adults can.

It appears as if reactive foods cause hyperactivity by increasing the levels of the stimulating adrenal hormones, and by decreasing levels of the calming neurotransmitter serotonin. Furthermore, certain reactive foods have direct pharmacologic effects upon brain cells. These direct reactions, which I discussed in Chapter 2, often affect mood and behaviour.

In my practice, I've seen a number of children improve in mood and behaviour when they eliminated their food reactions. Some of these children had been labelled as having ADHD, and a few of them were on the most common medication for ADHD, Ritalin. Some were able to discontinue Ritalin if they adhered closely to their new diets.

Studies confirm the role of food reactions in ADHD. In one study of 76 children with ADHD, 100 per cent improved after eliminating food reactions, and 28 per cent achieved complete cessation of symptoms.

Although most people think of ADHD as a childhood disorder, many people carry this problem into adulthood. This may indicate that adult ADHD is sometimes caused by food reactions that do not improve with the passage of time. It may also indicate that ADHD can be developed in adulthood, possibly because of food reactions.

Besides eliminating reactive foods, children and adults with ADHD should take essential fatty acids. Some ADHD patients respond well to them. This supplementation is especially important if the patient also has a skin problem, such as hives or eczema, or if the patient has hay fever or asthma. Skin problems, hay fever, and asthma also often respond well to essential fatty acids, such as the omega-3 and omega-6 oils. In the entry on eczema, I describe the treatment of an 11-year-old boy who had problems with eczema, weight control, and emotional impulse control (which is closely related to ADHD). All of these problems cleared up when he stopped eating reactive foods and started taking essential fatty acids.

It is also often helpful to naturally support brain function with nutrients that increase levels of neurotransmitters. These nutrients include the B-complex of vitamins, lecithin, zinc, and 5-HTP. Consult your health practitioner for guidance on dosages.

Hypoglycemia

Hypoglycemia is a serious disorder that can make your life miserable, and harm your health. Food reactions are a notorious cause of hypoglycemia, or low blood sugar. They cause it because of their effects upon adrenal hormones, the thyroid, and the pancreas (which produces insulin). I have already discussed hypoglycemia and don't want to be repetitive, so please see pages 96 and 290.

The symptoms of hypoglycemia are somewhat similar to those of food cravings, partly because low blood sugar is usually a major component of food cravings. People with hypoglycemia don't feel just a normal sensation of hunger before meals. They feel weak, irritable, anxious, and ravenously hungry. If these symptoms apply to you, you should review the pages on hypoglycemia and make a special effort to eliminate your food reactions.

Insomnia

Insomnia has many causes, but I believe that one of the most common causes is food reactions. Many of my patients on the False Fat Diet complained of insomnia when they first consulted with me. Of these patients, the majority reported a moderate to excellent improvement in insomnia after going on the False Fat Diet.

Food reactions cause insomnia primarily by disrupting the normal balance of hormones and neurotransmitters. Food reactions increase the stimulating hormone cortisol, which stays in the system longer than adrenaline, and they also depress levels of the calming neurotransmitter serotonin. In addition, direct reactions, discussed in Chapter 2, have a variety of effects upon brain cells and can cause insomnia.

Allergic addiction to reactive foods can also trigger insomnia, when food cravings and their accompanying malaise strike during the night. If the person suffering the food craving does not eat at this time, the sense of malaise and agitation can last virtually all night long. It's common for people with this problem to raid the refrigerator in the middle of the night.

Insomnia tends to increase as we age, because production of the primary sleep hormones, melatonin and serotonin, decreases as we age. Melatonin and serotonin are closely associated; therefore because food reactions decrease serotonin, it's possible that food reactions may also decrease levels of melatonin. Little research, however, has been done on this.

The most common treatment for chronic insomnia is use of sleeping pills, tranquilizers, and anti-depressants, which increase serotonin levels. This approach can be helpful, but it's better to build serotonin levels naturally, with supplements such as 5-HTP (see the entry on fibromyalgia). Other nutrients that can exert a calming effect are lecithin (which contains the nutritional precursor for the neurotransmitter acetylcholine), magnesium, calcium, and niacinamide. In fact, niacinamide, a form of niacin, has been called 'the poor man's Valium.' Appropriate daily dosages for most people may be 50–100 mg of 5-HTP (taken at bedtime); 2,000–3,000 mg of lecithin; 400–600 mg of magnesium; 600–800 mg of calcium; and 100–500 mg of niacinamide (at bedtime). It can also be very helpful to take 1–3 mg of melatonin at bedtime (only available on prescription in the UK – consult your doctor).

Irritable Bowel Syndrome

Irritable Bowel Syndrome, or IBS, is a relatively common disorder among people with chronic, severe food reactions. It's estimated that a third of all visits to gastrointestinal specialists are for IBS.

IBS is characterized by common digestive tract problems, including diarrhoea, constipation, gas, and abdominal cramping. Many of these symptoms are directly related to poor digestion. Therefore, the most common treatment for IBS is dietary modification and avoidance of reactive foods.

The most frequent food triggers of IBS are milk and other dairy products. The second most common trigger is animal fat. Animal fat may cause problems even in people who aren't reactive to it, because it contains a chemical called cholecystokinin, which can cause contractions in the intestines. The other common dietary causes of IBS are sugar (especially fructose), citrus fruits, and the cruciferous vegetables, such as cauliflower and broccoli.

The most compelling recent theory on IBS is that it is caused by a deficit of the neurotransmitter serotonin. The primary supporting evidence of this theory is that IBS often strikes people who have other disorders that are caused by a serotonin deficit. One of these disorders is fibromyalgia; 70 per cent of fibromyalgia patients have IBS, and 65 per cent of IBS patients have fibromyalgia. Other low-serotonin disorders that are common among IBS patients are migraines, food cravings, anxiety, and depression. Premenstrual syndrome, which is characterized by low serotonin, is also linked to IBS-type symptoms. In a study of PMS patients, 34 per cent of women who did *not* have chronic IBS reported IBS-type symptoms when they had PMS.

Because of these indications that IBS is linked to low serotonin, IBS patients should try to build their serotonin levels. One important way to do this is by avoiding reactive foods. Another is by taking approximately 50–100 mg of 5-HTP daily (see the entry on fibromyalgia). People with IBS should also try to improve their digestion with a high-fibre diet. They should, in addition, take a digestive enzyme tablet with each meal, and take probiotics (providing approximately 5–10 billion organisms of acidophilus and bifidobacteria). It may also help to take mild herbs that promote digestion, such as peppermint oil in capsule or leaf tea, or ginger root capsules or tea. Take as directed before meals or drink a cup of ginger-peppermint tea between meals or away from meals. Peppermint oil should be taken in enteric-coated capsules, one or two times daily between meals, to allow it to reach the intestines.

Mood Disorders

Mood disorders, particularly depression and anxiety, are among the most common symptoms of food reactions. Mood changes occur because of disruption of hormonal and neuro-transmitter balance. I have already discussed mood disorders in detail, so please review Chapter 4.

When my patients go on the False Fat Diet, improvement in mood almost always occurs among people with existing anxiety and depression. On occasion, patients are able to discontinue their use of anti-depressants and anti-anxiety medications.

Some physicians believe that food reactions are even implicated in a certain small percentage of psychotic disorders, including profound depression and schizophrenia. I have never encountered this in my practice, but I know doctors who have. Their accounts of these cases are fascinating. If you are interested in the brain allergy approach to serious mental disorders, you may want to consult a physician associated with the Orthomolecular Health/Medicine Society, based in San Francisco (see Resources and Referrals).

Sinusitis

Sinusitis, or sinus infection, occurs frequently among people with food reactions. This happens because the tissue swelling and excess mucus caused by food reactions often interfere with proper drainage of the sinuses.

Food reactions also contribute to sinusitis by exacerbating hay fever. Food reactions often push people past their allergic thresholds and make them more reactive to allergens such as pollen or dust. These airborne allergens frequently congest the nasal passages, block drainage, and result in infection.

Food reactions that exacerbate candidiasis, or yeast over-growth, which can irritate and inflame the mucosal tissues in the nose and sinuses, can also lead to sinus infection.

People often take antibiotics for sinus infections, and this is often a viable short-term treatment, even though it may require repeated courses. Antibiotics do interfere with in-testinal flora, however, and thereby increase food reactions and candidiasis. Therefore, if you take antibiotics, you must replenish the healthy bacteria in your intestines by taking pro-biotic capsules or by eating yogurt that contains probiotics (if you are not reactive to dairy). In many people, though, yogurt increases mucus production, so it's generally wiser to ingest probiotics in capsule or powder form.

Another effective nutritional therapy for sinus infections is to take supplements that increase immunity, such as vitamin C (2–5 g daily), vitamin A (10,000–30,000 IU daily), garlic (500–1,000 mg daily), and echinacea and goldenseal (200–500 mg each daily, for no more than three weeks at a time; take one week off, resume if you need to).

Homeopathic medications also often help clear sinus in-fections. These medications, which are gentle and free of side effects, can speed healing significantly. Many brands are now readily available. Homeopathic nasal sprays can also help.

Some herbal therapies can help alleviate blockage. Ephedra, or Ma-Huang, is a natural decongestant similar to pseudo-ephedrine, but is less stimulating. If you use ephedra, take no more than 100–200 mg daily, in equally divided dosages (early in the day, such as morning and after lunch, to avoid inter-fering with sleep). Ephedra should not be used by people with heart conditions or high blood pressure, because it may cause overstimulation. Nor should it be taken in extremely high amounts, such as a gram or more at once. Several years ago, a number of people took extremely high dosages of ephedra in order to produce a stimulating, drug-like high, and this unwise use resulted in illness and even several deaths.

Another way to help overcome sinus congestion and infection is to irrigate the nasal passages with a mild saline solution made with warm water and table salt. To start with, try it with only ¼ teaspoon of salt per cup of warm water, and don't go higher than ½ teaspoon. If the solution has too much salt, it will be uncomfortable and might irritate nasal tissues. Use only the amount of salt that is comfortable. To perform a nasal irrigation, pour some of the saline solution into a cupped hand, inhale some of it into both nostrils, hold it for a few moments, then expel it. Repeat the process. Often this completely clears congestion and allows you to breathe freely. To help the solution reach all of your sinus cavities, you should sometimes bend over briefly after you inhale the solution, as if you were touching your toes.

Decongestant inhalers temporarily relieve the stuffiness of sinus congestion, but if you use them for more than two or three consecutive days, they will have a rebound effect and make tissue swelling worse. Therefore, it's smart to use a saline inhaler, which doesn't contain decongestants. Many of the saline inhalers now contain small amounts of eucalyptus oil and menthol, which help you breathe freely without the risk of rebound congestion. One of my patients, a 39-year-old man, had been virtually addicted to nasal sprays for almost twenty years before he began his False Fat Diet. Currently, he is still off these addictive sprays and is breathing freely.

Oral decongestants, such as pseudoephedrine and antihistamines, may help promote drainage by opening clogged passages. But they can prolong infections if they are overused, by drying the nasal passages and sinuses of mucosal flow. A moderate amount of mucus flow is valuable, because it carries away bacteria and brings immune substances to the site of the infection.

As you can see, the False Fat Diet, which can help relieve or prevent all of these many disorders, is not just a weight-loss diet. It is a health-promoting diet that can be valuable for virtually anyone.

Practically everyone has one of the aforementioned conditions – or is at risk for contracting one of them.

Now it's time to move on and implement this diet into your own life. You'll be amazed to see how easy it is. And after you start the diet, you'll be astonished at how rewarding it can be. When you begin living a life that's free from food reactions, you'll feel better and you'll look better – for the rest of your life.

PART TWO

HOW TO DO THE
FALSE FAT DIET

6
FINDING OUT YOUR OWN
FALSE FAT FOODS

Now that you know *WHY* this diet will work and how *much* it can help you, you have only one thing left to learn: how to implement the diet into your own life.

The good news: that's the easy part! There are no further scientific principles to learn and no complicated menus to plan. You simply have to determine your own false fat foods and eliminate them from your diet.

Eliminating your false fat foods will require discipline. But within just a few days, you will be past your allergic addiction to your reactive foods, and that will make them *much* easier to resist. In fact, you'll be able to easily resist foods that you used to crave.

These foods will no longer have power over you. *You will have power over them.*

In this chapter, I'm going to tell you how to determine your own reactive foods. As soon as you know this, you'll be well on your way to a healthier, slimmer life.

There are two ways to determine your false fat foods:

- a medical blood test, or
- an elimination diet, in which you temporarily eliminate suspected reactive foods, and then reintroduce them, to see if they cause symptoms.

I believe, as do most physicians who specialize in this area, that the most accurate system is to combine *both* of these methods. That way, each of the two methods serves as a double check on the other and their margin for error is extremely small. However, it is quite acceptable to just do the elimination diet.

First, let's look at the elimination diet method. It's an excellent place to begin because it's *free*, it can be started *immediately*, and it is usually quite *accurate*.

Then we'll take a look at medical tests for food reactions. Many patients prefer to begin their False Fat Diet with a medical test, because it *eliminates the detective work* of an elimination diet, and because it gives the patient a set of *written guidelines* – something in black and white. Furthermore, the medical tests usually take only a week or two to process.

You can't go wrong either way. And if you combine the methods, you'll be sure to succeed.

How to Do an Elimination Diet

The theory behind an elimination diet is simple: if you eliminate all reactive foods from your system for 7 to 10 days and then reintroduce them one by one, you'll notice symptoms when you eat a reactive food. One reason you'll be likely to notice symptoms is because you'll be especially sensitive to these foods, once they've been cleared from your system.

As a rule, food reactions occur within a few hours of eating a reactive food. If you don't react by at least the following morning after you eat a suspected reactive food, you probably won't have a reaction. However, on occasion it can take up to three days to experience a delayed food reaction (which may be more subtle than an immediate reaction). Therefore, when you do reintroduce foods, you should reintroduce them gradually, at a rate of no more than one or two new foods every day. If you reintroduce foods too quickly, you might become confused. The ideal is to add one food every two days, especially if you seem to be having reactions.

There are various ways to do an elimination diet. Some

ways are more strict than others, because they eliminate a greater number of foods. The most strict way, for example, is a fast, in which you consume nothing but fruit and vegetable juices. The least strict way is to just eliminate a few of the most common allergens, such as wheat, milk, and sugar, at once. The more strict ways are generally more accurate than the least strict ways, because they reduce the detective work. However, the more strict ways can be harder to stick to.

When I place patients on an elimination diet, I generally tell them about these different approaches and let them choose the one that feels right for them – which is usually the one they can stick with.

The approach that *sounds best to you* is the approach you should choose.

I'll now tell you about my different approaches, starting with the *lease* strict.

The Limited Elimination Diet

The least strict approach is the Limited Elimination Diet, in which you eliminate just a few of the most commonly reactive foods, *plus* any food that you eat virtually every day.

The three most commonly reactive foods are **wheat, milk,** and **sugar**.

Wheat and milk are notoriously reactive foods, for two apparent reasons. One reason is that both of these foods were introduced into the human diet at a relatively late stage of our evolution. People didn't eat wheat and milk until after the advent of agriculture, about 10,000 years ago. During the 2.6 *million* years prior to that, as the human body gradually evolved, people lived mostly on wild fruits, vegetables, nuts, and game meat, like rabbit and woolly mammoth. According to many nutritional researchers, humans are best suited to a diet that excludes the relatively new food sources of cultivated grains and dairy products. This non-grain, non-dairy diet is sometimes called the Paleolithic diet, or hunter-gatherer diet.

The other reason that wheat and milk are hard to digest may be because we eat them *too often* and exhaust our body's ability to digest them adequately. As I've mentioned, the more often you eat any one food, the more difficult it can be to digest that food.

Whatever the reason, an extraordinary number of people are reactive to wheat or milk or both. Most of my food reaction patients are reactive to at least one of them.

Sugar is another reactive food. It causes far fewer classic food allergies than either wheat or milk, but it is still often very disruptive to the metabolism. It wreaks havoc with insulin levels and often triggers hypoglycemia. Therefore, I usually recommend that people avoid it as much as possible, especially during the first weeks of their diets.

When you eliminate these commonly reactive foods, you also have to eliminate the many processed foods that contain them. If you're reactive to milk, you should also eliminate cheese, butter, cream, ice cream, and yogurt. You should also check food labels for **casein**, **lactalbumin**, and **whey**, and avoid them, too.

If you're reactive to milk, you might also be reactive to eggs, because both eggs and milk contain similar proteins. The *ovalbumin* protein in eggs is quite similar to the *lactalbumin* protein in milk.

If you're reactive to wheat, you should check food labels for wheat germ, bran, couscous, durum, graham flour, farina, and semolina, and avoid them. Furthermore, if you're reactive to wheat, you might also be reactive to barley, rye, or oats, because these grains all contain a highly reactive substance called gluten. Gluten may be the substance in wheat that causes your reaction. Gluten is the cohesive, high-protein, sticky element – the glue that helps hold grain together.

If you avoid all of these forms of wheat and milk, it will mean passing up most processed foods. For a complete list of the common processed foods that contain wheat and milk, see the food lists in Part Three. As you'll note, milk is hidden in a great many foods, including doughnuts, biscuits, waffles, and soufflés. Wheat is also hidden in many processed foods, such as creamed soups, bologna, sweets and chocolate bars, and gravies.

Besides wheat, milk, and sugar, you should also *avoid any*

food you eat virtually every day, You should especially avoid foods you eat several times each day. For most people, this means avoiding one or more of the Sensitive Seven most commonly reactive foods: **wheat, dairy, sugar, eggs, corn, soya,** and **peanuts.** People often eat one or more of these foods many times each day in various forms. For example, even if you don't eat whole corn on a given day, you might still consume corn syrup or corn oil in a dozen different foods, including ketchup, margarine, salad dressing, sweets and chocolate, jam, grape juice, bread, fizzy drinks, and peanut butter. (For the complete list, see Part Three.)

Therefore, it's important for you to become an ardent reader of labels. **You cannot gain power over food if you don't know what you're eating.** (My book *The Staying Healthy Shopper's Guide* may be helpful.)

Not all of the foods that people eat every day, however, are among the Sensitive Seven foods. A great many people have their own unique, frequently eaten foods. One of my patients with severe food reactions, for example, recently received the results of her food reaction test from a medical lab and discovered that the only food she was highly reactive to was mustard. Most people don't eat mustard very often, don't really love it, and don't react to it. This patient, however, loved mustard and ate it several times each day, on everything from French fries to pizza.

It was hard for her to quit eating mustard, but once she began to overcome her food reaction symptoms – weight gain and nightly insomnia – it became much easier, because the sacrifice was well worth the multiple rewards. Also, once she had the chemicals from mustard out of her system, she lost her intense craving for it.

If you use the Limited Elimination Diet, you should avoid your suspected reactive foods for at least one week. Then eat one of them and wait at least a day for symptoms to appear. If no symptoms appear, you are probably not reactive to that food. If you suspect that you are *not* reactive, you may begin to eat the food again, but you should remain alert for reactions.

When you're monitoring yourself for reactions, don't take antihistamines or any other allergy medications. They can mask symptoms and ruin the accuracy of your elimination diet and food challenges.

As you monitor yourself for symptoms, remember that a wide range of symptoms may occur – anything from bloating and swelling to headaches, congestion, itchiness and hives, and insomnia. For the full list of problems that food reactions cause, review Chapter 5.

Some patients keep a simple diary of what they eat and how they react physically and mentally to foods. This basic list can be a very helpful tool.

The Limited Elimination Diet is relatively simple, but it can sometimes be misleading, because it leaves so many foods *in* the diet. To make it work, you have to be a good detective. For example, if you eliminate just sugar, wheat, and dairy but are actually reactive to only eggs and oats, you might spend several extra weeks doing medical detective work. As you search for the real culprits, you may become confused by the recurring symptoms that you suffer from eating eggs and oats.

Therefore, it's often actually *easier* to eliminate a wider range of foods. This will increase your chances of eliminating the foods you react to and will ultimately make your detective work simpler.

If you are reluctant to eliminate a wider variety of foods because you're afraid of going hungry, remember that you can eat practically as much of your remaining foods as you want. This phase of the diet is not the time to worry about losing adipose tissue. It's the time to *determine your reactive foods*. After you've figured them out, *then* you can focus your efforts on fat loss. But if you *fail* to accurately identify your reactive foods, you may *never* lose fat.

Remember, too, that during the first few days of your elimination diet, you'll probably lose a significant amount of false fat. Be satisfied with *that* slimming process, and don't push yourself to lower your caloric intake markedly.

Don't forget that you will be on this eating plan for the long haul, and that you'll need to find ways to stay comfortable and full. Don't go hungry. This is not a crash diet. It's an eating strategy. If you're patient and smart, you can use this strategy to gain a power over food that will last for the *rest of your life*.

A sample one-week menu plan on the Limited Elimination Diet directly follows this chapter (see pages 178–84).

The Sensitive Seven Elimination Diet

This approach is probably the most popular of the various elimination diets I recommend, because it's not terribly difficult and it's usually quite effective. It is very similar to the Limited Elimination Diet, but it's more strict. Instead of eliminating just wheat, milk, sugar and any food you eat every day, you eliminate all of the Sensitive Seven most commonly reactive foods: **wheat, milk, sugar, soya, peanuts, corn,** and **eggs.** *You also eliminate any food that you eat every day.*

In addition, many patients eliminate oats, yeast, and chocolate, because reactions to them are common. Some patients also eliminate oranges (especially young people, who tend to be more reactive to this fruit).

Like all of the elimination diets I place patients on, this one consists of at least *one week* of sensitive food avoidance, followed by the reintroduction of foods one at a time. For details on exactly how to enact the elimination diet process, review the information on it in the preceding section (the Limited Elimination Diet).

As you can see, eliminating the Sensitive Seven foods will mean significantly reducing the amount of processed food you eat. This is good! Reducing the number of processed foods you eat is one of the smartest things you'll ever do. Some processed foods are healthy, but most of them aren't. For the most part, processed foods are *fattening, reactive,* and *low in nutrients.* They're usually loaded with extra fat, extra sugar, high-calorie fillers, and chemicals.

Processed foods tend to trigger allergic addiction, because they almost always contain at least one of the Sensitive Seven foods, and often several. A package of pre-cooked noodles with sauce, for example, might contain peanut oil, corn syrup, wheat bran, milk whey, egg solids, soya protein, and sugar. Furthermore, it might also contain MSG and a number of other allergenic chemicals that enter the body as indigestible macromolecules. The packet of noodles may look harmless and sound healthy: 'Low fat! High fibre! Vitamin enriched!' But it's a veritable time bomb of reactive foods. It will almost certainly touch off food cravings in the *majority of all reactive people*. They'll eat it, enjoy it, and then be hypoglycemic and hungry again in just a few hours – and not know why. They'll crave something like milk-laden, sugary ice cream, or a whole wheat roll or bagel with butter. But to keep from feeling guilty, they'll probably eat *low-fat* ice cream or spread *low-fat* margarine on their bagel. Almost immediately, though, they will begin to feel bloated with false fat and will soon add another layer of adipose tissue. And they will ask themselves '*What went wrong?* I ate a low-fat, high-fibre, low-calorie dinner and a healthy snack! *Why am I fatter?*'

> *Most processed foods are absolutely*
> *loaded with the Sensitive Seven.*

The alternative to processed foods, of course, are unprocessed, whole foods: fresh fruits, vegetables, fish, poultry, nuts, rice, beans, and any number of other wholesome, real, non-reactive foods. *These* are the foods that will make you slim and healthy.

A sample one-week menu plan on the Sensitive Seven Elimination Diet begins on page 174.

The Total Elimination Diet

This elimination diet consists of eating just a very *few* foods, all of which are notably non-reactive. A classic Total Elimination Diet consists primarily of lamb, pears, apples, walnuts, salmon, butter beans, and steamed chard or kale, because these foods cause reactions in very few people. Other foods that may be included, if they are not usually consumed regularly, are: lettuce, almonds, sunflower seeds, rice, sesame seeds, yams, green beans, cucumbers, celery, radishes, garlic, parsley, pine nuts, and pistachios.

Most people, however, can also add one or two more foods without causing reactions. The safest foods to add are a couple of fresh fruits and vegetables, or some chicken, turkey, or fish. It's generally wise, though, to avoid grains, citrus fruits, and the frequently reactive vegetables that compose the nightshade family, such as potatoes and tomatoes. It's also wise to avoid shellfish.

Of course, you must also avoid any food that you tend to eat every day, even if it's a typically non-reactive food.

The general principle of the Total Elimination Diet is to eat as few different foods as possible and to eat foods you usually don't eat.

The beauty of the Total Elimination Diet is that it makes your detective work very simple. Because you're eating only a few foods, it's easy to link reactions to specific foods.

The difficult element of the Total Elimination Diet is that it's restrictive and can be monotonous.

However, some people enjoy the simplicity of the Total Elimination Diet. People who lose their food cravings for the first time in their lives almost always love their new power over food, and often celebrate this power by paring down their diets to a bare minimum. They get pleasure from their spartan regimen, just as a finely tuned athlete takes pleasure from a hard workout. Furthermore, after they eliminate their food cravings, they feel significantly less hungry than usual.

A sample one-week menu plan on the Total Elimination Diet begins on page 167.

The Juice Fast Elimination Diet

This is the most strict way to begin the False Fat Diet, but it can also be the most rewarding. This is the method I used myself when I first developed the False Fat Diet. I enjoyed my short juice fast because it gave me energy and mental clarity, and after the first day, I wasn't hungry.

The juice fast is ideal for uncovering food reactions, since it strips the diet down to so few foods. When a food is reintroduced and causes a problem, it's easy to pinpoint the offending food.

One advantage of the juice fast over the Total Elimination Diet is that the juice fast is even better at eliminating toxins. Fasting is a superb way to stimulate the release of toxic debris, even when it is deeply embedded at the cellular level. Fasting releases toxins from the body's tissues and cells through the liver, kidneys, colon, lungs, bladder, sinuses, and skin.

Besides eliminating toxins, fasting also rids the tissues and membranes of excess mucus. Excess mucus commonly contributes to a variety of congestive illnesses, such as colds, sinusitis, and bronchitis, because germs grow best in mucus. Juice fasting is generally better than fasting with just water, because it more efficiently stimulates the clearing of wastes and more effectively supports energy.

Because of these actions, fasting is a powerful therapy that has been used by natural healers for centuries. I have supervised the fasts of hundreds of patients who have used juice fasting not just to determine reactive foods but also to help overcome a variety of troubling medical conditions, including high blood pressure, chronic sinusitis, allergies, back pain, joint pains, headaches, constipation, and skin conditions.

If you do employ a short juice fast to begin your diet, avoid orange and grapefruit juices, since citrus is the most commonly reactive fruit. The exception is lemon juice, which tends to be non-reactive for most people.

Every spring, I like to do a 7- to 10-day detoxification juice fast in which I drink 8 to 12 glasses a day of a tasty concoction I call the Spring Master Cleanser: two tablespoons of fresh lemon or lime juice, one tablespoon of pure maple syrup, one-tenth of a teaspoon of cayenne pepper, and eight ounces of spring water.

Because juice fasting is such a powerful detoxifier, it frequently causes temporary 'detox' symptoms such as headaches, irritability, bad breath, skin odour, skin eruptions, and a white coat on the tongue. These symptoms, which are a sure sign that your metabolism is healing, pass in a couple of days, and are generally replaced with a very pleasant sense of calmness and satisfaction. Detox symptoms, however, can also occur with other types of elimination diets.

Fasting is safe and healthy for most people, but it should be avoided by people with certain medical conditions, including low blood pressure, cardiac arrhythmias, impaired immunity, peptic ulcers, cancer, abnormally low weight, mental illness, or chronic fatigue. It should also be avoided by pregnant or lactating women, and by pre-operative or post-operative patients.

If you begin your False Fat Diet with a juice fast, you'll probably quickly lose false fat because you'll almost certainly be avoiding your reactive foods. You may also lose true fat because you won't be consuming many calories. You should enjoy this quick slimming effect, but I urge you not to become focused on losing adipose tissue at this time. Remember, this is a *detective* phase, *not* a crash-diet phase. Forget about fat. Focus on *knowledge*. In the long run, *knowledge about your own body* will be your single best weapon in your fight against fat.

Also, don't forget that if you do significantly lower your caloric intake during a juice fast, your metabolism will react with the starvation response and will hoard the calories you eat. Therefore, when you go off the fast, be careful to eat a relatively light diet to avoid a rebound weight gain. It's smart to end your fast by first reintroducing just a few whole, whole-some, hypoallergenic foods, such as fresh fruits, steamed vegetables, and other juices (diluted by half with water).

See my Juice Fast sample menu on pages 166-7.

Those are the various approaches that I generally recommend to patients who do an elimination diet.

When you start your False Fat Diet with an elimination diet, you simultaneously begin the first phase of your diet, the Cleansing Phase. This is a wonderfully rewarding phase of the diet, during which many people shed several pounds of edematous swelling and bloating and achieve a slimmer, trimmer shape. Often they feel better than they have in years – more alert and free from the many symptoms caused by food reactions and toxicity.

The Cleansing Phase is also a time of change, adjustment,

and healing, which can cause detox symptoms, including headaches, food cravings and irritability. You can do a number of things to decrease these uncomfortable symptoms, however, and I'll tell you about them in Chapter 7. Read that chapter before you begin your elimination diet. It will make the whole process easier for you.

Now let's look at the other method of finding out your own false fat foods: **medical testing**. A great many patients prefer to start their False Fat Diets with a blood test for food reactions, mostly because it's the simplest and fastest way to discover reactive foods.

Even if you do a medical test, though, it's still wise to do a restrictive elimination diet, in case there was an error in your test. Even with medical testing, however, it is helpful for the first week or two to exclude any commonly eaten foods *and* the Sensitive Seven, because these can also cause reactions and false fat, which may not be picked up by tests. Overall, the ideal would be to do medical tests for the good information they will give you *and* still follow the elimination diet and cleansing programme to begin with.

Take a look at the next section and decide for yourself if medical testing sounds appropriate for you.

Medical Testing for Food Reactions

There are a number of ways to find an allergy test. The recommended way is via your doctor, who will refer you to an allergy clinic for a free blood test. Your blood sample will be sent to a testing laboratory that will send the results back to your doctor. There are also a number of private laboratories and homeopathic clinics, some of whom advertise on the Internet, that will conduct tests direct. Occasionally, medical food reaction testing can be inaccurate, as are many other medical tests. Most of the time, though, it is quite helpful. Errors in the tests are mainly false negatives, the failure to spot a food reaction. Less common are false positives, an indication of a reaction where none actually exists.

If you decide to have a medical blood test, you'll still need to do a moderate amount of elimination-diet testing. For one thing, you probably eat more than 100 different foods, even though you may eat some quite rarely. For another, as previously mentioned, there is always the chance of an error in your test. You may get a false positive, telling you to avoid a food you're not really reactive to, although this is uncommon. More common is the likelihood of getting a false negative, in which the test indicates that you may eat a food that you do react to. This may occur if you haven't had recent exposure to a food and your antibody levels drop. No medical test is perfect.

Furthermore, food reactions frequently change; just because you're reactive one month doesn't mean you'll always be reactive. One of the great things about the False Fat Diet is that it helps people recover from food reactions.

By the same token, though, new food reactions can also *begin* at any time, especially if you start to eat any one food too frequently. New reactions can also begin if your general health starts to decline or if you take antibiotics or steroids or if you have problems with digestion or in your GI tract. Therefore, even if you do a food reaction test, you should still be alert for unexpected symptoms.

Nonetheless, I think laboratory tests are of considerable value because they quickly provide information that might take you a month or more to gather on your own. Furthermore, many patients are motivated to cut out these foods by seeing their food reactions confirmed technologically.

Investing time and even money in your own health is always one of the smartest investments you can make. Your health is not only the foundation of your earning power, but is also the wellspring of your joy and strength.

Now let's look at the various types of medical tests you can do. There are two types that I think are most effective for determining reactive foods. We'll start with these two, then take a quick look at other methods that may help. The two types I prefer are the **ELISA Test** and the **Cell Reactive Test**.

PATIENT'S FOOD REACTION SUMMARY

Highly Reactive Foods (3+)

Cheese	Cow's milk	Gluten	Pineapple
Corn	Egg white	Lactaclburnin	Wheat
Cottage cheese	Egg yolk	Oat	Yogurt

Moderately Reactive Foods (2+)

Alfalfa sprouts	Beet	Cauliflower	Papaya
Apricot	Broccoli	Goat's milk	Peach
Asparagus	Cabbage	Lamb	Rye
Barley	Carrot	Nectarine	

Slightly Reactive Foods (1+)

Apple	Corn gluten	Lemon	Spinach
Avocado	Courgette	Lettuce	String bean
Beef	Cranberry	Olive	Sunflower seed
Blueberry	Cucumber	Orange	Tomato
Brewer's yeast	Garlic	Oyster	Walnut
Buckwheat	Grape	Peanut	White potato
Cane sugar	Grapefruit	Pear	
Celery	Green pepper	Pork	
Chocolate	Kidney bean	Rice	

Nonreactive Foods (0)

Almond	Crab	Pecan	Shrimp
Baker's yeast	Halibut	Pinto bean	Sole
Banana	Honey	Plum	Soya
Butter bean	Lentil	Raspberry	Strawberry
Chicken	Lobster	Red snapper	Sweet potato
Clam	Mushroom	Salmon	Trout
Cod	Onion	Sardine	Tuna
Coffee	Pea	Sesame	Turkey

The ELISA Test

This is one of the more popular and accurate tests for food reactions. The ELISA, or Enzyme Linked Immuno-Sorbent Assay, determines which foods you react to and how badly you react.

Lab technicians determine this by adding a special enzyme to your blood sample, along with extracts of different foods. When they add a food extract that you're reactive to, the enzyme produces a noticeable change in the colour of your blood. The more the colour changes, the more reactive you are to that food.

The colour change occurs because of a chemical reaction with IgG or IgE antibodies. These antibodies, as you probably remember, mistakenly attack foods that they perceive as foreign invaders.

The only real problem with the ELISA test is that it reveals *only* food reactions that are caused by these antibodies' mistaken attacks on foods. Although these are the most *frequent* causes of food reactions, they are not the *only* causes. As I mentioned in Chapter 2, food reactions can also be caused by circulating immune complexes (antibodies bound to food antigens), by direct cellular reactions, and by the drug-like pharmacologic actions of some foods. These three causes, however, are less common.

Even though the ELISA test misses some of these causes, it's still an excellent test, since it does reveal the most common causes of food reactions.

If one of your false fat foods does slip past the ELISA test, you can still identify this reactive food with the elimination diet method. If a food reaction occurs even though you've avoided every food your test told you to avoid, you should eliminate the foods you ate around the time of the reaction. Then reintroduce these foods after 7 to 10 days of strict avoidance, one by one, to find the culprit.

The patient of mine who took this test, Tony, a 49-year-old man, was found to be very reactive to dairy products, but only with delayed IgG reactions. His only immediate IgE reaction to a dairy product was to mozzarella, and even that was just a reaction of 1 on the scale of 1 to 3. He was also quite reactive to eggs, corn, gluten, oats, and wheat.

Tony, like many other patients of mine, had tried hard for most of his life to eat a healthy diet, but he hadn't been eating the foods that were right for *him* as an individual. Before his test, Tony had been eating a lot of yogurt, granola, whole wheat bread, and vegetables. According to many dietary recommendations, this type of low-fat, nutrient-rich diet, high in complex carbohydrates, is ideal. For Tony, though, the diet had been far from ideal and had needed fine-tuning. When he eliminated wheat, milk, eggs, oats, and corn, he began to feel much better. He lost weight, recovered from chronic sinusitis, recovered from severe chronic heartburn, and recovered from chronic insomnia. His recovery from insomnia was particularly heartening, because he'd already been treated at one of the country's leading sleep disorder clinics, to no avail. He was really amazed, and I was very pleased.

Furthermore, Tony discovered that if he avoided his most troublesome foods – those with a 3 rating – he could cheat by eating some of the less reactive foods, without suffering symptoms.

I have ordered ELISA tests for hundreds of my patients over the years, and have generally been quite satisfied with the results.

The test is not infallible, but it invariably offers excellent insight into each patient's own unique metabolic needs.

There is another type of test similar to the ELISA test called the RAST test, or Radio Allergo-Sorbent Testing. This test employs a radioactive material to reveal mainly IgE antibodies, although it can test IgG as well.

Now let's look at the other most effective test for food reactions, the cell reactive test.

Tony thought he was eating a healthy diet. But it wasn't healthy for him.

Cell Reactive Food Tests

Cell reactive, or cytotoxic, tests have one primary advantage over ELISA tests: they identify food reactions other than immune-related IgE and IgG antibody reactions. This test also measures the less common adverse pharmacologic reactions.

To perform a cell reactive food test, laboratory technicians observe samples of your blood under a microscope as they add various food extracts one by one. The technicians look for toxic reactions. The toxic reactions the technicians look for include changes in the size and count of white blood cells and the clumping together of blood cell platelets.

This analysis is somewhat subjective, though, so there is some margin for error. Even so, one of the best cell reactive tests, the ALCAT test, appears to be quite reliable. In one study of the ALCAT test, performed by a London hospital, the accuracy rate was 83 per cent, and in another double-blind trial of the test, the accuracy rate was 96 per cent.

The ALCAT test has been used successfully by many doctors for more than ten years. The acronym ALCAT stands for Antigen Leukocyte Cellular Antibody Test.

Some ALCAT tests examine more foods than others. The least comprehensive test is a relatively inexpensive 10-food panel, and the most comprehensive includes a panel of 100 foods, 10 additives, 10 food colourings, and 10 chemicals.

Like the ELISA test, the ALCAT cytotoxic test is not infallible, so even if you take it, you should still be alert for symptoms. If symptoms occur, use the elimination diet method to determine what food caused the problem.

Although the ELISA and cell reactive tests are the most accurate tests for food reactions, other tests are also sometimes used. Let's take a quick look at them. They might be of help to you.

Scratch Tests

This is the type of test that is most widely used by conventional allergists, but it has a serious drawback: it identifies only immediate, IgE allergies, which are often so obvious that people recognize them without a test. Scratch tests don't reveal the much more common delayed IgG reactions, nor do they reveal immune complex or pharmacologic reactions. Therefore, they are quite limited as a measure of food reactivity.

A scratch test is quite useful, though, for diagnosing reactions to inhalant allergies, such as those caused by pollen. Most people who seek medical treatment for allergies have inhalant allergies, and that is why this test remains so popular among conventional allergists. Diagnosing food reactions is still a relatively new endeavour among most allergists, and many allergists simply haven't kept up with the emerging body of research on the best tests for food reactions. Many of them still tell patients that food reactions are not a common problem.

To perform a scratch test, a doctor makes small, shallow scratches on your skin, and then touches them with food extracts or with other suspected allergens. If you have an IgE reaction to any allergen, your skin will develop a slight swelling and redness. The process generally does not cause significant discomfort.

The scratch test is sometimes helpful as a back-up for other tests. If you take an ELISA or cell reaction test, and it shows that you have an IgE reaction to a food, you may want to get a scratch test to confirm the diagnosis.

However, some researchers believe that the scratch test often generates false negatives, telling people that they aren't reactive when they really are. It can also generate false positives when histamine is at a high concentration in the bloodstream.

I usually do not recommend this test for food reactions, but it is helpful for inhalant allergies.

Experimental Food Reaction Tests

There are several other tests that are occasionally used to determine food reactions, but their accuracy has not been as well documented in medical literature. Therefore, these tests are considered unproven, or experimental. They include sublingual tests, pulse tests, and kinesiology tests.

Sublingual testing consists of placing food extracts under a patient's tongue and then watching for symptoms, such as wheezing, itching, congestion, or changes in moods and energy levels. This type of testing is sometimes interesting, but it relies on the subjective perceptions of both patient and doctor, and is not very scientific. Furthermore, it identifies only immediate reactions. Because of its considerable limitations, I don't use it.

Pulse testing is less subjective, but is still far from definitive. To perform this test, a patient takes his or her own pulse, and then eats a moderate to large portion of a suspected reactive food. For best results, this should be done first thing in the morning, on an empty stomach. The patient waits fifteen minutes, then takes his or her pulse again. If the pulse increases significantly – by 10 to 15 beats per minute – it can indicate a food reaction. This test is sometimes useful as an adjunct to other, more accurate tests, such as the ELISA test, cell reactive test, or elimination diet method.

Kinesiology testing is also unscientific, but it can be interesting as a back-up test. The best way to do this test is to have it performed by a practitioner who is familiar with it, such as a chiropractor or naturopath. The doctor will place a sample of a suspected reactive food directly against your skin and will then test your muscle strength, usually by pressing down on your outstretched arm. If you are able to resist more forcefully when the food is *not* touching your skin, it can indicate reactivity. This test is relatively subjective and is poorly documented in medical literature. Oddly, though, it sometimes works.

Now you know everything you need to know to get started. You just have to choose between a laboratory test or the elimination diet method. As I mentioned, there's no right or wrong choice. They both work, and the *best* method is to employ both approaches.

The main thing is *just to start*. That's the key to any journey. And this will be one of the most exciting journeys of your life!

Your first step is the Cleansing Phase. You'll find it highly rewarding. It may make you feel better than you have in years.

First, though, you may want to take a look at some sample elimination diets. These guidelines will help you decide which elimination diet is best for you.

SAMPLE ELIMINATION
DIET MENU PLANS

B ECAUSE THE FALSE FAT DIET IS THE MOST HIGHLY individualized of all current diets, *there is no one single menu plan that is appropriate for all people.*

As a dieter, you are on a unique, solitary quest to determine your own particular food reactions. Therefore, you must find your own special, individualized combinations of foods *that most effectively make you healthy and trim.*

To recap, the best way to determine your own individualized version of the False Fat Diet is with an elimination diet, in which you eliminate suspected reactive foods and then gradually reintroduce them to see if they cause reactions. The other way to determine your food reactions is with a medical blood test. But even patients who do a blood test should *still* undertake the detective work of an elimination diet to be sure that their test results were correct.

As you determine all of your own reactive foods, *your elimination diet gradually becomes your permanent, long-term diet.* Even your permanent diet can change, though, because food reactions often disappear after a food is eliminated for several months. As you successfully add foods that do not cause reactions, your diet will increase in variety and become more satisfying. This new, emerging diet will consist of the *smart food choices that will serve you well for the rest of your life.*

Following are four sample menu plans for the types of elimination diets that I have described: (1) the Juice Fast Elimination Diet, (2) the Total Elimination Diet, (3) the Sensitive Seven

Elimination Diet, and (4) the Limited Elimination Diet.

Of these four types, the most strict are the Total Elimination Diet and the Juice Fast Elimination Diet. The Juice Fast is particularly strict. These two approaches are relatively difficult to follow for an extended period. However, they are excellent ways to *begin* the False Fat Diet. The Juice Fast, in particular, will yield spectacularly fast results for most people, since it is such a pure, low-calorie diet.

Sometimes patients like to begin their False Fat Diet with several days of one of the more strict approaches, such as the Juice Fast or the Total Elimination Diet, and then ease into a less strict approach, such as the Sensitive Seven Elimination Diet. This is a sensible way to begin.

As a rule, the more strict approaches, which are harder to stick to, yield faster, more dramatic results. Patients lose weight at an accelerated pace, and generally get a very clear, accurate picture of their food reactions.

The following menu plans are intended only as guidelines or suggestions. You may be able to devise menu plans that more appropriately meet your own individual needs, desires, and available foods and juices. When you do vary from the menu plan, though, you should *retain the general spirit of the menu plan* by substituting only similar foods in similar amounts.

The Juice Fast Elimination Diet

This diet is the most strict form of an elimination diet and is very low in calories, usually averaging less than 1,000 calories per day. It is not appropriate as a long-term eating plan. Because this diet is so low in calories, it may trigger the body's starvation response, causing it to hoard calories. Therefore, you should go off this diet gradually, to avoid rebound weight gain.

This is the best diet for detoxification and the most certain to yield fast, gratifying results. The diet consists of essentially the same regimen every day, so only one day is outlined here.

After several days on the Juice Fast, or perhaps a week,

most people eliminate the majority of toxins in their bodies and begin to feel great. When this happens, they are usually ready to move on and begin reintroducing foods to see if they react to them. Foods are reintroduced one by one, as the patients remain alert for negative reactions. Some people are reactive to certain juices, so be alert for any negative reactions. If you experience a reaction, eliminate the juice that caused it.

Sometimes, though, instead of reintroducing foods one at a time, patients switch to one of the other types of elimination diet, such as the Total Elimination Diet. This is quite acceptable, but it does make it somewhat harder to spot reactions, because several new foods are reintroduced at once. It may be helpful to keep a journal to track your reactions.

SAMPLE MENU, JUICE FAST ELIMINATION DIET

This menu may be repeated each day.

Breakfast

Master Cleanser Lemonade: 2 tbsp fresh lemon or lime juice, 1 tbsp pure maple syrup, a pinch cayenne pepper ($\frac{1}{10}$ tsp), and 225 ml spring water. Also early in the morning: 1 cup of herbal tea, such as peppermint, ginseng or hot lemon water.

NOTE: Master cleanser can also be drunk throughout the day. You should have at least three glasses throughout the morning, which will cleanse and energize you. After each glass of this lemonade, you will want to rinse your mouth and teeth with plain water to protect them from irritation or calcium/enamel loss (the citric and ascorbic acids in the lemon can pull calcium from the teeth).

Snack

Fruit juice (fresh-squeezed, from lemon, lime, apple, pear watermelon, or cherry) (420 ml) or more Master Cleanser. Ideally, use organic and in-season fruits when available. Grape, orange, and pineapple should generally not be used because they tend to be more commonly reactive.

Lunch
  Vegetable juice (from fresh carrots, beetroot, celery, spinach, or wheat grass) (420 ml)
Snack, early afternoon
  Vegetable juice (not tomato) (420 ml)
Snack, later afternoon
  Fruit juice or vegetable juice (420 ml)
Dinner
  Vegetable juice or warm broth (not tomato) (420 ml)
Snack, early evening (if desired)
  Vegetable juice (420 ml)
Snack, late evening
  Herbal tea, such as peppermint, chamomile, or licorice

The Total Elimination Diet

This is the second most strict form of elimination diet, after the Juice Fast Elimination Diet. It is a superb way to start the False Fat Diet, because it eliminates almost all foods that may be reactive. Also, it is lower in calories than either the Sensitive Seven Elimination Diet or the Limited Elimination Diet, both of which average about 2,200 calories per day. *The Total Elimination Diet averages approximately 1,500 calories per day.* Thus, it is only moderately higher in calories than the Juice Fast.

The Total Elimination Diet is so low in calories because it is comprised *mostly of vegetables*, which are generally low in calories, compared to almost all other foods. Because vegetables are high in bulk, fibre and nutrients, however, the Total Elimination Diet actually can be quite filling and nutritious.

Because the Total Elimination Diet is filling and satisfying, many patients find that they can stick with it for a relatively long time – often for a month or so. At 1,500 calories per day, the Total Elimination Diet is similar in caloric content to many other weight-loss diets. However, it tends to be far easier to stick with than other weight-loss diets, because of its unique, powerful ability to end food cravings.

Some patients begin their False Fat Diets with a few days

(or more) of the Juice Fast, then make the transition to the Total Elimination Diet. They then often gradually switch to one of the less restrictive elimination diets. During this entire time, they gradually try new foods, to see if they cause reactions.

To follow is a one-week programme. To help yourself know what foods you can eat during this week, you might want to make a list of foods mentioned on page 152 that you know are safe for you – and also that you eat only rarely. You may also want to add to this list other vegetables that are generally non-reactive, such as cabbage, bok choy, broccoli, and greens such as mustard cress, spring greens, and nettles. But skip using soya sauce or tamari on your greens! For your salads, why not add some cleansing greens, such as radicchio, endive, and watercress. Try the Seasonal Vegetable Medleys on page 318.

Sample Menu
Day 1

Breakfast
- Pear (1)
- Hot rice cereal, 90–270g, cooked, with 1 tsp maple syrup
- Hot herbal (or green) tea

Snack
- Raw or toasted sunflower seeds (45g)

Lunch
- Chicken breast (1) with sea salt and pepper (preferably cayenne, the healthiest pepper) or other non-soya seasonings. Black pepper is irritating and often an allergen.
- Steamed Swiss chard, with garlic and salt

Snack
- Walnuts or almonds (5–10) or a handful of sunflower seeds
- Iced (or hot) herbal tea

Dinner
- Vegetables stir-fried in 1–2 tsp olive oil (may include carrots, beetroot, celery, turnips, butter beans, kale, and onions (540–720g)
- Steamed rice (cooked rice with 1 part rice to 2 parts water),

served with the stir-fry, with 25g walnuts, seasoned with salt, pepper, and garlic
- Lettuce salad, with 2–3 tsp olive oil and apple-cider vinegar

Snack
- Pear (1)
- Hot herbal tea

Day 2

Breakfast
- Apple (1)
- Rice cake (2–3) or 90–270g cooked rice or cream of rice (prepared without milk or cream)
- Hot herbal tea

Snack
- Rice cake with walnuts, almonds, or almond butter

Lunch
- Split Pea or Haricot Bean Soup (420 ml) (see page 331)
- Swiss chard salad, with raw radishes, 1 tbsp vinaigrette dressing (equal parts olive oil and balsamic vinegar, and a dash of sea salt). (If the chard is young, you may like it raw, but if the leaves are bigger and the stems thicker, try them steamed.)

Snack
- Walnuts (5–10) or 10–20 unsalted pistachios or pine nuts

Dinner
- Turkey breast, barbecued, baked, or roasted
- Steamed carrots with parsley
- Raw kale salad, with 1 tbsp olive oil and vinegar. (If the kale is young, you may like it raw, but if it's older, you'll want to steam it to make it tender.)

Snack
- Baked acorn or butternut squash (½ squash, with 1 tsp honey, as glaze) or one apple

Day 3

Breakfast
- Banana (1), sliced, and topped with 5–10 crushed almonds or walnuts, and 1 tsp maple syrup
- Hot herbal or green tea

Snack
- Carrot sticks (8)
- Vegetable juice (not tomato) (225 ml)

Lunch
- Steamed vegetables (may include kale or chard, carrots, onions, and squash)
- Steamed rice (90–180g)
- Iced (or hot) herbal tea

Snack
- Pear (1)
- Almonds (5–10)

Dinner
- Lamb (or a salmon dish) roasted with small whole onions and rosemary or thyme; seasoned with garlic and salt (1 serving)
- Lettuce salad with 1 tbsp vinaigrette dressing
- Yam (sweet potato), baked, with 1 tbsp honey glaze or 1 tsp olive oil

Snack
- Rice cake with 1 tsp of almond butter, or 1 banana
- Hot herbal tea

Day 4

Breakfast
- Cantaloupe melon (½) (wait 15–30 minutes before eating rice cakes)
- Rice cakes (2), with 1 tsp apple or pear butter
- Hot herbal tea

Snack
- Apple juice (225 ml)

Lunch
- Steamed vegetables (360g) (may include onions, turnips, carrots, butter beans, Swiss chard), seasoned with garlic salt and 1–2 tsp olive oil or flaxseed oil. Rotate most vegetables to at least every other day.
- Steamed rice (90 g), or a protein, like 60–110 g of fish or poultry
- Iced (or hot) herbal tea

Snack
- Lemonade, made with fresh lemon and 1 tsp maple syrup, or Master Cleanser (see page 166)

Dinner
- Chicken breast, barbecued or roasted, with roasted sesame seeds
- Lettuce salad, with 1 tbsp vinaigrette dressing
- Steamed or stir-fried (in ½ tsp olive oil) green beans

Snack
- Walnuts (5–10) or slice apple

Day 5

Breakfast
- Pear (1)
- Cream of rice cereal
- Hot herbal tea

Snack
- Carrot sticks (5–7)
- Iced herbal tea

Lunch
- Vegetable soup (420 ml). (Use only vegetables listed for elimination diet, cooked in water with 1–2 tbsp of seasoning such as parsley, basil, pinch of sea salt, and olive oil.)
- Rice cakes (1–2)

Snack
- Raw or roasted sunflower seeds (45 g)
- Apple juice (225 ml)

Dinner
- Baked salmon, with carrots, onions and courgettes
- Lettuce salad, with 1 tbsp oil and vinegar dressing
- Steamed rice (90–180 g)

Snack
- Rice cake with 1 tsp apple butter
- Hot herbal tea

Day 6

Breakfast
- Lemonade, made with fresh lemon and 1 tsp maple syrup
- Wait thirty minutes before you eat: rice cake with 1 tsp

almond butter
Snack
- Baked apple (1) with 1 tsp honey, and 3–5 chopped almonds. (You can core the apple before baking and pat the honey-almond mixture inside.)

Lunch
- Chicken breast, hot or cold
- Swiss chard salad (raw or steamed), with shredded beetroot, sliced radish or jicama, thin slices of cucumber, and 1 tbsp vinaigrette dressing

Snack
- Almonds or walnuts (5–10) or unsalted pistachios or pine nuts (10–20)
- Carrot or vegetable juice (225 ml)

Dinner
- Steamed vegetables (or stir-fried with 1 tsp olive oil), topped with crushed nuts, salt, pepper, garlic, and parsley
- Steamed rice (180 g)
- Fresh or steamed kale salad, with 1 tbsp oil and vinegar dressing

Snack
- Hot nut milk, with 1 tsp maple syrup (see page 286)

Day 7

Breakfast
- Hot cream of rice cereal, with 1–2 tsp maple syrup or honey
- Hot herbal tea

Snack
- Raw vegetable sticks (carrots, celery, cucumber, or courgettes) (5–10)

Lunch
- Turkey, sliced (175 g), hot or cold
- Lettuce salad, with carrots, 1 tbsp vinaigrette dressing
- Iced herbal tea

Snack
- Hot apple cider or raw apple

Dinner
- Lamb or chicken stew, with peas, beans, carrots, and squash, seasoned to taste

- Rice (90–180 g), steamed
- Fresh cucumbers, sliced and marinated in apple-cider vinegar, garlic, and salt

Snack

- Baked apple, with 1 tsp honey or maple syrup

The Sensitive Seven Elimination Diet

This eating plan is among the most popular among patients on the False Fat Diet, because it eliminates all of the Sensitive Seven most commonly reactive foods: **dairy products, wheat, corn, eggs, soya, peanuts**, and **sugar**.

The daily menu plans average approximately 2,200 calories.

This eating plan should result in the quick loss of *false fat* among people whose food reactions are confined to the Sensitive Seven group. If you are also reactive to foods other than the Sensitive Seven, you should eliminate them, too. In addition, you should eliminate any food that you have been eating almost every day.

Your loss of adipose tissue in this eating plan will depend upon several factors. Among the most important is your activity level. If you are very active, and exercise an hour or more each day, you may lose several pounds each week on this eating plan. If you are moderately active, and exercise every other day, you may lose a pound or two each week. If you are inactive, and don't exercise at all, you may not lose weight, and might even gradually gain some weight.

In addition, men will tend to lose adipose tissue on this eating plan more quickly than women, because men generally have a higher percentage of muscle, and usually burn fat more efficiently.

Another factor that will determine your rate of weight loss is your size. Both men and women will lose weight more quickly the more overweight they are. If you are a big, heavy person, you will tend to lose more weight on this eating plan than a small, lighter person. If you are inactive, or if you are a woman, *you may need to eat somewhat less food than this eating plan calls for*, in order to lose weight. You can do this by reducing portion sizes, or avoiding some of the foods the plan calls for.

After at least one week on this eating plan, you may begin to reintroduce suspected reactive foods, as you begin your food 'challenges.' When you add one of these foods to your diet, you could subtract another food, to keep from adding calories, or just eat a little less. You could also add puréed vegetable soups or a 'cream' of vegetable soup blended with a very loose oatmeal instead of milk or cream. You could also eat a lighter lunch or dinner on some days, or just drink juice at those times.

SAMPLE MENU
Day 1

Breakfast
- Hot cream of rice cereal, with 1–2 tsp honey and 2 tbsp rice milk (small bowl)
- Fruit salad (225 g, with banana, apple, raisins)
- Hot tea

Snack
- Rice cake or rice bread with 1 tbsp almond butter or 1 tbsp all-fruit spread
- Fruit juice (225 ml)

Lunch
- Tuna salad, with sliced celery or onion and 1–2 tbsp vinaigrette dressing
- Curried (or seasoned) green beans (90 g)
- Spelt or rice bread (1 slice), with 1 tsp non-dairy (non-soya) butter/spread, such as apple or pear butter

Snack
- Carrot and celery sticks (5–10)
- Almonds (5–10) or sunflower seeds (20–40 or 1 handful)

Dinner
- Stuffed Bell Pepper (omit the tempeh/soya) (see page 315, or Rich Veggie Soup (420 ml) (see page 329)
- Green salad, with 1 tbsp vinaigrette dressing
- Iced herbal tea

Snack
- Honey Sundae (see page 341) (must use non-dairy, non-soya ice cream!) or a piece of fruit

Day 2

Breakfast
- Cold cereal (make sure it's wheat-free) or cream of rice with rice milk or apple juice. You may use 1 tsp natural sweetener, such as maple syrup, *if* you're not using apple juice.
- Hot herbal tea
- Sunflower seeds (25 g or small handful)

Snack
- Frozen banana, coated with carob and chopped almonds; or one apple (easier)

Lunch
- Chicken vegetable soup
- Green salad with 1–2 tbsp olive oil and vinegar (or lemon) dressing
- Rice cake (1–2)

Snack
- Popcorn, with 1 tbsp sprayed or drizzled olive oil and salt

Dinner
- Potato-Crusted Salmon (see page 301)
- Green salad with 2 tbsp dressing (non-allergenic, or lemon and olive oil)
- Asparagus (1 serving), steamed or lightly sautéed, with seasoning

Snack
- Non-dairy/non-soya ice cream (90 g) or apple and 2 dates

Day 3

Breakfast
- Non-wheat pancakes (4 medium-sized pancakes), with 1 tbsp maple syrup and 1–2 tsp non-dairy, non-soya butter
- Hot herbal tea

Snack
- Apple (1)
- Walnuts (5–10)

Lunch
- Broccoli Soup (see page 330)
- Steamed rice (180 g), with 1 tsp olive oil or ½ tsp sesame oil, salt, and pepper
- Iced herbal tea

Snack
- Rice cake with apple butter (1 tsp)

Dinner
- Grilled Swordfish with Pineapple Mustard (see page 310)
- Sweet potato, with 1 tsp olive oil and 1 tsp honey
- Green salad with Avocado Dressing (see page 332)

Snack
- Baked apple, with cinnamon, raisins, and 1 tsp honey

Day 4

Breakfast
- Fruit salad (rotate apples and other fruits, such as pears, bananas) with cinnamon and 4 chopped almonds or cashews (350–400 g)
- Spelt or rice bread (1 piece) with 1 tsp almond butter
- Hot tea

Snack
- Sunflower seeds

Lunch
- Cold chicken breast (no skin)
- Green salad with 1 tbsp vinaigrette dressing
- Baked potato with 1 tsp olive oil, sprinkle of sea salt, and pinch of red pepper. May add a quarter of an avocado, sliced.

Snack
- Vegetable juice (fresh carrot, tomato, or vegetable mixture) (225 ml)

Dinner
- Sea Bass en Papillotte (see page 309) or baked salmon
- Steamed broccoli, with 1 tsp olive oil, garlic, salt, and lemon juice
- Steamed rice (90 g)
- Green salad with Avocado Dressing (see page 332) or vinaigrette

Snack
- Apple and 2 dates

Day 5

Breakfast
- Breakfast Rice (350 g) (see page 325)
- Hot herbal tea

Snack
- Rice cake (2) with 1 tbsp almond butter and 1 tbsp fruit spread

Lunch
- Sliced turkey (110 g)
- Wilted Spinach Salad (see page 339)
- Iced herbal tea

Snack
- Lemonade, with maple syrup (225–350 g)
- Almonds (10–15)

Dinner
- Grilled Salmon on a Bed or Braised Lentils with Baby Artichokes (see page 306)
- Baked acorn squash, with 1 tsp olive oil and ½ tbsp honey
- Salad greens, with 1 tbsp balsamic vinegar

Snack
- Non-dairy ice cream (90 g), or hot apple cider

Day 6

Breakfast
- Grapefruit (1), with 1–2 tsp honey or maple syrup
- Spelt or rice toast with 1 tsp almond butter (1 piece)

Snack
- Hot herbal tea
- Wheat-free crackers or oatcakes (3–5) or walnuts (5–10)

Lunch
- Split Pea or Haricot Bean Soup (see page 331)
- Green salad, with 1 tbsp vinaigrette
- Iced herbal tea

Snack
- Apple (1)
- Pumpkin seeds (10–20)

Dinner
- Snapper Mexicana with Tropical Fruit Salsa (see page 309) or pan-seared chicken, Mediterranean-style (see page 301)
- Baked sweet potato, with 1 tsp olive or flaxseed oil
- Steamed baby peas and pearl onions (180 g), with 1 tsp olive oil, and a dash of salt, garlic, and pepper

Snack
- Pumpkin Pie with Oat Crust (1 piece) (see page 343)

Day 7

Breakfast
- Hot buckwheat or oat cereal, with 1 tbsp rice milk and 1 tsp honey
- Hot herbal tea
- Apple or ½ banana

Snack
- Sunflower seeds (45 g or 1 handful)
- Fruit juice (225 ml)

Lunch
- Lentil soup, or hearty bean soup
- Green salad, with 1 tbsp Basil Balsamic Vinaigrette (see page 331)
- Rice cake, with Butter-Free Veggie Spread (see page 335)

Snack
- Raw vegetable pieces with 1–2 tbsp Avocado Dressing (see page 332)

Dinner
- Red Snapper on Black Bean Relish (see page 302)
- Garden Tomatoes with Balsamic Vinaigrette (see page 319)
- Baked potato with 1 tsp olive or safflower oil, salt and pepper

Snack
- Cashew or Almond Butter Cookies (2) (see page 346)
- Hot herbal tea

The Limited Elimination Diet

This is the least strict type of elimination diet. It eliminates only **wheat**, **dairy products**, **sugar**, and **any food you eat**

virtually every day. Some people who are reactive to dairy products are also reactive to eggs, because they contain a similar protein, so eggs have also been eliminated from the 7-day sample menu prototype of the Limited Elimination Diet.

Like the Sensitive Seven Elimination Diet, the guidelines for the Limited Elimination Diet call for about *2,200 calories per day*. At this level of caloric intake, active or large-framed people will probably lose adipose tissue, but inactive, small-framed people might *not* lose much fat and could even gain weight. If you are inactive or not more than 10 pounds overweight, you may need to reduce portions in order to lose true fat.

Some patients are drawn to this version of the elimination diet because it sounds easier. However, the Limited Elimination Diet will be easier for you *only* if your reactions are confined to the foods the diet restricts. For example, if you're also reactive to soya, which is allowed in the Limited Elimination Diet, eating it will make your diet much harder. You'll be much more vulnerable to hunger, food cravings, mood swings, and all the other symptoms caused by food reactions.

Therefore, you should be especially alert on the Limited Elim-ination Diet for food reactions. If you experience them, figure out which food caused them. If you are having trouble figuring it out – because you are eating such a wide variety of foods – it may be wise to switch to a more restrictive elimination diet, such as the Total Elimination Diet or the Sensitive Seven Elimination Diet.

Once you're free from your reactive foods, you'll probably experience significantly *less* hunger, even though you may be eating *fewer* calories.

SAMPLE MENU
DAY 1

Breakfast
- Oatmeal, with 1–2 tsp honey and 2 tbsp soya or rice milk
- Spelt bread toast, with 1 tsp non-dairy or nut butter*

---

*Many non-dairy butters and margarines are made with soya. If you know soya is not a trigger for you, you can try one. If it is an allergen for you, try almond butter.

- Hot herbal tea

Snack
- Banana Bread (1 slice) (non-wheat) (see page 345)

Lunch
- Prawns with Lentil Salad (see page 308)
- Green salad, with 1 tbsp oil and vinegar dressing
- Carrots and peas, lightly stir-fried in 1 tsp olive oil, seasoned with tamari, garlic, pepper, and sweet basil

Snack
- Vegetable sticks (8–10), with 1 tbsp Avocado Dressing as dip (see page 332)
- Iced herbal tea

Dinner
- Spiced Butternut Squash Bisque (420 ml) (see page 328)
- Green salad with Basil Balsamic Vinaigrette (see page 331)
- Rice cake (1–2)

Snack
- Fruit Sorbet (page 342)
- Hot herbal tea

Day 2

Breakfast
- Tofu squares with diced spring onions, sautéed in tamari, 1 tsp olive oil, and red pepper; or Breakfast Rice (see page 325)
- Spelt bread toast, or rye bread (1 piece) with 1 tsp non-dairy butter (avoid if using rice dish)
- Hot herbal tea

Snack
- Cashews or almonds (5–10)
- Lemonade, made with fresh lemons and 1 tbsp maple syrup

Lunch
- Chicken vegetable soup (280–420 ml)
- Sliced fresh tomatoes, seasoned, or green salad with 1 tbsp vinaigrette, or both
- Iced herbal tea

Snack
- Carrot juice (225 ml)

- Celery stick (1) filled with 1 tbsp natural peanut or almond butter

Dinner
- Pan-seared or baked squares of salmon with flavour of choice (see page 301)
- Steamed rice (90 g) with Sweet and Sour Sauce (see page 333)
- Green salad, with Avocado Dressing (see page 332)
- Fresh corn on the cob, with 1 tsp non-dairy butter and salt and pepper

Snack
- Fruit (Cherry) Cobbler (1 piece) (see page 348)
- Hot herbal tea

Day 3

Breakfast
- Fruit salad, with apple butter as dressing, sprinkled with almonds and cinnamon
- Rice cake (1–2), with 1 tbsp apple butter
- Hot herbal tea

Snack
- Apple juice (225 ml)
- Almonds (5–10)

Lunch
- Chicken breast, cold, or pan-seared chicken with vegetables (see page 301)
- Green salad with 1 tbsp vinaigrette
- Steamed green beans (90 g)

Snack
- Courgette Cake (1 piece) (see page 345)

Dinner
- Seasonal Vegetable Medley (see page 318), water sautéed or stir-fried in 56 ml vegetable stock and 30 ml white wine (if desired) and served with 1 tbsp olive oil, seasoned to taste (served over rice), topped with 10 crumbled, roasted cashews or almonds
- Steamed rice (180g)
- Green salad, with 1 tbsp Avocado Dressing (see page 332)

Snack
- Cashew or Almond Butter Cookies (2) (see page 346)
- Hot nut milk (see page 286)

Day 4

Breakfast
- Cream of rice hot cereal, with ½ banana, sliced, and/or 1–2 tbsp of honey or maple syrup, and 1 tsp non-dairy butter
- Spelt bread toast, with 1 tsp all-fruit spread
- Hot herbal tea

Snack
- Apple (1)
- Walnuts or almonds (5–10)

Lunch
- Chicken stew (simmered with vegetables) or Blackened Tofu Steaks (see page 316)
- Green salad, with 1 tbsp vinaigrette
- Iced herbal tea

Snack
- Carrot and celery sticks, with 1 tbsp Green Onion Dressing as dip (see page 332)

Dinner
- Grilled sole or halibut, marinated in tamari, garlic, lemon, and pepper
- Green salad, with 1 tbsp Italian dressing
- Steamed broccoli, topped with sesame seeds and 1 tsp non-dairy butter

Snack
- Honey Sundae or Chocolate Pudding (see page 341)

Day 5

Breakfast
- Cold non-wheat cereal, in goat's milk (or soya or rice milk), with ½–1 tsp date sugar or honey
- Hot herbal tea

Snack
- Rice cake (1 or 2) with 1 tbsp almond butter and 1–2 tsp all-fruit spread

Lunch
- Black bean soup (420 ml) or Mexican Salad Bowl (see page 340)
- Spelt bread (1 slice), with 1 tsp non-dairy butter
- Green salad, with 1 tbsp oil and vinegar dressing
- Cashew or Almond Butter Cookie (1) (see page 346)

Snack
- Fresh vegetable juice
- Almonds (5–7)

Dinner
- Maple and Orange Marinated Pork Loin (see page 312) or Tofu Brochettes (see page 317)
- Asparagus, steamed (1 serving) with 1 tsp non-dairy butter
- Green salad, with 1 tbsp balsamic vinaigrette dressing
- Baked potato (1), with 1 tbs non-dairy butter or olive oil or ¼ avocado (mashed or sliced) and chives

Snack
- Non-dairy ice cream or an apple and 2 dates

Day 6

Breakfast
- Hot rice and raisin cereal, with 1–2 tsp maple syrup and 1 tsp non-dairy butter, or
- Spelt bread toast, with 1 tsp non-dairy butter and/or 1 tsp all-fruit spread
- Hot herbal tea

Snack
- Pear (1)
- Almonds (5–10)

Lunch
- Gazpacho (420 ml) (see page 329)
- Baked sweet potato or yam, with 1 tbsp non-dairy butter
- Iced herbal tea

Snack
- Banana or fruit freeze or apple or orange

Dinner
- Baked turkey breast, rubbed with garlic, pepper, and olive oil
- Stuffed acorn or butternut squash (½ squash), with 1 tbsp non-dairy butter

- Green salad, with 1 tbsp Basil Balsamic Vinaigrette (see page 331)
- Mushrooms sautéed in 1 tsp olive oil and 1 tsp tamari,* with pinch of cayenne pepper, 1 tsp chopped parsley or basil

Snack
- Non-dairy ice cream (90 g) or a piece of fruit

Day 7

Breakfast
- Non-wheat pancakes (4 pancakes), with 1–2 tbsp maple syrup and 1–2 tsp non-dairy butter, and fruit topping (e.g., strawberries, bananas, or blueberries)
- Hot herbal tea

Snack
- Toasted or raw pumpkin seeds (45 g)
- Fruit juice (280 ml)

Lunch
- Beef barley or Rich Veggie Soup (see page 329) (280–420 ml)
- Green salad, with 1 tbsp vinaigrette
- Non-wheat crackers (4)
- Iced herbal tea

Snack
- Vegetable sticks (carrot, cucumber, celery), with 1 tbsp Avocado Dressing (see page 332)

Dinner
- Seared Sea Scallop and Tiger Prawn Salad with Curry Vinaigrette (see page 307)
- Baked potato, with 1 tbsp non-dairy butter, salt, and pepper (if desired)
- Green salad, with 1 tbsp Italian or vinaigrette dressing
- Cauliflower, steamed, with salt and pepper, and 1 tsp non-dairy butter

Snack
- Cherry pie (see recipe for non-wheat crust on page 346)

---

*Tamari contains soya, so only use if you know you are not sensitive to soya.

7
THE CLEANSING PHASE

LAURA, A PATIENT OF MINE, CALLED MY OFFICE ON THE second day of her False Fat Diet. Her voice sounded tight and reedy, irritable – as if she'd been fighting with someone. She had. She'd been fighting with herself.

She desperately wanted to stay on her diet, she told me, but part of her was resisting. The resistant part of her *didn't feel good*, and was crying out, 'Give up! It's not worth it! You can't do it!'

This reaction is common. During this first phase of the diet, the body cleanses itself of reactive food chemicals and other toxins, and this biochemical makeover is hard for some people. *But nothing good is ever easy!*

The False Fat Diet requires *change*, and some people just can't handle that. They want to cut some calories, trim some pounds, and retain all their old habits.

But that's not how the body works.

If you want to look better and feel better, you've got to *live better*. You've got to make the smart, tough choices that will change your own life. It's up to you: change or don't change. But don't expect your body to change unless *you* change.

Change, however, need not be painful. If you handle it correctly, change can be exciting. Handling it correctly, though, means learning how to *stay in control* of the discomfort and disorientation that change often brings.

The changes that Laura was experiencing had caught her off-guard, even though she and I had previously discussed the symptoms that might arise during her diet's one-week Cleaning Phase. Laura had begun her diet with a weekend juice fast, and this strict approach usually causes the most uncomfortable symptoms. A juice fast accelerates the elimination of toxins from the body, and the faster toxins leave, the more discomfort they cause. After the weekend juice fast, she'd transitioned to a juice and fruit diet, which is still quite strict and rapidly eliminates toxins.

'If it's any consolation,' I told her, 'the people who are the most uncomfortable at first usually end up with the *most improvement*. Right now your body is telling you that you need to do a *lot* of healing, and the smartest thing you can do is to pay attention to the wisdom of your body and make the changes that it's demanding. But if you want to,' I said, 'you can decrease your symptoms just by going off your juice and fruit diet and doing a less strict type of elimination diet.'

She thought about it. 'I'd rather just get it over with,' she said. 'These feelings will go away in a few days, won't they?'

'Yes, they probably will,' I said. 'Tell me exactly what you're experiencing.'

'Well, I don't feel hungry, like I thought I would. I don't really feel like eating at all, because my stomach is sort of queasy. I've been going to the bathroom a lot, and I feel a little jittery. Didn't sleep well last night. Around midnight, I felt like I was dying for some ice cream or some cereal and milk, even though I wasn't actually hungry. This morning, I had a headache, but it went away.'

'That's a good sign,' I said. 'The worst may be over. Right now, you're experiencing two things. The first is withdrawal from allergic addictions. From your chart, it appears that dairy products are your biggest problem. That's why you craved ice cream last night. The other thing you're experiencing is detoxification; your body is throwing off toxins that may have been in your system for months or even years.'

'But I didn't think I'd *have* many toxins in my body,' she said plaintively. 'I don't smoke or drink, and I don't eat junk food.'

'For you, *milk* is junk food. It's practically poison for you.'

Then I told her what to do to feel better. I have a two-part strategy: (1) **Speed the exit of toxins** to get the detox process over as quickly as possible. (2) **Support and comfort the body** during the Cleansing Phase, with a variety of measures, to make the process as pleasant as possible.

I went over these two strategies with Laura, and will tell you about them. First, however, let's take a quick look at what kind of symptoms you should expect during your Cleansing Phase and why they will occur.

You'll definitely want to handle the Cleansing Phase properly, because it will likely be the most challenging part of your False Fat Diet. Some of my patients have had a hard time during their first few days, because they didn't take full advantage of the correct detoxification measures. It was a mistake for them.

You don't want to make the same mistake. You want to succeed! Here's how.

What to Expect

If you have been eating reactive foods for most of your life, you may now have, in effect, 70 trillion rubbish bins for cells. Your cells are probably crammed full of necrotic debris from partially assimilated foods and environmental toxins. In addition, your cells and tissues may contain food dyes, pesticides, herbicides, rancid fats, and other poisonous chemicals. Your cells and tissues are probably so congested with toxins that many of them are literally dying from *cellular suffocation*.

As if that's not bad enough, your organs of elimination are probably in even worse shape. For years, your eliminative organs may have struggled to evacuate all the harmful things you put into your body, but they probably weren't able to keep up. As a result, your colon may be riddled with pockets of waste that have been there for too long, and your liver may be swollen or possibly even fatty from abuse of alcohol and chemicals in foods. The nephrons in your kidneys may be inflamed, and your lymph glands may be clogged with backed-up poisons.

I know that this sounds like a dire assessment, but this type

TOXIC CONDITIONS

Skin rashes	Atherosclerosis
Bad breath	Depression
Constipation	Anxiety
Sinus congestion	Itchy, red eyes
Insomnia	Asthma
Backache	Allergy
Headache	Angina pectoris
Joint pain	Chronic cough
Stiff neck	Runny nose
Sore throat	Hives

of toxic congestion is astonishingly common. After all, three out of four Americans die of degenerative diseases, such as cancer and cardiovascular disease, and these diseases don't come out of thin air. Toxic congestion is a major element in many forms of cancer and cardiovascular disease. In fact, given the extent of toxic congestion that exists in most people, it's a testimony to the regenerative powers of the body that we're able to be as *healthy* as we are for as *long* as we are.

Consider the list of conditions that are most often caused by toxic congestion above. As you can see, there is a significant similarity between these *toxic conditions* and some conditions that are often caused by *food reactions*. That is because food reactions are, in a sense, toxic reactions. When you eat a reactive food, your body thinks that it's been attacked by a toxic invader, such as a bacteria. Your body tries to isolate and deactivate the presumed toxin, partly by surrounding the reactive food molecules with water, which results in swelling. Sometimes the reactive food molecules are quickly eliminated, but sometimes they become lodged in tissues and cells.

Within cells, the reactive food molecules, as well as other toxins, may damage the function of the cell. If this condition is widespread, as it often is, it can cause dysfunction and discomfort throughout the body.

The *most discomfort*, however, occurs when a large volume of toxins are dislodged from the cells and begin to *leave the body*. This generally overwhelms the organs of elimination and detoxification, resulting in toxins circulating around the body, searching for an exit. That is why any type of detoxification, including the Cleansing Phase of your diet, can be uncomfortable.

During your Cleansing Phase, your cells will begin to expel their toxic materials. As you begin to burn stored fat, even *more* toxins will be released, because most toxins are stored in fat cells. As toxins are released, they may become backed up in your system. They will become especially congested in your organs of detoxification and elimination: your *colon*, *kidneys*, *lymphatic system*, *liver*, *lungs* and *respiratory tract*, and *skin*.

If these toxins enter your bloodstream and travel to your head, they may cause a headache or result in itchy, watery eyes or congested sinuses. If they try to exit from your skin, they may cause a rash, a blemish, or allergic eczema. In your oral cavity, toxins being eliminated may cause irritated or bleeding gums or a thick, foul-smelling coat on your tongue. In your lungs, they may cause bronchial congestion, as your lungs secrete extra mucus to surround them. In your kidneys, they may cause soreness or frequent, malodorous urination. In your liver, they may cause swelling and a feeling of abdominal fullness and upset. In your lymph glands, they may cause enlargement and tenderness. In your colon, they may cause diarrhoea, constipation, swelling or bloating.

When these organs and glands become congested with toxins, they will function far less efficiently. This will cause an even *greater backlog* of toxins. It may also harm the other, non-eliminative functions of certain organs. In the liver, for example, a toxic backlog can impair the liver's ability to break down fat and regulate hormones.

Therefore, it is critically important to *accelerate the elimination of these toxins*. If you don't do this, you may feel discomfort for an extended period of time and be tempted to abandon your diet.

At the same time that toxins may begin to temporarily clog your system, you may also begin to experience the first uncomfortable symptoms of *allergic withdrawal* from your reactive foods. As you'll recall, these symptoms are somewhat similar to the symptoms that cigarette smokers feel when they stop smoking. You may feel cravings, irritability, headaches, and a general sense of malaise.

Many of the symptoms of *allergic withdrawal* will feel quite similar to the symptoms caused by the *elimination of toxins*. Both of these forces cause mood changes, aches and pains, insomnia, and other uncomfortable feelings. When the two forces combine, some patients definitely feel under the weather for a couple of days.

However, you can *fight* these uncomfortable symptoms and win. After all, the feelings are very temporary and are usually relatively mild.

Furthermore, if these feelings do become severe – which occurs mostly among people with severe food reactions – it's a sure sign that your life will soon be *much* better: the harder the healing, the greater the cure.

Now let's look at my cleansing programme for fighting off these feelings, and getting past them as quickly as possible.

The cleansing programme consists of:

1. gastrointestinal tract cleansing;
2. supplementation;
3. herbal therapy;
4. increased water consumption; and
5. physical therapies, such as exercise and saunas.

This cleansing programme is quite similar to the detoxification programme I described in my 1997 book, *The Detox Diet*. When used carefully, this programme is extraordinarily powerful. Also, it's generally quite pleasant. Many patients enjoy it as a positive, healthful way of pampering themselves.

The Cleansing Programme

Gastrointestinal Tract Cleansing
The GI tract is a vital primary exit site for toxins. When you begin to expel toxins from your cells, billions of them will enter your bloodstream, travel to your liver, and then be

routed by your liver to your intestines, for elimination. When they arrive, you must eliminate them from your intestines as quickly as possible. If they linger, they may become reabsorbed by your body and will continue to cause discomfort. Also, as long as they're in your intestines, they will predispose you to bowel problems, such as diarrhoea, gas, inflamed mucosal membranes, bloating and constipation.

In addition, if you have been eating reactive foods, processed foods, and other unhealthy foods over a long period of time, you may already have physically impaired your lower intestine, or colon. The walls of your colon may be encrusted with waste. Also, small pockets in the colon wall, called diverticula, may have developed. These pockets can become painfully inflamed, causing diverticulitis. Many other problems with your colon may also have occurred, including loss of muscle tone, loss of proper shape, ulceration, narrowing, and dysfunction of the colon's mucosal membrane. These are *not* rare conditions. *Most* people have at least one of these problems. Older people, or unhealthy young people, may have several of them.

Because poor health of the colon is so prevalent, many people have serious medical problems in their colons. Irritable bowel syndrome, characterized by pain, gas, and frequent diarrhoea, strikes an estimated one out of five people at some time, and colon cancer is among the most common forms of cancer.

However, there are many methods of improving the health of your colon, all of which will speed elimination of toxins and help you feel better during your Cleansing Phase.

One of the best things you can do for your colon is to avoid certain foods, most of which you'll be avoiding anyway at the outset of your diet. These foods often congest, clog, and irritate the colon. They include: milk, cheese, sugar, gravies, butter, meats, eggs, coffee, black tea, chocolate, ice cream, white flour products (including pasta, pastries, and many processed foods), and alcohol. Even if you're not reactive to them, you should still avoid them for a week or two – or longer, if you like, since you don't need most of these foods to be healthy.

Nutrients that help *heal* the colon and stimulate its function include: L-glutamine; vitamins B$_5$, A, C and E; the minerals zinc and selenium; and the omega-3 and omega-6 fatty acids. Reasonable daily dosages for most people are: 500–1,000 mg of L-glutamine, 50–100 mg of vitamin B$_5$, 5,000–10,000 IU of vitamin A, 2–4 grams of vitamin C, 400–800 IU of vitamin E, 15–30 mg of zinc, 200–300 mcg of selenium, and 2–4 capsules of essential fatty acids, such as flaxseed or other omega 3/6 oils. Dosages should be divided evenly throughout the day and may be taken with meals.

It's also quite important to eat a high-fibre diet and to drink a lot of water. One of the best sources of fibre is psyllium seed, a bulking material that expands to 5 to 10 times its normal size in the moist environment of the colon. Psyllium seed products are readily available, in brand names such as Metamucil. Metamucil, however, contains sugar, but other, similar products do not.

Herbs can also stimulate colon function and heal the colon. Herbs that stimulate the colon and have a laxative action are senna, barberry root, peach leaves, and cascara sagrada. Herbs that help heal the colon are peppermint, goldenseal, aloe vera, and rhubarb root. At your health food shop, you can probably find a good formulation that will contain many of these herbs. If you use a formulation, take it as directed. If you use individual herbs, take them as directed on the packaging. Because the herbs are typically non-toxic if taken in the directed dosages, you may continue to take them for as long as they help you to feel better. However, it is generally wise to refrain from taking the laxative herbs for more than 3 to 4 consecutive weeks, because continual use of any type of laxative can create dependence upon it for normal bowel function. Furthermore, you should remember that even though most herbs have far fewer side effects than pharmaceutical medications, they are still powerful medicinal substances and should not be used haphazardly.

Certain juices also stimulate colon function. These include the juices of apples, prunes, black cherries, celery, carrots and spinach.

Mild stimulation of the colon can be helpful, but you should not overdo it. Ideally, you should have two or three bowel movements per day during your cleansing; more than that may be harmful. On the other hand, though, I do not agree with the conventional wisdom that one bowel movement per day is ideal; I believe this is outdated thinking.

As a rule, patients who have begun to eliminate their false fat foods experience an immediate reduction of gas in their GI tracts. This is gratifying for them, since gas is a significant contributor to abdominal bloating, often adding two to three inches to the waistline. On occasion, though, when people begin to heal from years of eating reactive foods, they will temporarily experience an increase in gas, as toxins exit from the colon. If this happens to you, certain herbs, which may be ingested as teas or taken in capsules, will help resolve the problem. They include fennel seed (which is sometimes given to infants as a natural colic cure), ginger, and aniseed. These herbs may be purchased from health food shops and should be taken as directed.

As you recover from your food reactions, you should note a marked, permanent decrease in gas, because incomplete digestion and fermentation of foods are the primary causes of gas. Gas will be decreased as the colon becomes healthier. A healthy colon products little, if any, flatulence.

Not gulping food, which can cause you to swallow air, will also reduce gas. Chewing your food well is the beginning of good digestion.

Bloating will probably decrease immediately, as gas subsides.

Possibly the single most important nutrients for colon health are acidophilus and bifidobacteria, the healthy probiotic bacteria commonly found in cultured yogurt. Probiotics break down foods and control unhealthy candida yeast colonization. If you need to avoid dairy products, take your probiotics from non-dairy sources, as a capsule, liquid, or powder. Take 2 to 6 capsules daily, supplying about 4 to 10 billion probiotic organisms.

If your colon remains sluggish or if you have a generally toxic, full feeling, it may be helpful to use an enema. This may be done with purified water or with a mixture that may contain probiotics or wheatgrass (if you're not reactive to wheat). Another option is to have a colonic irrigation performed by a health professional. This procedure does not usually cause discomfort, and some of my patients report that afterwards they feel energized and noticeably cleaner. Detoxification will give you a clear mind, a good mood, and a feeling of vitality.

Abdominal exercises also help colon function. These include the modified sit-ups called stomach crunches. Do 10 to 20 in the morning and evening, as a start, and more as you get stronger. Another good exercise consists of simply pulling your abdomen in forcefully, 10 to 20 times in a row.

You can also improve your colon health by giving yourself a brief abdominal massage in the morning, shortly after arising. To do this, while lying on your back, slowly massage your intestinal area in a clockwise direction.

Another extremely important organ for you to support and stimulate during your Cleansing Phase is your liver. Your liver is your most important organ of detoxification, since it routinely extracts chemical toxins from your blood. Besides eliminating toxins, it also neutralizes them, rendering them harmless.

If your liver is not functioning well, or if it has more toxins than it can handle, *you will not feel good.* You'll be irritable, tired, queasy, or headachey.

To nurture your liver, first stop poisoning yourself. Stay away from alcohol, tobacco, recreational drugs, chemicalized foods, environmental pollutants, and animal fat.

Then you should start to *heal* your liver. Certain herbs will help. They include dandelion root, goldenseal, prickly ash bark, safflower herb, and yarrow flower. The most effective herb, though, is milk thistle, or *silymarin*. Numerous medical studies show that milk thistle helps the liver regenerate its cells, and even helps recovery from some liver diseases.

At a health food shop, you should be able to find a formulation designed especially for the liver. It will contain milk

GI TRACT CLEANSING FOR THE COLON

Nutrients

(Take in evenly divided dosages, 2 to 3 times daily.)

- L-glutamine (500–1,000 mg/day)
- Vitamin B_5 (50–100 mg/day)
- Vitamin A (5,000–10,000 IU/day
- Vitamin C (2–4 grams/day)
- Vitamin E (400–800 IU/day)
- Zinc (15–30 mg/day)
- Selenium (200–300 mcg/day)
- Omega 3/6 oil (2–4 caps/day)

(These nutrients may be taken during just the Cleansing Phase or may be continued throughout the diet, if desired.)

Bulking Agents

- Psyllium seed products (take as directed)
- Water (6–8 large glasses throughout day)

Laxative Herbs

(Choose one or find a herbal combination. Take as directed on packaging.)

- Barberry root
- Peach leaf
- Cascara sagrada
- Senna leaf

Healing Herbs

(Choose one or find a combination.)

- Peppermint
- Goldenseal
- Aloe vera
- Rhubarb root

(Laxative herbs should be taken for no more than 3 to 4 consecutive weeks, to avoid dependence. Healing herbs may be taken indefinitely, throughout the False Fat Diet, except goldenseal, where a week break should be taken every 3 to 4 weeks.)

Avoid

- Dairy products
- White flour
- Alcohol
- Chocolate

(These foods may be added, in moderation, after the conclusion of the Cleansing Phase, if they do not cause food reactions.)

Physical Therapies

- **Enemas**
- **Exercise** (including 10–20 stomach crunches or more, two times daily)

FOR LIVER HEALTH

Nutrients
(Take in evenly divided dosages, 2 to 3 times daily. Some
of these nutrients may already be included in your colon
cleansing programme or your general detoxification
programme.)

- B-complex vitamins (50–100
  mg/day) (especially B_3 and B_6)
- Vitamin A (5,000–7,500 IU/day)
- Vitamin C (2–4 grams/day)
- Vitamin E (400–1,000 IU/day)
- Zinc (15–30 mg/day)
- Calcium (600–850 mg/day)
- Selenium (200–300 mcg/day)
- L-cysteine (250–500 mg/day)
- Alpha-lipoic acid (50–100
  mg/day)

Juices
(Drink 4–6 total glasses of juice daily, throughout the
Cleansing Phase. After the Cleansing Phase, intake could
include 2–4 glasses daily.)

- Beetroot
- Carrot
- Celery
- Cucumber
- Lemon
- Spinach

Herbs
(A number of liver-supporting herbal formulas are available.
Take as directed on packaging. They should include several
of the following ingredients.)

- Milk thistle (most important herb)
  for liver, appropriate in dosages
  of 200–400 mg daily)
- Dandelion root
- Goldenseal root
- Prickly ash bark
- Safflower herb
- Yarrow flower

Avoid

- Alcohol
- Tobacco
- Drugs
- Pollutants
- Chemicals
- Animal fat

Physical Therapies

- Coffee enemas
- Massage, abdominal and lymphatic

thistle, along with other herbs and nutrients. Take this formulation as directed for at least 2 to 4 weeks and during any cleansing periods or after drinking alcohol.

Certain juices also help regenerate the liver and stimulate the release of bile by the gallbladder. They are the juices from beetroot, carrots, lemons, and spinach. You may drink 4 to 6 glasses of juice daily, throughout the day.

A common therapy for liver detoxification is a short retention enema with a mild coffee solution. The caffeine from the coffee travels directly from the colon to the liver, via the large portal vein, which connects the two organs. It stimulates liver activity and quickly eases the flu-like feeling of toxicity that sometimes arises during the Cleansing Phase. This therapy is used in some progressive cancer treatment programmes, to help ease the extreme toxicity that often accompanies the breakdown and elimination of cancer cells. Some of my patients report that this procedure leaves them feeling energetic and refreshed, and has helped them to overcome their uncomfortable feelings of toxicity.

Supplements can also help the liver to function better. The most effective are the B-vitamins (especially B_3 and B_6), as well as vitamins A, C, and E, and zinc, calcium, selenium, and L-cysteine (an amino acid that supports detoxifying enzymes, such as *glutathione peroxidase*). Appropriate daily dosages for most people are 50–100 mg of the B-vitamins, 5,000–7,500 IU of vitamin A, 2–4 grams of vitamin C, 400–1,000 IU of vitamin E, 15–30 mg of zinc, 600–850 mg of calcium, 300 mcg of selenium, and 250–500 mg of L-cysteine. Dosages should be divided evenly throughout the day and may be taken with meals.

It may also be helpful to get a massage and ask the masseuse to focus on abdominal and lymphatic massage.

Supplementation – the Key to Cellular Cleansing

True cleansing of the body – the type that can really change your life – starts from the inside out. For total rejuvenation, you must begin to purify your body at the cellular level. That's the only way to rid yourself of the reactive food chemicals that are causing your cravings, false fat, and feelings of distress.

Fortunately, cellular regeneration isn't nearly as hard as it may sound. The human body is almost magically regenerative. Your cells expel toxins every single moment. Furthermore, every cell in your body replicates itself on a regular basis – as often as every few days. Even slow-growing bone cells are completely replaced every six months. Therefore, if you start to clean out your cells today, you can have a much purer body in a matter of days, and a whole new you in six months or less.

Supplements are a superb way to cleanse your body from the inside out, because they provide the concentrated nutrients that help the cells to expel toxins, and rebuild themselves.

During the Cleansing Phase of your diet, your supplement-ation will focus on three goals: (1) speeding detoxification; (2) easing uncomfortable symptoms; and (3) avoiding depletion of nutrients.

In the preceding section, I mentioned some supplements that are good for the colon and liver. Some of the supplements I mentioned, such as vitamin C, have such far-reaching effects that they will also help with your overall detoxification and cell rejuvenation efforts.

Among the best supplements to accelerate detoxification in cells throughout your body are those that will shift your body's acid-alkaline balance to a relatively more alkaline condition. Alkalinity aids detoxification by making cell walls somewhat more permeable, which increases the exit of toxins and the entrance of healing nutrients.

Furthermore, alkalinity tends to decrease the body's response to food reactions.

The supplements that will most effectively shift your body to an alkaline condition are *potassium* and *magnesium*. You may take 100 mg of each mineral three times daily, with meals, throughout your Cleansing Phase. Also, chlorophyll-based green juices, such as green algae drinks or spirulina, will help create alkalinity. Plain baking soda will also induce alkalinity.

Among the foodstuffs that create alkalinity are vegetables

(especially green vegetables), fruits, sea vegetables/seaweed, millet, buckwheat, and raw seeds. The acid-forming foods, which should generally be avoided during detoxification, include meat, fish, eggs, beans, most grains, and nuts.

Other supplements will help ease the discomfort that can accompany detoxification. Most of the supplements that can do this are the ones that have a mild natural sedating effect. Calcium and magnesium are both excellent for soothing frayed nerves, and so are certain herbs, such as valerian root. The herb willow bark is a natural form of aspirin, and may help relieve minor aches and pains, and headaches. The amino acid glutamine powerfully inhibits cravings for sugar and alcohol and may therefore help make you feel more comfortable.

Certain homeopathic medications are also excellent at calming the nervous system and relieving feelings of stress and malaise. These products, available at most health food shops, state on the label the conditions that they help. Many people find relief from formularized *combinations* of homeopathic remedies. Also, some herbs help with anxiety and stress. They include valerian, kava, and Siberian ginseng.

During the Cleansing Phase, you must also avoid nutrient depletion by taking a few basic supplements. This is especially important if you are on one of the strict elimination diets, such as the Juice Fast, since a restricted diet can be low in nutrients. If you become nutritionally depleted, you will feel more uncomfortable. Also, your food cravings will probably be worse, because you'll crave the nutrients that certain foods contain.

Moderate intake of antioxidants during the Cleansing Phase will help protect your body from the free radicals and other toxins that will be cast off. During the *next* phase of your diet, False Fat Week, your supplementation programme will *increase* as you begin to take nutrients that will stimulate fat burning, build muscle, and heighten energy. During the Cleansing Phase, however, your supplement programme will be relatively limited and simple. The daily supplements I generally prescribe during this phase (usually taken in two doses) are:

- Vitamin C, 1–4 grams
- Vitamin A, 5,000–7,500 IU
- Beta-carotene (or mixed carotenoids), 15,000–30,000 IU
- Vitamin E, 400–1,000 IU
- Zinc, 15–30 mg
- Selenium, 200–300 mcg
- B-complex vitamins, 50–100 mg
- Calcium, 600–850 mg
- Magnesium, 300–500 mg
- Potassium, 300–500 mg
- Algae (blue-green, chlorella, or spirulina), 4 to 6 tablets or capsules

Obviously, the dosages that I recommend are higher than the conventional Minimum Daily Recommendations, or MDRs. MDRs are designed mostly just to *avoid illnesses*, not to achieve healing and regeneration. For that task you will need higher amounts. Please consult your doctor before embarking on any programme of supplements.

The supplements should be taken when you eat or when you drink your juice. None of these nutrients should upset your stomach, but high dosages of vitamin C and magnesium may cause mild bowel irritation in some people. If you experience diarrhoea, you may need to decrease your dosage of either vitamin C or magnesium or both.

The regenerative power of the body is remarkable. You can have a whole new you in six months or less.

Reactions to Supplements

It's fairly unusual, but some people can also react to the nutritional supplements that they ingest. This can be difficult to sort out from food reactions. If you are reactive to certain foods, however, you may also react to the supplements that contain them. Many natural supplements are created from food extracts; however, most supplements are synthetic nutrients and herbal extracts made in the laboratory.

It's also possible to react to the fillers and binders used to make up the tablets, as well as to other additives and food colourings used within and on the coating. Children's vitamins commonly contain synthetic food colouring and sugars unless the manufacturer is conscientious about creating cleaner, non-toxic products.

Although reactions have been rare in my many years of experience with placing people on supplement programmes, some immediate and long-term reactions have occurred. These are usually mild and might include gastrointestinal upset or nausea (usually an immediate concern, especially with the multiple vitamins that contain 20 to 30 ingredients), constipation or diarrhoea, headaches, skin rashes, fatigue or anxiety, and mood alterations. While any products might be the culprit, the most likely ones are multivitamin/minerals and other combination formulas and stronger herbal combinations. High amounts of calcium, vitamin C, and magnesium can cause loose bowels, and the latter two can cause sleepiness. For more specifics on this area, I have discussed each vitamin, mineral, and many other nutrients extensively in *Staying Healthy with Nutrition* (1992).

If you suspect that you are having a reaction to one of your supplements, you can try to guess which product it might be, and then avoid it and see if there is a difference, much as you would do for a suspected food. Or, depending on the kind and severity of the reaction, you may need to stop the supplement programme completely and take a week or two off to see if symptoms clear. Then, as you reintroduce the supplements one by one, watch for any reactions just as you would watch for food reactions after the elimination diet.

Herbal Therapy for Cleansing

I have prescribed herbal therapy for many years, and am now gratified that many conventional doctors have begun to

NATURE'S CLEANSING HERBS

(Choose one or two from the category in which you need help.)

Blood Cleaners
Echinacea
Dandelion
Yellow dock
Oregon grape

Bowel Stimulants
Cascara sagrada
Buckthorn
Senna leaf
Licorice root

Diuretics
Parsley
Yarrow
Cleavers
Juniper berries

Skin Cleansers
Burdock
Goldenseal
Cayenne pepper
Ginger root

Antibiotics
Garlic
Prickly ash
Echinacea
Propolis

Mucus Reducers
Echinacea
Goldenseal
Garlic
Yarrow

Take as directed. Usual dosages are 1 to 2 droppers of liquid extract or 2 to 3 capsules or tablets, once or twice daily, before or after eating.

Sample Cleansing Formulation
(Multiple herbs combined in one capsule.)

Garlic
Cayenne pepper
Licorice root
Milk thistle
Dandelion root

Echinacea root
Ginger root
Cascara sagrada
Peppermint leaf
Goldenseal root

Take as directed. A usual dosage of a formulation is 2 to 3 capsules or tablets, twice daily.

appreciate this form of medicine. Herbal medication is generally milder than pharmaceutical medication, with fewer side effects. Furthermore, it can be very effective; in fact, more than a third of all pharmaceutical medications are derived from herbs.

The herbs listed opposite are those I most commonly prescribe during the Cleansing Phase to help detoxification. I recommended these same herbs in my recent book *The Detox Diet*.

Use these herbs judiciously, according to your individual need for them, as you would other over-the-counter medications. You probably won't have *all* of the various conditions that these herbs address, such as constipation or excess mucus, so you will probably not need to take all of them. If you do have one of the conditions, you may not need all of the herbs that help the condition. A single herb may solve the problem. Often, though, combinations of herbs are more effective than single herbs. Because these herbs are safe and gentle, you may try different combinations, to see which ones work best for your own unique metabolism and lifestyle.

You may be able to find a good herbal detox formulation at your health food shop. Using a formulation is a smart approach, because it makes ingestion of the proper herbs much easier. Look for a formulation that contains many of the herbs on this list.

If your health food shop does not have an appropriate formulation, you may wish to purchase one from a mail-order company. These companies tend to serve consumers who are relatively sophisticated about natural medicine, and usually offer a wide variety of high-quality formulations. Also, their products are usually less expensive than those sold in stores. (See Resources and Referrals).

Increased Water Consumption

The kidneys filter approximately 1,500 litres of blood every day – or 1 litre every minute – and eliminate much of the body's toxic waste. During your Cleansing Phase, your kidneys will eliminate many of the toxins and reactive food chemicals that are now lodged in your cells. Therefore, it's important to drink extra water during this phase, to aid the removal of these waste products.

If the kidneys are not regularly flushed with water, they will fall prey to toxic buildup, and may begin to send toxic materials back into the bloodstream. This is a relatively common occurrence among many people. Toxic buildup can also result in inflammation of the kidneys and even infection. It can also contribute to the formation of kidney stones, and can cause gradual deterioration of the kidneys.

Toxic congestion of the kidneys is also relatively common, partly because many people simply don't drink enough water. I generally recommend that patients on the False Fat Diet drink 8 to 10 large glasses of water daily, and as many as 10 to 12 large glasses during the Cleansing Phase. This usually causes increased urination, which is helpful during this phase, since the kidneys are often overloaded with toxins.

The water you drink should be pure, because even mildly polluted tap water can cause more problems than it solves. I generally recommend filtered or bottled spring water. Some doctors recommend distilled water, but I believe it may alter the body's biochemical/electrical balance.

The water should be drunk mostly between meals, because extra fluid at mealtime can dilute your digestive juices and weaken digestion.

On the False Fat Diet, you will be trying to lose much of the retained water, or swelling, that food reactions cause, and you may therefore be reluctant to drink *extra* water for fear of retaining it. However, this will not happen. The opposite will happen: *drinking extra water is likely to reduce your swelling*.

This occurs for several biochemical reasons: (1) drinking extra water will help you excrete cellular sodium, which causes water retention. (2) Drinking extra water decreases two hormones that cause water retention (aldosterone and anti-diuretic hormone). (3) When the body chronically receives *too little* water, it begins to hoard water, in somewhat the same way that the body hoards calories during starvation. Furthermore, studies have indicated that water restriction actually increases the laying down of fat. Therefore, it's *extremely* important to drink plenty of water, especially during the Cleansing Phase.

I rarely prescribe prescription diuretics to patients, because they can cause too much water loss and occasionally result in dehydration.

*Drinking extra water actually helps
you lose water weight.*

Physical Therapies for Detoxification

The most comprehensive physical detoxification therapy is exercise, because it exerts the widest range of effects. (1) It increases toxin excretion through perspiration. (2) It stimulates flow of toxins through the lymphatic system. (3) It increases toxin discharge from the lungs, through deep breathing. (4) It improves hormonal and neurotransmitter function by increasing the production of stimulating norepinephrine and the calming, feel-good endorphins. (5) It reduces stress and muscular tension.

During the Cleansing Phase, I don't recommend that patients try to lose weight with exercise. That strategy comes later, during the Balance Programme. During the Cleansing Phase, patients use exercise simply to *feel better*. If you haven't exercised for some time, you may have forgotten how rejuvenating and pleasurable exercise can be. If so, you owe it to yourself to set aside 30 to 60 minutes every day to be physically active. You'll soon find that physical activity is one of life's true joys. Children, who are full of life and rich with vitality, love nothing more than the exuberance of activity. You can recapture that spirit! It's inside you, waiting to be re-ignited.

Any exercise can be valuable: walking, jogging, swimming, cycling, gardening, golf, tennis, aerobics, or weight training. Do the one that sounds like fun. If it's hard at first, stick with it. Every day it will become less difficult and more fun.

Another excellent physical detoxification measure is use of a sauna or steambath. Sweating releases innumerable toxins, because the skin is the largest organ of elimination. Every pore of your body can be used to rid yourself of the toxins that are making you feel bad. Most people eliminate almost half as much water from sweating as they do from urinating, and this perspiration can be a significant outlet for toxins.

Sweating is an especially powerful way of excreting the

toxins from alcohol, drugs, cigarettes, and pesticides.

When you first launch your cleansing programme, it's very possible that your perspiration will have an unpleasant odour, indicative of toxic excretion. As your programme progresses, though, the odour should diminish considerably and eventually cease entirely.

Some of my patients enjoy the cleansing procedure of niacin/sauna therapy, in which they combine the capillary-expanding effects of niacin with the pore-opening effects of a sauna. To do this, take enough niacin to produce a niacin flush, which will make your skin pink and warm for about 20 minutes. To achieve a niacin flush, take at least 50 to 100 mg about an hour after a light meal. Some people may require up to 400 mg. Then take an extended sauna, stopping periodically to cool off and replenish your fluids and electrolytes. It's also generally wise to drink as much water as desired while in the sauna. This is a powerful therapy and should be avoided by people with pre-existing medical problems, weakness, or fatigue.

An alternative to a sauna is a steambath, which can be even more helpful, because inhaling the hot steam will help clear the nasal passages, sinuses, and lungs. Ideally, it should be done with filtered water, to avoid chlorine. Another good alternative is a hot bath, preferably with one or more cups of Epsom salts, which help to draw out toxins. To extend the period of sweating from a hot bath, you can wrap yourself in a sheet, blanket, or heavy bathrobe when you get out of the bath.

Another effective way to open your pores and facilitate the elimination of toxins through the skin is to brush your skin, while dry, with a skin brush, or loofah, which can be purchased at a health food shop. Brush – not scratch – your entire body lightly until you feel a warm glow. Then take a hot shower or bath to remove the dead skin you have loosened. At the end of your shower, you may want to alternate the water temperature between warm and cool, to tone the muscles that control dilation of pores.

Another important organ of detoxification is the lungs. Typically, the lungs excrete almost 20 per cent of the water that you lose every day, and this water carries toxins. Other toxins are also eliminated when you cough up mucus or blow your nose.

The best way to clean the lungs is with aerobic exercise. However, it's also helpful to do yoga deep-breathing exercises, such as Slow Deep Breathing. To do this, take as deep a breath as possible, extending your belly for maximum intake of air. Then exhale slowly and repeat, for approximately 3 to 5 minutes, several times daily.

Another way to eliminate toxins through your airways is to irrigate your nasal passages periodically with water. To do this, cup your hands under a tap, fill them with water, and then inhale some of the water into your nose. Blow the water out forcefully, and it will carry away mucus and toxins. After your nose and nasal passages are cleaned out, inhale some of the water all the way into your throat and expel it through your mouth. This will cleanse the entire nasal area and may significantly improve sinus drainage. This procedure can also be done with a mild saltwater solution or in the shower. Some people find this process to be mildly uncomfortable, but most patients don't mind it at all. Furthermore, almost all patients find it to be very effective, especially during pollen season, when the nasal passages are prone to congestion. It can be very helpful in preventing and helping to relieve infected or inflamed sinuses. Cleaning the nasal passages with water is safe and non-invasive and may be performed as often as desired.

To further drain your sinuses, inhale forcefully through your nose – as if you had a runny nose – drawing mucus into your throat. Then spit it out. Repeat this until you can breathe freely. If you are quite congested, you may have to repeat this procedure 10 to 20 times or more, until your nasal passages are clear and clean. This procedure works best when performed concurrently with the nasal irrigation.

A final form of physical therapy that can help is massage. The most appropriate form of massage during the Cleansing Phase is massage that focuses on the lymphatic system. If the glands are notably swollen, you may be able to do this yourself, simply by rubbing the swollen glands gently, to relieve congestion of toxins. Other forms of massage – such as Swedish

THE CLEANSING PHASE PROGRAMME

GI Tract Cleansing
- Nutrients
- Bulking agents
- Herbs
- Avoidance of certain foods

Supplements
Vitamins C, A, E, B-complex,
  beta-carotene, zinc,
  selenium, calcium
  magnesium, potassium

Increased Water Consumption
- 10–12 large glasses of water daily
- Herbal diuretics: parsley yarrow, cleavers, juniper berries
- Juice diuretics: watermelon cranberry, celery, wheatgrass

Liver Cleansing
- Nutrients
- Juices
- Herbs
- Avoidance of certain foods
- Physical therapies

Herbal Therapy
- Blood cleaners
- Diruetics
- Antibiotics
- Bowel stimulants
- Skin cleaners
- Mucus reducers

Physical Therapies
- Exercise
- Sauna, steambath, hot bath
- Niacin/sauna therapy
- Dry skin brushing
- Deep breathing
- Nasal irrigation
- Massage

massage – can also help, by providing relaxation and comfort and by helping your body feel more balanced.

Another practical technique that often helps at this time is to clean your home thoroughly. Make your home sparkle! Make it beautiful! Get rid of things you don't want and organize the things that you keep. This house-cleaning will mirror the internal housecleaning that you are doing in your own body. It will reinforce your sense of renewal, and it will remind you every day of how much cleaner and healthier you are.

By the same token, the Cleansing Phase is also a good time to clean house spiritually and emotionally. Try to rid yourself of any poisonous emotions that may be making you tense or rigid. Just as you are learning to create a healthy physical flow in your body – nutrients in, toxins out – you should learn to go with the flow spiritually and emotionally. The power of the entire universe is flowing constantly – from season to season, night to day, change to change – and if you can tap into this flow, your personal power will increase immeasurably. On the other hand, if you hang on to your rigidity, you'll never feel comfortable in the state of flux that characterizes all healing.

One of the best ways to learn to go with the flow is to meditate. To do it, find a quiet place, sit comfortably, close your eyes, adopt a calm, passive attitude, and breathe deeply. Try not to think about anything. Quiet your thoughts by repeating a single, soothing word or phrase, such as 'peace'. When thoughts intrude, let them go and return to your calming phrase. After 10 to 20 minutes, you'll feel amazingly refreshed.

A Summary of the Cleansing Phase

That's the entire cleansing programme! As you can see, it's simple but powerful. I urge you to engage in it whole-heartedly, because it can really make you feel great.

You don't need to do every single aspect of the cleansing programme, but the more you do, the better you'll feel. To make this programme easy to remember, there's a summary of it on pages 210–11.

Most patients get such a lift out of the cleansing programme that they want to continue to do it even after the cleansing week is over. The cleansing procedures are especially helpful when fat burning begins, since so many toxins are stored in fat cells.

A sample daily schedule of a Cleansing Phase programme is on page 210. As I've explained, this element of your False Fat Diet, much like the other elements, should be individualized in order to best fulfil your own unique needs. Therefore, this schedule is only an example and may be tailored to fit your own lifestyle. Even if you do only a little more than half of these suggestions, you will support your cleansing.

This short, one-week period of cleansing and detoxification

SAMPLE DAILY SCHEDULE FOR
THE CLEANSING PHASE PROGRAMME

This is based on waking up at 7.30 a.m. If you normally arise earlier or later, you can adapt this protocol to fit your schedule.

7.30–7.50 a.m.   Drink a large glass or two of water; one could have the juice of half a lemon to support cleansing and digestion.Take 15 to 20 minutes of quiet reflection, organization of your day, and abdominal massage. Be positive and think good thoughts.

7.50 a.m.   Take 2 to 3 capsules of a cleansing herbal formula with an additional capsule of milk thistle and 1 to 2 capsules of probiotics.

7.55–8.15 a.m.   Do 5 minutes of stretching and 10 to 15 minutes of aerobic activity.

8.15 a.m.   Drink one large glass of fruit juice, diluted with some water (¼–½ water).

8.20 a.m.   Perform 3 to 5 minutes of dry skin brushing.

8.25 a.m.   Take a hot bath or long shower. Nasal irrigation can be done in the shower or with saline before, or alternatively can be done in the evening.

8.35 a.m.   Breakfast with herbal tea.

8.50 a.m.   Supplements: vitamins C, E, A, B-complex, zinc, selenium, and L-cysteine.

9.00 a.m.   On to your work, household chores, errands, and your life.

10.00 a.m.   Take 2 capsules of dandelion root (or other liver herb, like milk thistle) with a glass of water.

10.30–11.00 a.m.   Drink a glass of water or juice – fruit or vegetable.

12 noon   Outdoors for some fresh air and some deep breaths. Rub your scalp, your back, or any area that calls to you or needs attention.

12.10–12.30 p.m.   Lunch with a glass of fresh vegetable juice or fresh veggies if available. Chew well.

12.30 p.m.   Supplements: vitamins C, B_6, B_3, omega 3/6 oils, L-glutamine, digestive enzymes if needed, and a capsule of calcium/magnesium.

12.35–1 p.m.   Take a good walk for 10 to 15 minutes, followed by 10 to 15 minutes of rest and meditation.

2.00 p.m.   Drink a large glass of water and do 5 minutes of deep breathing and recharging. Rub your shoulders, neck, and head.

3.00 p.m.   Drink one large glass of fresh fruit or vegetable juice.

3.30 p.m.   Have a light snack if needed, like a piece of fruit or some nuts or seeds. Take antioxidant supplements beta-carotene, E, selenium, zinc, L-cysteine, and some C, or a packet of Emergen-C powder in some water or juice.

4.00 p.m.   Drink a large glass of water.

4.15 p.m. (or after work)   Niacin/sauna therapy (with 100–250 mg niacin) or steam or exercise programme. This is helpful to do 2 to 3 times a week when you can fit them in your schedule.

5.00 p.m.   Drink a glass of water and some juice or herb tea.

6.00 p.m.   Have dinner and then take supplements: digestive enzymes, hydrochloric acid for protein meals, omega 3/6 oils, glutamine, and a multiple vitamin if that is used.

6.45 p.m.   Take a leisurely walk.

7.00 p.m.   Drink a glass of water and 1 to 2 capsules of goldenseal or other appropriate herb.

7.30 p.m.   Nasal irrigation if needed, or light self-massage or exchange with a companion.

8.00 p.m.   Drink water with 2 to 3 capsules of a cleansing herbal formula.

8.55 p.m.   Take vitamin C and 1 to 2 capsules of calcium/magnesium; this helps with relaxation and sleep.

9.00 p.m.   Do 10 to 20 minutes of meditation. If you get tired, go to sleep. If not, go look at the stars, listen to some music, or organize tomorrow.

In general, during cleansing week, you may want to lighten up on watching television, reading newspapers, or whatever habits you have that may be unhealthy or give you stress. This is a time to nurture yourself.

can mark the beginning of a whole new life for you. You are leaving behind all the old nutritional habits that have weighed you down and held you back. These habits – eating reactive foods, and eating chemicalized, empty foods – were literally poisonous to your system.

By the end of the Cleansing Phase, most of these poisons will be out of your system. You're probably going to feel better than you have in years!

But there's *much more* to look forward to. The next phase of

THE FALSE FAT DIET

WEEK ONE THE CLEANSING PHASE	WEEK TWO FALSE FAT WEEK	WEEK THREE THE BALANCE PROGRAMME
1. Begin elimination diet or begin allergy-free diet after taking blood test.	1. Continue elimination diet or allergy-free diet.	1. Continue elimination diet or allergy-free diet.
2. Begin taking supplements (to prevent nutrient depletion).	2. Begin taking new supplements that support weight control.	2. Continue supplement programme.
3. Begin detoxification measures.	3. Begin to confront psychological factors of eating.	3. Continue food reintroduction challenges.
4. Begin light exercise programme, or continue existing one.	4. Begin food reintroduction challenges.	4. Increase exercise programme.
		5. Begin stress management programme.

your diet is False Fat Week, in which you'll lose more of the bloating and swelling that have long made you look and feel far more overweight than you really are. When your body starts looking and feeling the way you always hoped it would, you're *really* going to get motivated!

Before we forge ahead, though, see the chart above that outlines the first, important 21 days on the diet, as you progress through the diet's three phases: the Cleansing Phase, False Fat Week, and the Balance Programme. The Balance Programme begins during approximately the third week of the diet and continues indefinitely as a maintenance programme.

8
FALSE FAT WEEK

Laura, my patient who'd felt like giving up during the first few days of her Cleansing Phase, practically floated into my office for her one-week follow-up visit. Her smile was luminous. 'Look at me!' she enthused. 'Have you *ever* seen a response like *this*?'

'You look great,' I said. And she did. She'd lost the puffy, saggy look that characterizes so many patients with food reactions. Her eyes sparkled – a sign that her system had detoxified – and her skin glowed.

Actually, though, I *often* see people respond as dramatically as she had. It's quite common for the body to change remarkably after a week of cleansing. In fact, it's unusual when the body *doesn't* change.

Laura, a 32-year-old homemaker who'd been about 20 pounds overweight when she'd started her diet, had lost 5 to 6 pounds, mostly by overcoming systemic reactive edema, or swelling throughout her body. She'd especially lost a lot of bloating in her abdomen. Some of this bloating had been caused by edemic swelling of gut tissues, and some had been caused by excess gas. She told me that she'd lost about two inches from her waist, and was wearing jeans that she hadn't been able to fit into for 5 years. Her face had also lost its fleshy, swollen look, so she looked younger and more attractive.

'How long did your cravings last?' I asked her.

'Less than a week,' she said. 'I was surprised at how quickly they went away. My main food reaction is to dairy products, and the first few days, I really missed them. Especially ice cream. But I bought some non-dairy pineapple sherbet and had a few bites when I felt like eating ice cream. Then, over the next few days, I started losing that sense of physical *need* for reactive foods that you and I talked about.'

'The need-to-feed reaction?'

'Yeah, the need-to-feed. I didn't realize how much *stronger* it is than just regular hunger.'

'It's not hunger at all, is it? Your stomach can be totally full, but you'll still have that craving for a special food. That happens to a lot of people at dessert time. Their stomachs are already full, but their body still feels a physical need for sugar or fat.'

'I know I've still got a long way to go,' she said, 'but I really feel pumped, like I'm definitely going to make it this time. I've dieted before, but this just isn't as *hard*.'

'That's because you're finally over your cravings.'

The need-to-feed reaction from
food cravings is far stronger than
mere hunger.

'So what's next? This is the official start of my False Fat Week. What's going to happen?'

I told Laura what would probably happen during her False Fat Week.

What Happens During False Fat Week

During False Fat Week, you will continue to avoid all of your reactive foods. You will remain on either your elimination diet or your allergen-restricted diet. Because you will be avoiding reactive foods and therefore losing false fat, you will continue to lose weight at a relatively fast pace – perhaps as much as 5 pounds per week or even more. Your rate of weight loss will depend partly on how heavy you were at the beginning of the diet. If you were quite overweight, with a considerable amount of false fat, you will probably lose weight faster than someone who was only moderately overweight.

Most of the weight you will lose will come from loss of swelling as reactive food chemicals are flushed from your body. As the chemicals leave, your body will no longer need to surround them with water, in order to protect you from foreign invaders. You will excrete most of this water through urination, and will probably notice that you are urinating significantly more than usual. You will also lose fluids through perspiration, especially if you are using saunas or hot baths for detoxification. At first your perspiration will probably have a noticeable odour and will be murky in appearance. Quickly, though, it will lose its musky odour and become increasingly clear.

Much of this water weight will come from your abdominal area, but it will also come from all of your bodily tissues. You may notice that your hands are less swollen, and that your rings do not fit as tightly. You may also lose swelling from your face and from under your chin, where fluid tends to collect. Some doctors also think that excess fluid retention contributes to the dimpling of cellulite, so you may have a reduction of cellulite from your thighs.

This loss of swelling will probably make you look more sleek and streamlined and feel lighter and more supple. Water weight is notorious for making people look fatter than they really are, and for making them feel heavy and lethargic.

As the health of your digestive tract improves, you will also probably lose the bloating that excess *gas* causes. Some of this gas, such as carbon dioxide, is odourless, but other types, such as hydrogen sulphide, are odourous. Some gas comes from fermentation of foods, and some comes from incomplete digestion. For several days, the residue of this gas may remain trapped in your colon, but it will gradually be released. As long as you continue to avoid your false fat foods (and also chew your food thoroughly), gas will probably not re-form to a significant degree.

You may also notice that even though you may be limiting your food intake to only juice, your normal pattern of bowel movements may not change. Toxic debris and backed-up waste materials may continue to exit from your body during this phase. However, if your normal pattern of bowel movements does decrease, you may feel better if you use mild herbal laxatives, on occasion.

Because you will probably still be excreting toxins during False Fat Week, you may still experience some detoxification symptoms, although significantly less than during the Cleansing Phase. The length of your detoxification period will depend to some degree on how overweight you were when you started the diet, and how many toxic habits you had. As long as you keep losing fat, you may continue to experience detox symptoms, since so many toxins are stored in fat cells. Therefore, it will be wise to continue at least a partial detoxification programme, including the use of herbs, throughout your diet. This will help relieve your established toxic buildup.

Continuing your detox programme will also help eliminate *new* toxins, hopefully before they become lodged in your cells. Ingesting or inhaling new toxins is unavoidable in modern society. If you eat a perfect diet, you'll still inhale some toxic pollutants. However, I recommend that you should *not even try* to eat a perfect diet. Perfectionism is just a form of rigidity. It's simply compulsive 'not eating,' and it's usually replaced with compulsive eating after it becomes too unpleasant. Your *real* goal should be to overcome compulsiveness of any kind. To overcome compulsiveness, don't try to be perfect – try to be good. Over the long run, good beats perfect every time.

Although you may still experience some toxic feelings, your overall sense of health and well-being will probably begin to soar during False Fat Week. You will probably have fewer of the symptoms caused by food reactions, such as headaches, sinus congestion, and low energy. Your cravings for your reactive foods will decrease further.

Therefore, you may enjoy False Fat Week, even though your diet might still be quite restricted (if you're doing one of the strict forms of the elimination diet). If you're not doing an elimination diet but are merely avoiding the reactive foods that your blood test called for – you might *really* enjoy False Fat Week. For you, False Fat Week might be all gain, no pain.

> *Perfectionism is just another form of rigidity. It's compulsive 'not eating', and is usually replaced by compulsive eating. Your goal should be to overcome compulsiveness.*

Accompanying your new feelings of *physical* well-being will probably be a welcome sense of *emotional* renewal. When patients feel the grip of food reactions begin to loosen, they often experience a tremendous sense of relief. They feel as if they have finally solved a lifelong puzzle. When this happens, many of my patients remark to me, 'So *this* is what was wrong!'

Not all patients, however, respond this quickly. *Everyone is different*, and some patients need several weeks for their diets to kick in and start paying off. Sometimes this happens to patients who have only *minor* food reactions; their symptoms are more subtle, and recovery from them may take more time to notice. This can also happen, however, to patients whose food reactions are quite *severe*; these patients require more time to be healed. Most patients, though, are in the mid-range of severity and experience notable improvement during False Fat Week.

This quick payoff is what *you* should expect to happen, but don't be discouraged if it doesn't. The long, slow path is often the best.

During False Fat Week, as you continue to avoid your reactive foods, you will begin to add new supplements to your nutritional programme. These supplements will make your efforts easier and your success more certain.

Now I'll tell you about supplements that really pack power and make weight loss a much more scientifically engineered experience.

Supplements for False Fat Week

Not even the purest, most nutrient-dense diet will be able to provide you with 100 per cent of the nutrients you'll need to rebuild your body and overcome your food reactions. To achieve this goal, you will need to flood your body with extra nutrients. Over time, these nutrients will help heal your organs, glands and tissues, and will help you create the kind of body you've always hoped you could have.

Before our modern industrial age began, it *was* possible to get enough nutrients from diet alone, but those days are over. Currently, even most healthy foods are generally lower in nutritional quality than foods once were. In their attempts to increase productivity, the agriculture and food processing industries have inadvertently stripped nutrients from foods, by engaging in practices such as: monoculture (the growing of only one crop per field); heavy use of fertilizers, herbicides, and pesticides; increased hybridization; chemical growth stimulation of animals; the decline of minerals in the soil; the growth of tough-skinned fruits and vegetables that will withstand the rigours of machine harvesting and processing; and the application of long-term food storage techniques. These practices have created foods that look healthy, glossy, and rich, but which are so devitalized and de-natured that they are almost as lifeless as junk foods.

This decline in nutrients has contributed to widespread nutritional deficiencies. The U.S. Department of Agriculture recently estimated, quite conservatively, that '48 per cent of all U.S. households do not fully meet the approved intake of one or more nutrients.'

It's probable that a lack of nutrients was a major contribution to your weight gain. In an unconscious attempt to ingest the nutrients you needed, you probably ate too many calories. For example, if you weren't getting enough vitamin C, you might have craved fruit and eaten too much of it, developing a reaction to it. Also, if you weren't getting enough nutrients, your nutrient deficiencies probably contributed to your food reactions. To digest and assimilate foods properly, you need a wide range of nutrients.

During your Cleansing Phase, you may have begun to take the nutrients I recommended for avoiding depletion. Now it's time to also start taking some nutrients that will help you *overcome your food reactions*. In addition, it's time to take some supplements that will 'turn up the heat' on your fat burning by *revving up your metabolism*.

First, let's look at the supplements that will help you overcome food reactions. The following list *replaces the list* of supplements I recommended to you during your Cleansing Phase. This new list not only protects against depletion, as did the Cleansing Phase, but also includes nutrients that help *prevent food reactions*.

I have recommended the following list of nutrients to food reaction patients for many years, and included this list adapted from my book *Staying Healthy with Nutrition*.

I've mentioned most of these supplements already, so I'll give you just some brief descriptions of some of them, to avoid repetition.

• **Vitamin C** is a superstar vitamin that strengthens cell walls and helps keep reactive food chemicals out of your cells. It also builds adrenal strength, which helps reduce allergic reactions.

• **Quercetin** reduces histamine release and stabilizes the cells that release histamine (mast cells). It also inhibits the inflammatory response.

• **Gamma linolenic acid**, or GLA, reduces reactive symptoms by helping balance inflammatory prostaglandins. It also promotes fat burning.

• **Niacin** releases histamine, which causes the 'niacin flush' and reduces the amount that can cause allergic reactions.

• **Hydrochloric acid**, or betaine hydrochloride, helps digest food, which prevents reactive food macromolecules from entering the system.

• **Digestive enzymes** help to break down foods more efficiently, which reduces risk of food reactions.

• **Lactobacillus** and other **probiotics** (including bifidobacteria) help stop food reactions by improving digestion. They also help control candida yeast colonization, which exacerbates food reactions.

ANTI-REACTION SUPPLEMENTS

To accomplish this plan, get a multivitamin-mineral combination with most of the following basic nutrients and antioxidants. You will need to supplement your multivitamin to get up to the levels you need with additional vitamin C and other antioxidants, quercitin, MSM, and the amino acids with additional L-cysteine for detoxification support, GLA oils, probiotics, digestive support with HCl and digestive enzymes, CoQ_{10} and bromelain (as an anti-inflammatory). These daily amounts are usually divided into two portions.

Nutrients	Daily Amounts
Vitamin A	5,000–10,000 IU
Beta-carotene	10,000–20,000 IU
Vitamin D	400 IU
Vitamin E	400–800 IU
Vitamin K	300 mcg
Thiamine (B_1)	50 mg
Riboflavin (B_2)	50 mg
Niacin (B_3)	100 mg
Niacinamide (B_3)	50–100 mg
Pantothenic acid (B_5)	250–500 mg
Pyridoxine (B_6) or	50–100 mg
Pyridoxal-5-phosphate* (if available)	50–100 mg
Cobalamin (B_{12})	50–100 mcg
Folic acid	400–800 mcg
Biotin	500–1,000 mcg
PABA	75–150 mg
Vitamin C	4–8 g
Bioflavonoids	250–750 mg
Quercetin	300–600 mg
Calcium	600–1,000 mg
Chromium	200–400 mcg
Copper	2–3 mg
Iodine	150 mcg
Iron	10–18 mg
Magnesium	300–600 mg

Nutrients	Daily Amounts
Manganese	5–10 mg
Molybdenum	250–500 mcg
Selenium (ideally solenomethionine)	200–300 mcg
Sulphur (as methylsulfonylmethane, or MSM)	500–1,500 mg
Silicon	50–100 mg
Zinc	30–60 mg
L-amino acids	750–1,500 mg
L-cysteine	250–500 mg
Gamma linolenic acid (GLA)	3–6 capsules or 240–480 mg
Lactobacillus (and other probiotics)	1–2 billion organisms
Coenzyme Q_{10}	30–60 mg
Hydrochloric acid (betaine hydrochloride)	10–15 g
(Take with meals containing protein and fat)	
Digestive enzymes (after meals)	3–6 tablets
Bromelain (between meals)	100 mg

* The active coenzyme of vitamin B_6

- **Chromium** stabilizes blood sugar and reduces cravings.
- **Magnesium** helps keep blood vessels flexible, which can reduce some symptoms of food reactions, such as headaches. It also has a calming effect.
- **Vitamin A** and **zinc** work together to normalize the antibody response to foreign invaders. They also help heal GI tract mucosa. **Vitamin E** protects tissue membranes and neutralizes toxins. They are part of the antioxidant formula.
- **Coenzyme Q_{10}** improves energy production in cells and reduces some food reaction symptoms.
- **MSM** (methyl-sulfonylmethane) helps reduce allergic reactions, and helps reduce inflammation of joints and tissues.

**THE BASICS: MINIMAL EFFECTIVE
SUPPLEMENTATION PROGRAMME**

Vitamin C   500–1,000 mg, 3–4 times daily (up to 6 g)
(after meals and at bedtime)

Quercetin   200–300 mg, 3 times daily (after meals with
vitamin C)

GLA   60–120 mg, 3 times daily (from either starflower or
evening primrose oil)

Niacin   50–100 mg, 2–3 times daily

Hydrochloric acid   5-grain caps (300 mg), 1–2 caps
(with protein meals)

Digestive enzymes   Caps or chewables, 1–2 caps, 3
times daily (3–6 daily) (after meals) (including enzymes
for proteins, fats and carbohydrates)

Probiotics   powers or caps, 1–2 caps or ¼–½ tsp
powder, 2 times daily (morning and evening) (strength is
in billions of healthful microbes per dosage)

Chromium   100–200 mcg, twice daily

Magnesium   150–300 mg, twice daily

Antioxidant formula   1 cap or tab, twice daily, containing
at least vitamins A, C, E, beta-carotene, selenium, and
zinc (might also contain L-cysteine, CoQ_{10}, lipoic acid,
and others)

MSM   500–1,000 mg, 2 times daily (after meals)

Enzymes

One category of supplements that deserves a more detailed
discussion is enzymes. *Enzymes help stop food reactions.* As
you'll recall, one of the primary reasons that your body fails to
completely digest foods – sending undigested food macromolecules into your system – is because you don't secrete
enough of the enzymes that break down foods. This lack of
enzymes is extremely common. In fact, it's estimated that
approximately 70 per cent of the world's population does not
secrete enough of the milk-digesting enzyme *lactase* to digest
dairy products adequately. This vast lactose-intolerant population includes a majority of African Americans, Native

Africans, Native Americans, Asians, Hispanics, and Jews of Western Europe heritage.

Studies have also shown that enzymes tend to decrease markedly as we age, which may be why most food reactions often begin in adulthood. In one study, a group of young people had *thirty times* as much of the starch-digesting enzyme *amylase* as a group of older people.

A lack of enzymes is very closely associated with gas after meals and bloating of the abdomen. Therefore, it is a significant cause of false fat.

One reason so many people have enzyme deficiencies is because cooking and processing foods kills the natural enzymes that foods contain that help you digest them. When you kill most of them, your own body must secrete all the enzymes needed to digest the food, which can exhaust the body's primary source of digestive enzymes, the pancreas. Studies indicate that when a person lives mostly on cooked foods, his or her pancreas tends to become enlarged. Therefore, it's smart to eat as many raw foods as possible. This will help your digestion immensely.

An additional cause of enzyme deficiency is simply that we tend to eat too much at a time. When we do this, our bodies can't secrete enough enzymes to digest all the food.

Another simple reason for enzyme deficiency is that we don't sufficiently chew our food. Many enzymes, especially starch-digesting enzymes, are present in saliva and must be mixed with food during chewing. A study at the University of Illinois revealed that up to 80 per cent of all carbohydrates are digested by the enzymes in saliva. In addition, many food molecules are surrounded by a hard shell of indigestible cellulose, which must be broken down by chewing. Therefore, it's important to chew your food until it is in a near-liquid, semi-solid form.

The three most common enzymes are *protease* (which digests protein), *lipase* (which digests fat), and *amylase* (which digests starch). I recommend that you take at least one supplement containing all three of these enzymes after every meal and large snack. This may greatly reduce your food reactions and will also help you overcome uncomfortable digestive symptoms, such as heartburn, gas or bloating.

Other enzymes help digest specific foodstuffs. For example, the enzyme *lactase* helps digest milk. Also, the enzyme *alpha-galactosidase* will help you digest beans, broccoli, and onions, which cause many people to develop gas. Most people assume that beans *naturally* cause gas, but that's not true. It's the inability to fully *digest* beans that causes gas.

You should take your enzymes just after you eat. It may also help to take a multivitamin with them, since many vitamins act as coenzymes, helping enzymes to do their work.

Before (or with) your meals, you might try one or two tablets or capsules of betaine hydrochloride to augment your stomach acid. This, too, will help prevent bloating, gas, and food reactions. If you feel any stomach burning, discontinue.

Taking enzymes and betaine hydrochloride is one of the best things you can do for your food reactions. I strongly urge you to try this approach. However, if you tend to have an overacid stomach, which can be aggravated by HCl, you may feel better if you reduce the amount you take.

ANTI-ALLERGY AND ANTI-FOOD-REACTION HERBAL FORMULA

Ma-Huang (ephedra)	Echinacea
Nettle leaf	Garlic
Licorice root	Horseradish
Gentian root	Cayenne pepper
Ginger root	Mullein leaf

Herbs

In addition to these *nutrients*, food reactions can also be decreased with careful, moderate use of *herbal medications*. Herbs tend to have a more hard-hitting, pharmacologic action than vitamins, minerals, and amino acids, so you should be cautious in your use of them.

The herbs listed above will help not only with pollen allergies, but also with food reactions. Furthermore, as you'll recall, pollen allergies can make your food reactions worse, by pushing you past your 'allergic threshold'. By the same token, food reactions can make pollen allergies worse.

Find a formula that contains some of these herbs and take as directed or create one that has some or many of these herbs. There should be lesser amounts (about a half to a third) of the very spicy herbs cayenne and horseradish. A typical dosage is 1 to 2 dropperfuls of an extract or 2 to 3 capsules of a powder, taken twice daily, usually away from food. For example, you might take one dose in the morning before or after breakfast and the second around dinner. Alternatively, you could take the second dose in the early afternoon to make sure the stimulating properties of this formula don't adversely affect your sleep.

With this formula, you are basically trying to support the lungs, cleanse the body of mucus and waste, reduce digestive allergic reactions, and improve digestive function, particularly by improving hydrochloric acid production. Here is what the individual herbs do.

- **Ma-Huang** (*Ephedra sinensis*) is a Chinese herb that supplies ephedra, a stimulant milder than caffeine that will help open airways, relieve congestion, and reduce IgE levels. There are other ephedra-containing herbs that don't work as smoothly as Ma-Huang. The actions of this herb are mimicked by the drug pseudoephedrine, or Sudafed. Ephedra also increases fat burning by stimulating the metabolism. *Use ephedra cautiously.* Too much can cause agitation, and a gross excess, taken all at once, can even cause heart failure. A few years ago, it became a teenage fad to take huge amounts of ephedra, to create a drug-like high, and several young people died from it.
- **Nettle leaf** supports the health of tissues and membranes, and reduces the allergic response.
- **Licorice root** is a soothing herb that has antihistamine and anti-inflammatory actions.
- **Gentian root** supports HCl and digestive enzyme production, and modulates immune function in the gut.
- **Ginger root** is a good cleansing, warming, and stimulating herb with some antihistamine and anti-inflammatory effects.

- **Echinacea** helps regulate the immune system so that it is not so likely to attack reactive food chemicals. It also lowers IgE levels.
- **Garlic** helps detoxification. It also boosts immunity.
- **Horseradish** is a cleansing and pungent root with immune-balancing effects.
- **Cayenne pepper** helps circulation and helps clear the excess mucus that is caused by food reactions.
- **Mullein leaf** is a soothing expectorant herb that helps strengthen the lungs and reduce allergies.

Metabolic Stimulation

False Fat Week is also the proper time to begin to introduce supplements that will help *improve your metabolic rate and increase fat burning*. Some doctors use fat-burning supplements as the primary modality of their weight control programmes, but I do not. I use them only as an adjunct to dietary and lifestyle change. I believe that using nutraceuticals as drugs without other lifestyle and dietary changes is a throwback to old-fashioned conventional 'magic bullet' medicine.

Nonetheless, as *adjunctive* modalities, they can be extremely effective.

The metabolism-enhancing nutrients that I most often prescribe are described below. Not all of these nutrients, most of which are amino acids, are appropriate for everyone, so please read the follow-up information carefully. These nutrients are powerful. Don't misuse them, and do consult your doctor first.

Here are what these nutrients do.

• **Carnitine** is an amino acid that will help move your fat molecules into your cells' energy-producing mitochondria, where they will be burned for energy. This nutrient is popular among athletes and people on weight-loss programmes. Studies indicate that it enhances weight loss.

• **Arginine** and **ornithine** are amino acids that help release fat that is stored so that it can be burned for energy. They do this primarily by increasing the production of human growth hormone, or HGH. HGH stimulates growth of bones and muscles, helps heal wounds, and metabolizes fat. Production of HGH drops rapidly after age 30, and virtually stops at 50. The use of injectable HGH is becoming a popular anti-ageing treatment.

• **Tyrosine** is an amino acid that acts as a natural appetite suppressant and is a precursor of a thyroid hormone. It also seems to help control depression and anxiety. It stimulates release of the hormone CCK (cholecystokinin), which induces a feeling of satiety.

• **Glutamine** and **phenylalanine** are also natural appetite suppressants. Glutamine is an amino acid that helps stop cravings, especially for sugar and alcohol, and helps release the hormone CCK that makes you feel satisfied after eating. If you don't have enough CCK, you will tend not to feel satisfied after meals. Phenylalanine, also an amino acid, helps control appetite, and also can be effective for chronic pain.

• **DHEA** is a natural adrenal hormone that forms the sex hormones, including testosterone and estrogen. It helps lock fat storage and can help build muscle. In many studies, it's been shown to promote weight loss. DHEA declines as we age. It is a powerful hormone and can only be taken under a doctor's care, after the doctor tests you for your existing DHEA levels. It should not be taken by men with enlarged prostates or prostate cancer, or by women with cancers of the breast or reproductive organs.

• **Choline** and **guggul** help to dissolve fat molecules in the liver. Therefore, they are known as lipotropics. Choline, found in lecithin, is also an excellent nutrient for enhancing memory (because the primary neurotransmitter for memory, acetylcholine, is made from choline). Guggul is a herb from the Asian pharmacopeia that has been proven in a number of studies to lower cholesterol and triglycerides and stimulate weight loss. It is currently not as widely available as some supplements, but some of the better mail-order supplement companies may supply it.

• **Chromium** appears to be the best nutrient for stabilizing blood sugar levels. It improves the absorption of glucose into cells and is excellent for preventing hypoglycemia. Many patients are far better able to control their eating habits when they take it. It also appears to help decrease 'bad' cholesterol, and increase 'good' cholesterol.

Because these substances are merely supportive medications, intended to be just *one part* of a complete programme, you need not take every one of them on a regular basis. Instead, you should try some of them to see which seem to best meet your own needs. Eliminate ones that duplicate the effects of others. For example, take just one of the natural appetite suppressants.

If you do take one or more of these supplements, you'll probably lose more weight and feel healthier. Of course, these supplements do not replace the most important element of weight loss: sensible eating. However, eating sensibly will be much easier for you now than it's ever before been, because you'll be largely free from food cravings.

Even so, some of my patients have continued to overeat even after they had overcome the physical, need-to-feed re-action of food cravings. This generally happened because they had an unhealthy emotional attachment to food. They relied on food to make them feel happy and to help solve some of their emotional problems, such as anxiety or boredom. If you have emotional attachments to food that make you overeat, you owe it to yourself to grow beyond them. After all, for the first time in your life, you'll be *physically* free to make smart food choices.

The Psychology of Overeating

During False Fat Week, you may smack headlong into your own worst enemy: yourself. I know that the *core* of your being wants to lose weight and be healthy; if this were not true, you would not be reading this page at this moment. But human beings are complex, multifaceted creatures, and we all have psychological aspects that sometimes prompt us to overeat.

In my clinical practice, I've found that the psychological aspects that make most people overeat generally fall into two categories. The first category is what I call learned food fallacies. These are ideas and concepts about food that are very popular but false. The second category consists of emotional eating – eating for reasons other than hunger.

If you can overcome these two psychological aspects of overeating – *and* continue to control your food cravings – you will gain tremendous power over food. Food will no longer dominate you. You'll dominate it.

Learned Food Fallacies

There are many fallacies about food, but in my practice, I mostly see five major fallacies. All of these are *learned* fallacies, and now it's time to *unlearn* them.

Fallacy 1. Food is love.

As children, most of us learn to equate the *food* our mothers give us with the *love* our mothers give us. But too often, we begin to think that their food *is* their love. It's not. *Food is not love.* Food is *food*. *Love* is love. As we grow older, we often eat the foods our mothers gave us to remind us of their love. But Mum's apple pie is not Mum – it's pie. If you want to feel your mother's love, think about her or call her up. Get the real thing, not the symbol.

Fallacy 2. It's a virtue to clean your plate.

Many of us were raised by parents who lived through the Great Depression and taught us that it is a sin to waste food. In addition, *everyone* knows that there are millions of starving people in the world. Therefore, many of us hate to waste food, even though we don't feel very guilty about wasting other valuable commodities such as electricity or petrol. Waste *is* wrong – but it's more wrong to waste your own body by overeating than to waste a few bites of food. Ask yourself: will *I* be better off with this food in *my body* or in the *dustbin*?

Better yet, *save* the food you're not hungry for. At a restaurant, get a doggy bag. At home, put it away for later, even if it's just a few bites. A couple of hours after dinner, you may remember the great sweet potatoes you had for dinner and feel like a snack. It's better to snack on a few bites of leftover sweet potatoes than on a bowl of ice cream – and you may much *prefer* the sweet potatoes to the ice cream.

Fallacy 3. I should be able to eat what everybody else eats.

The corollary to this fallacy is: and everybody *else* eats pizza and milkshakes. The truth is, everyone is different, and there's no more reason for you to eat what other people eat than there is for you to live where other people live. You're *you*, and you're unique. *Millions* of Americans, for example, eat diets very different from the 'standard' fattening American diet, and *billions* of people in other countries eat vastly different diets. Conformity is not a right. It's not even smart. Be who *you* are. Eat what *you* need. And don't assume that everyone who eats rich, reactive food gets away with it. For example, in pasta-loving Italy, wheat allergy is so common that most people are routinely tested for it.

Fallacy 4. Healthy food isn't fattening.

It is if you eat too much of it. I had a patient who was reactive to spinach, craved it, and sometimes ate as many as four cans of it over an evening – which added up to over 400 calories, as many calories as a piece of cake and ice cream. Of course it's smart to eat healthy foods, but if you think you can stuff yourself with them and not get fat, you're wrong. I especially see a lot of people eating too many complex carbohydrates (which is just a fancy name for starch). They think that whole wheat bagels can't possibly add up to many calories. They can. Be *moderate* or be fat.

Fallacy 5. Only fattening food tastes good.

I often hear the phrase 'Fat is flavour.' I also often hear patients say that dessert is their downfall – as if dessert must necessarily consist of some typical fat-and-sugar concoction. Once you clean up your diet and eliminate your food cravings, you'll be amazed at how good *wholesome* food tastes. A great way to unlearn this fallacy is to start eating non-dessert foods for desserts and snacks. Instead of pie for dessert, have a piece of fruit and a few nuts. Slice the fruit, arrange it nicely on a plate, and even sprinkle a touch of sugar or a few drops of honey on it if you need to accentuate the flavour. It will taste *good*. And you'll *feel* good. You'll soon learn to prefer this to an allergen-laden, rich dessert that gives you heartburn, makes you congested, and makes your abdomen swell with false fat.

If any of these fallacies have been part of your attitude toward food, I strongly urge you to realize that they are *just not true* and are very harmful.

Now let's look at the other major personality trait that causes overeating. It consists of what I call emotional eating. Emotional eating – eating for reasons other than hunger – is rampant in our society. It's terribly destructive, and you probably won't be able to become slender and healthy if you engage in it.

Emotional Eating

Most people engage in emotional eating at only three times: when life is good, bad, or indifferent. In other words, they eat (1) to celebrate or to reward themselves, (2) when they're upset or stressed out, or (3) when they're bored.

The catch, obviously, is that life is almost *always* either good, bad, or indifferent. Therefore, if you indulge in emotional eating, you'll almost always have an excuse to eat.

The antidote to emotional eating is to face life head-on and *deal* with life's ups and downs and its boredom. This is easier said than done, but it certainly *can* be done, especially if you are finally unencumbered by the burden of food cravings.

Of the three different times that people engage in emotional eating, the most common time is when life is difficult. Many people eat when they're unhappy or under stress. However, this is a *learned* response, not a natural instinct. The natural, biological response to sadness, anger, or fear is *not* to eat. This primarily occurs because the body's fight-or-flight response, which is activated by negative emotions, shifts energy away from the organs of digestion.

Over time, though, we learn that eating can take our minds off our problems, and this prompts some people to start using food as a drug. When we indulge in this type of emotional eating, we very frequently go into a virtual trance, unconsciously spooning bite after bite into our mouths until suddenly we're staring at the bottom of an empty food container. Going into a trance-like state, of course, was exactly what we felt we needed, since it temporarily took our minds off the real problem.

Sometimes we do this kind of eating when there's nothing really wrong in our *current* lives, but we still feel bad about the past. Millions of people temporarily escape from painful memories by eating. They stuff down their pain from past grievances or unhappy childhoods by stuffing down food.

Eating to escape from unhappiness is doubly destructive when we come out of our eating trance and then feel *guilty* about it. Guilt just compounds the problem, since it makes us feel even worse. Many people respond to their unconscious food binge with guilty self-hate, which just makes them want to escape again into *another* binge of unconscious eating. This vicious cycle is extremely common. I've heard dozens of patients describe it.

There is a way out of this trap, but it's not easy. It consists of tackling your problems, instead of hiding from them. You've probably tried to do this before, and maybe you've failed. Try again! This time, your willpower won't be chained down by food cravings. When just your *mind* is telling you to eat – instead of your mind *and* your body – you'll have much more power to resist. This time, you may well succeed.

Don't expect to have superhuman strength, though. Life is tough, and sometimes you're going to hide behind food. Everybody does. Even slender people. But when you do overeat or go on a food binge, don't beat yourself up over it. That will compound the error. Forgive yourself. Understand yourself. And start over with a clear conscience.

Eating to celebrate is less common than eating to escape. Still, this happens all the time. In fact, virtually every holiday and celebration in our culture includes a feast or a treat.

It's *good* to use eating for pleasure, for a simple reason: eating *is* inherently pleasurable. I don't think it's at all healthy to be ascetic about eating and to refuse to enjoy it. Life is meant to be enjoyed – it's meant to be *lived*. The problem comes when you *limit* your pleasure and celebration to *just* food. There are dozens of other ways to celebrate and enjoy life, and if you exclude them and focus just on food, you're probably going to get fat.

Instead of focusing mostly on *food* for pleasure, branch out. Indulge in life's full cornucopia of pleasures: music, nature, sports, conversation, family time, movies, sex with someone you love, art, reading, meditation, massage – anything that feels good and doesn't harm your body.

If you learn to branch out, you'll also be far less likely to eat when you are bored – because you won't be bored nearly so often. Occasional boredom is inevitable, though, so be conscious of it and refrain from trying to alleviate it with food. Most boredom will occur when you're barely even aware of it, during a dozen small moments throughout the day. When this happens, you may find yourself wandering to the refrigerator or pantry, opening it, and standing in front of it until you find something to nibble on. This is not a terrible thing to do *if* you choose a snack that's healthy, low in calories, and non-reactive, such as a carrot stick or a few nuts. If you're *not* very careful, though, this kind of emotional eating can be disastrous.

The *opposite* of emotional eating is simply to *eat when you're hungry* – and that's the type of eating you should do.

Furthermore, you should *stop eating* when you're no longer hungry. Eat until you're satisfied – not until you're full. Being full is very close to being stuffed, and it's just not healthy. Your body does not thrive when you have that feeling of a full, tight stomach that makes you want to loosen your belt or go lie down. After eating, you should still feel light and full of energy.

The best way to maintain that light, supple, satisfied feeling is to avoid unconscious, trance-like eating. Whenever you eat, whether it's a meal or a snack, try to *be aware of every bite*. Taste it. Savour it. Enjoy it.

A few years ago, I had lunch with Dr Dean Ornish, the noted author and creator of a famous low-fat heart disease programme. When the dessert tray rolled by, I asked Dr Ornish how he resisted rich desserts. He told me that with his background in meditation, he was able to take just one or two bites of dessert, focus *completely* on the taste, and feel satisfied.

While it's important to enjoy food, though, you should always be aware of the effect it will have on your body. Don't just zone out and forget about the effect that food has on your biochemistry. Ask yourself: 'Will this make me feel *good* later? Or will it make me feel *bad*?'

If you know it will make you feel bad later, take one more bite, enjoy the taste, and then stop eating.

You'll now have the power to do this. From this point on, if you avoid your reactive foods, you will not be a food addict, powerless to stop.

Enjoy stopping! It is the act of a powerful person.

Enjoy your power.

After you've begun your expanded programme of supplements and have started to examine your own psychology of eating, there will be only one more thing for you to do during False Fat Week: your first food challenge.

Let me tell you how to do it.

THE KEY TO WEIGHT CONTROL

- When you're hungry – eat.
- When you're not hungry – don't eat.
- Choose healthy foods.

Your First Food Challenge

If you began your False Fat Diet with an elimination diet, it's probably time to begin to reintroduce foods and challenge your system to see if you react to any of them.

The time to start dong this is *shortly after you've begun to feel better*. When you start to feel better, you will know that you have cleared most of the reactive food chemicals out of your body. If you *haven't* begun to feel better, it means your body is still detoxifying. If you start reintroducing foods while you're still toxic and uncomfortable, it will be very hard to tell if you're having a reaction. You won't know if your symptoms are from the new food or from lingering reactions to reactive food chemicals that are still in your system.

Therefore, you might be able to do your first food challenge just a few days after you start the diet, or you may have to wait as long as ten days to two weeks. An average time to begin food reintroduction is after about one week on a diet free of reactive foods.

Your first food to reintroduce should probably be one that you are not very likely to react to, such as a fruit or vegetable. One reason for this is that you'll be more likely to pass the challenge and will therefore be able to broaden your diet. Most people are anxious to quickly reintroduce as much variety to their diets as possible. Another reason to do this is because you will want your system to remain as clean as possible, free from reactive food chemicals. If you challenge yourself with a highly reactive food, such as milk, you might start feeling uncomfortable symptoms again. This may feel discouraging and will also slow down the food reintroduction process. Every time you react to a food, you may have to wait for at least a day for that food to leave your system; in some cases, it may take up to four days for the food to leave your system completely.

Doing a food challenge is easy. To do it, eat a moderate amount of the food by itself on an empty stomach. Then wait for a reaction.

There are three basic time periods in which the reaction will be most likely to occur: within the *first hour*, within the next *four to six hours*, or by the *next morning*. In my clinical practice, almost 90 per cent of food reactions occur during this time. As I've mentioned, they can occur up to three or four days after the food is eaten, but this is uncommon. These very delayed reactions tend to be reactions from circulating immune antibodies, and those are the least common type of food reaction.

As you wait for a reaction to occur, be aware of subtle changes in your body. Monitor yourself for the wide range of symptoms that food reactions can cause: heartburn, gas, headaches, irritability, bloating, nasal congestion, anxiety or depression, muscle aches, insomnia, hives or skin rashes, impaired concentration, food cravings, and swelling in your extremities. If *any* of these occur, it probably means that you are reactive.

If more than one symptom occurs or if any one symptom is severe, you are probably *very* reactive to that food.

The symptoms that may occur the morning after you eat the food might be slightly different. You might feel as if you had a minor hangover, or you might feel congested, as if you were coming down with a cold.

If you don't have any reaction, wait several days and then try the food again. This time, eat a larger amount of it. If this larger amount doesn't cause a reaction, you are probably not reactive to that food.

By the end of False Fat Week, you will almost certainly look better. You will most likely have lost the puffy, pouchy appearance that made you look far more overweight than you really are. What a relief that will be!

But the best is yet to come. The next phase of your diet will be the Balance Programme: a flat-out attack on your fat. From here on, most of the weight you will lose will come from adipose tissue. As this true fat begins to melt off your body, you're going to feel like a new person!

Now let's move on, and find out how you can recapture your fitness.

9
THE BALANCE PROGRAMME

'MY WEIGHT LOSS IS STARTING TO CHANGE,' SAID LAURA, my patient who'd been discouraged during her Cleansing Phase. 'The weight loss here,' she said, patting her abdomen, 'has levelled off. But now I'm starting to lose weight in my hips and thighs.'

'That means you've already lost most of your false fat and are starting to lose true fat,' I said.

She beamed and exclaimed 'Yes!' as she punched her fist into the air.

Laura, like so many of my patients, had a typically positive response to the False Fat Diet. She looked very different from the puffy, wan person I'd seen just a couple of weeks before. Much of the edematous false fat had drained away from her midsection, face, hands and feet, and from under her chin. In addition, her stomach had flattened, due to decreased gas, and also due to a decrease in the yeast fermentation of sugars that had bloated her gut.

She was also noticeably more animated and had more energy. The reactions she'd previously had to dairy products had not only ballooned her shape but had also sapped her vitality.

The third week on the False Fat Diet is called the Balance Programme. This phase is a sensible, medically sound regimen that helps you balance your lifestyle. It begins shortly after you have lost most of your false fat. It is a blueprint for a healthy way of living and is designed to last for the rest of your life.

There's nothing complicated about the Balance Programme. It simply consists of (1) a *good diet*, (2) *exercise*, and (3) *stress management*. When people eat well, stay active, and control their stress, they almost always begin to feel great and lose weight.

Occasionally, of course, some of my patients do fall out of balance and start to eat too much, work too feverishly, worry too often, or exercise too little. This sometimes happens during holidays, during family crises, or during brief illnesses. However, patients who have been on the Balance Programme for even a short time tend to bounce back quickly from their occasional imbalances. One primary reason they readjust quickly is because *balance feels good*. It's almost addictive.

The other primary reason that patients on the False Fat Diet tend to return easily to balance is because they are finally *biochemically capable of it*. When patients with moderate to severe food reactions first begin the False Fat Diet, they usually have imbalanced biochemistries that make them worry too much, sit around too much, eat too much, and stay too busy with tasks that don't really need to be done. However, after patients start their diets and begin to *heal their own biochemistries*, these underlying personality and behavioural traits often begin to disappear, and it's far easier for these patients to address problems or challenges in their lives.

For example, I recently had a food reaction patient named Robert who was obsessed with his job and driven to succeed. Unfortunately, this obsession was reinforced by almost everyone in his life, including his co-workers, his parents, and his wife, who thought that it was the key to his success. He proudly described himself as a workaholic. Even though no one brags about being an alcoholic, millions of people boast about being workaholics. Robert regularly rewarded his work binges with food binges, and was about 40 pounds overweight. The foods he most often binged on – ice cream, doughnuts, and pie and coffee – elevated his adrenaline and cortisol levels, as reactive foods do in many people. This left him with so much nervous energy that he often worked even when he didn't have to. In effect, he was using work as a drug to calm himself, just as he was using food as a drug to reward himself.

However, when Robert eliminated his false fat foods, he calmed down considerably. He overcame a bad case of chronic insomnia and didn't feel jittery nearly so often. His anxiety level dropped precipitously, and he gradually let go of his workaholism. He eventually discovered that he could get as much work done by staying relaxed and not agonizing over every little detail. His food binges stopped. He started spending more time with his wife and friends and played more tennis and golf. His life became more balanced, and he became healthier and slimmer – and more successful than ever.

I don't think Robert's breakthrough could have happened if he hadn't changed his diet. Diet, for most people, is the foundation of balance. A good diet free of reactive foods and other toxins makes physical activity feel like fun, and makes stress management far easier by reducing the biochemical stressors that bombard the brain and nervous system.

In fact, I sometimes illustrate the Balance Programme to patients in the following way, to indicate how dietary change is the foundation of a healthy, balanced lifestyle.

THE BALANCE PROGRAMME
FOR SUCCESSFUL WEIGHT MANAGEMENT

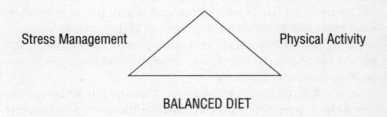

Stress Management   Physical Activity

BALANCED DIET

Now, I'm going to tell you what to expect as you begin your Balance Programme and what you will need to do. The principles are simple. You can easily learn them in a week and they will work well for you for the rest of your life.

What to Expect

As you begin the Balance Programme, continue to avoid all of your reactive foods. If you're on an elimination diet, it may take you a month or more to determine all of your reactive foods, using the food challenge method. If you did a blood test, you'll already know your reactive foods.

You will also *add two new principles* to your diet at this time: *rotation* and *metabolic typing*. Rotation simply means adding *variety* to your diet in order to avoid overeating any particular food. As you'll recall, eating any one food too often can create a new food reaction to it. Therefore, it will be wise for you to frequently rotate foods in and out of your diet, so that you don't eat the same food every day for a week or more.

Metabolic typing is a system of determining the best type of *general* diet for your *own unique metabolism*. For example, some people thrive on vegetarianism, while others need occasional animal protein, such as beef, poultry, eggs, and fish. I'll give you a questionnaire that will help determine your general metabolic type.

You'll also continue to take the anti-reaction supplements that I listed in Chapter 8, and you'll continue with your periodic detoxification. Hopefully, you'll be able to scale back on your detoxification, since your body will probably be significantly less toxic than it was at the beginning of your diet. However, any time that you begin to experience feelings of toxicity, you should clear the toxins from your system. This may occur regularly as you lose adipose tissue, since toxins are primarily stored in fat cells.

In addition to your dietary programme, you'll add two new *non-dietary* practices to your Balance Programme: *physical activity* and *stress management*. Both of them are critical for long-term health and for maintaining your optimal weight. I usually don't address either of these elements in the diet's first couple of weeks, because I don't want to overwhelm people. By now, though, you should be ready for them. *For permanent weight loss, physical activity and stress management are absolutely essential*.

Although both of these practices will help you continue to

lose weight, you should not expect to lose weight nearly as *quickly* as you did during the Cleansing Phase and False Fat Week. During those two phases, most of your weight loss came from false fat, which leaves the body quickly. During the Balance Programme, most of your weight loss will come from the burning of true fat, or adipose tissue, which leaves the body much more slowly.

It's important to be patient and not try to starve yourself into quick loss of adipose tissue. If you do, you'll activate your body's starvation response, and your body will begin to hoard calories. Trying to lose adipose tissue too quickly is one of the worst mistakes a dieter can make. Of course I know that we live in a fast-forward culture, in which we want everything to happen quickly. The beauty of the False Fat Diet, though, is that it achieves fast *weight* loss from loss of *false fat*, without triggering fast loss of *adipose tissue*. This satisfies most people's desire for quick results without sabotaging long-term success.

If you want to *accelerate* your weight loss, do it with exercise, rather than extreme caloric restriction. Extra exercise will not trigger the starvation response. Furthermore, it will not just burn fat, but will also improve your mood, boost your metabolic rate, increase your muscle mass, and aid your detoxification. Even so, don't overdo it. If you merely substitute compulsive exercise for compulsive eating, you'll never find the comfortable middle ground that will help you stay slender for ever.

I generally advise patients to try to lose about 1 pound of adipose tissue per week. That is approximately the maximum that can be lost through dieting without triggering the starvation response. To some people, this sounds slow, but it's not. It's really only slow compared to the foolish claims of crash diets that are often trumpeted in the tabloid press: 'Lose 20 Pounds in Ten Minutes!'

If you lose 1 pound each week, you'll lose about 25 pounds in six months, in addition to all the weight you lose by overcoming your edemic swelling. In nine months, you could sensibly and realistically lose about 35 to 40 pounds, and in a year you could lose over 50 pounds, if you have that much to lose.

Therefore, now that you're in the extended phase of this diet, don't think about how slender you'll be at the end of your initial 21 days on the False Fat Diet – think about how slender you'll be at the end of your first year. *That's what matters*.

Now let's look at each of the three elements of the Balance Programme, starting with the programme's foundation: diet.

The Balance Programme Diet

As always, the single most important dietary element is to *avoid your own reactive foods*. Don't lose sight of this simple principle. It is the heart and soul of the False Fat Diet.

If you began your diet by doing a blood test, you should avoid all of your reactive foods for at least *3 months*. If your blood test said you were *extremely* reactive to certain foods, avoid them for *6 months*. After 3 to 6 months, you can begin to eat your reactive foods occasionally to see if they still cause reactions. Some of them probably will, but some won't. The foods that have caused you the *most* severe reactions in the past will probably remain the most troublesome. Many of these will be foods that cause an *immediate* IgE-mediated reaction. Foods that cause immediate IgE reactions can remain problematic for years. Frequently they remain reactive forever.

You will be likely, however, to recover much sooner from reactions to foods that had caused *delayed* reactions. If a food doesn't cause a reaction until an hour or more after you eat it, you will probably be able to eventually add it back to your diet. These delayed, IgG-mediated reactions are much easier to recover from than immediate IgE reactions.

Many patients do a new, follow-up blood test after about a year, to see if their food reactions have changed. This is helpful, but you may want to monitor your own ongoing reactions to foods.

For the *rest of your life*, you should try to remain aware of your reactions to various foods. When you eat something, don't just ask yourself, 'Does this taste good?' Ask yourself, '*How does this make me feel?*'

* * *

If you began your False Fat Diet by doing an elimination diet, you will still be doing food challenges as you begin the Balance Programme. These challenges may continue for at least several more weeks. In fact you may still occasionally be challenging particular foods for a very long time, simply because it may be a long time before you eat a certain food. For example, you might eat cranberries only at Christmas, so you might not challenge them until then.

However, you should be able to challenge *most* of the foods you commonly eat within a few weeks. You can challenge up to at least one new food each day, so it won't take long to test the majority of foods that comprise your normal diet.

Remember to test new foods one at a time, preferably on an empty stomach. As I've mentioned, most reactions will occur *within one hour*, or *after 4 to 6 hours*, or *by the following morning*. If a food seems to cause a symptom, try it again in a week or two, to make sure it's really a problem.

Any food can cause a reaction, but be especially suspicious of the Sensitive Seven: dairy products, wheat, corn, soya, peanuts, sugar, and eggs. Be equally wary of highly processed, chemicalized foods.

Don't become discouraged if you don't always get a clear-cut, obvious, good-or-bad response to a food. Your response will sometimes fall into a grey area. When this happens, you'll just have to do more detective work. Food reactions can shift, waxing and waning. This happens because the human body is constantly changing and adapting, and is subject at any one time to many different forces, such as stress, seasonal changes, and airborne allergens and chemicals. Any of these forces can alter your reaction to a food. Therefore, you should not expect the same black-and-white reactions every single time you eat a particular food. That's just not how the body works. It is not simply a predictable, mechanical apparatus. Be glad you're not a machine! Your humanity, with all its complications and confusion, is your saving grace. Don't ignore it. Embrace it! Learn about your own unique body and how it reacts to food and the world around you.

As you settle into your long-term diet, try to rotate foods in and out of your daily diet. This will help prevent new food reactions, since habitual consumption of foods can cause re-actions. It will also help ensure you take in a wide variety of nutrients. In addition, it will help keep you from eating processed foods, since so many of them contain the same common, reactive foodstuffs, such as wheat, milk, corn syrup, eggs and sugar.

Ideally, after you eat a particular food, you should wait 3 to 4 days before you again rotate it into your diet. That will allow all of the chemicals in that food to leave your body, which will help prevent the development of a new food reaction. This long waiting period can be difficult, however, and is frequently not necessary. Often, it's sufficient just to skip one day. Many people can even eat the same food several days in a row, as long as they don't eat it every single day for weeks or months at a time.

In general, you should observe longer waiting periods for the foods that once caused you the worst problems. For example, if you previously had a strong reaction to wheat, but then overcame it, you should be cautious about eating wheat too frequently. If you eat it five days each week or even every other day, your reaction may return. On the other hand, if you formerly had only a mild reaction to wheat, you might easily get away with eating it every couple of days for the rest of your life. Many patients find that as they overcome their reactions, they can eat almost anything, as long as they don't eat it too often.

The most important thing is to avoid eating the same food three to four times every day. Many people, for example, eat wheat products at practically every meal, and also in between meals.

It's also smart to avoid regularly eating foods that are in the same food family. Virtually every food is in a family of similar foods, and sometimes even a family member can cause a re-action. For example, the poultry family contains not just chicken, but also turkey, duck, goose, and pheasant. Therefore, if you're avoiding chicken on a particular day, it's smart to also avoid turkey and other family members.

Some of the food families are rather hard to discern. The

plum family, for instance, includes not just plums and prunes, but also cherries, peaches, apricots, nectarines, and even almonds. For a complete list of all the food families, see Part Three.

Some allergy specialists are very strict about rotation diets, but I'm not. I try not to burden patients with difficult, complicated programmes that they can't follow. I want *results*, and believe that if a programme isn't practical, it will eventually fail.

Rather than insist upon a strict rotation diet, I simply advise patients to *avoid reactive foods as much as possible* and to *eat a wholesome, varied diet*, free of junk food and processed foods. This approach is simple but extremely effective.

Furthermore, as I've mentioned previously, you should not even *try* to be perfect. *Nobody's perfect*, and people who try to be just set themselves up for failure. As my friend and colleague Bethany Argisle has often remarked, 'Reduce your excesses, but not excessively.'

When you do cheat on your diet, though, and eat a reactive food, don't go overboard. Don't tell yourself, 'Well, I've fallen off the wagon, so I might as well eat whatever I want.' That is the kind of all-or-nothing thinking that makes people fat. The key to successful cheating is:

- **Don't cheat too *often*.**
- **Don't eat too *much* when you *do* cheat.**

When you *do* cheat, don't waste time feeling guilty about it. As I mentioned earlier, guilt is a counterproductive emotion that harms your self-image and makes you *far more vulnerable* to a food binge.

As a rule, the *best* time to cheat is on a special occasion. If you limit your cheating to just a few special times, you won't have very much opportunity to cheat. Furthermore, if you give yourself permission to cheat on special occasions, you won't feel deprived. You'll be able to look forward to your occasional breaks from the diet, and will feel like a normal human being eating a normal, pleasant diet.

A special occasion, for some people, might be a regular

Saturday night dinner, either at a restaurant or at home. For others, special occasions might mean your birthday or holidays such as Christmas.

It's important not to create *too many* special occasions. For example, it's fine to eat whatever you want at Christmas, but if you allow yourself to cheat for several weeks and on into the New Year, you're going to get in trouble. Similarly, if you eat whatever you want all weekend, instead of just on Saturday night, you'll probably get fat.

Also, remember that when you do cheat, you might biologically re-ignite your food cravings. If this happens, *be aware of it* and do whatever it takes to overcome the cravings. Overcoming the cravings may require extra supplements, extra detoxification – and extra willpower.

In fact, some of my patients find that it's actually easier for them *not* to cheat, since they know that cheating can reawaken old food cravings. This approach might sound like perfectionism, but it's really not. These patients are not trying to be perfect, they are just taking the path that works best for them.

In addition to rotating your foods, another superb way to ensure optimal nutrition is to determine your own metabolic type. Let's take a quick look at what this is.

Metabolic Typing

Over the past 25 years, a number of cutting-edge nutritional researchers have determined that different people need *different general diets*. The primary difference appears to be that some people seem to thrive on essentially vegetarian, high-carbohydrate diets, while others appear to require animal protein and a low-carbohydrate diet.

There are several reasons why these differing needs exist. One reason is that people have different ancestors and therefore have different genetic traits. Some people, for example, are descended from ancestors who lived in cold climates and who depended upon meat. People with this genetic heritage tend to require moderate amounts of meat. Other people, however, are descended from ancestors who lived in warmer climates and who depended mostly on fruits and vegetables. People with this genetic heritage tend to do better on a more vegetarian diet.

Besides genetic heritage, other factors that appear to influence metabolic type are: the rate of digestion and oxidation of food; the relative acidity or alkalinity of the body; and the body's general metabolic rate.

As a rule, *natural vegetarians* tend to be people with warm-climate ancestors, a comparatively slow rate of digestion, a relatively alkaline body pH, and a comparatively fast metabolic rate.

In general, *natural meat-eaters* are people with cold-climate ancestors, a relatively fast rate of digestion, an acidic body pH, and a slow metabolic rate.

A fundamental principle of metabolic typing is that people who digest food *quickly* are healthier when they eat foods that break down *slowly*. If these people eat quickly digestible food – especially breads, cereals and other grains – they're liable to oxidize the food too quickly, and run out of energy. When they eat slowly oxidized foods, though, such as meat and heavier proteins, they receive a stable supply of food energy.

Similarly, people who digest food *slowly* tend to be healthier when they eat food that breaks down *quickly*. If these people eat heavy food that is hard for them to break down, this food tends to sit in their stomachs, congesting their organs of digestion and elimination. When they eat quickly oxidized foods, though, such as grains, fruits and vegetables, they receive a stable, usable supply of food energy.

As I mentioned, people who *digest food quickly* often tend to have a relatively *slow* general rate of metabolism. These people tend to be calm and have steady levels of activity, instead of having Type A fight-or-flight personalities. As you probably remember, the organs of digestion just don't work well when people are in the fight-or-flight mode. When that type of aggressive, fast-metabolism mode predominates, the organs of digestion tend to shut down. You've probably noticed that when you get excited or nervous, you lose interest in food and have relatively more indigestion when you do eat. Some people experience this keyed-up, excitable feeling practically all day long, and it decreases their ability to digest food.

Neither metabolic type is superior. Each has advantages and disadvantages. For example, excitable, Type A people tend to be more slender, but also have an increased tendency to burn out from stress. Calm, Type B people have more of a tendency to be overweight, but they also tend to have better endurance and often feel more content than excitable people.

Once you determine your metabolic type, you should try to live in accord with it by eating the general type of diet you naturally thrive on. If you're a natural vegetarian, for example, you should try to generally avoid meat.

However, it's very important *not to overdo it*. Try to achieve balance. Natural vegetarians who eat *too* lightly can virtually destroy their bodies. I see this happen all too frequently. People who thrive on a mostly vegetarian diet, including a small amount of fish or chicken, sometimes begin to avoid meat entirely and even begin to eat only *very light* vegetarian fare, such as green salads, sprouts and fruits. These people tend to become depleted, weak, and depressed. Often they become too thin. Frequently, they then begin to eat too many carbohydrates, to bolster their low energy. This often makes them overweight and also contributes to their food reactivity. By the time they finally consult me, their bodies are usually soft and puffy and they feel exhausted. Often, they're quite confused about their lack of vitality and their obesity, because they believe that they have been eating a classic health food diet. These people would have stayed healthier if they had balanced their natural propensity for vegetarianism by eating a small amount of meat, poultry, or fish.

Only a relatively small percentage of people are pure vegetarians, who should eat virtually *no* animal protein.

By the same token, some people are natural meat eaters who take that trait too far. Sometimes this type of person will eat bacon for breakfast, chicken for lunch and steak for dinner. This heavy consumption of meat often overwhelms their organs of digestion and assimilation, and they then often begin to develop high blood pressure, high cholesterol, and excess adipose tissue. These people would have been healthier if they'd balanced their natural carnivorous tendencies with more consumption of fruits, vegetables and grain.

A very small percentage of the population thrives on a very heavy consumption of meat. This metabolic type is even more rare than that of pure vegetarians.

The key, of course, is *balance*. Extreme diets are rarely healthy, even when they're composed of individually healthy foods.

Let me provide you with a short questionnaire (see pages 250–1) that will help you determine your own general metabolic type.

As this questionnaire indicates, many people who are prone to being overweight require a moderate amount of meat (including fish, fowl, beef, and pork). I believe that the recent popularity of high-protein diets among overweight people supports the concept that many overweight people thrive on a relatively high-protein, high-vegetable, low-carbohydrate diet, which includes animal proteins.

Until recently, though, the most popular diets for weight control were diets high in complex carbohydrates and low in meat – and these diets just didn't work for millions of overweight people. Many of the people who failed to thrive on these high-carb plans were probably people who digested food quickly and needed the stable energy supply that's provided by slowly oxidized animal protein.

As a general rule, most people who require a moderate amount of meat have good digestive systems, are calm and rational, and have superior stamina. They tend not to enjoy exercise as much as more driven, Type A people, and often love good food.

If this sounds like you, it would probably be wise for you to eat a moderate amount of animal proteins, unless your spiritual beliefs prohibit it. If your spiritual beliefs don't allow meat eating, you still should try to eat a higher amount of relatively heavy non-meat proteins, such as soya, dairy, eggs, and nuts (unless you're reactive).

It's extremely important, though, not to eat too *much* meat, because some meats *can be very high in calories, chemicals and saturated fat*. Some fatty types of beef and luncheon meats are especially high in calories and should be eaten in moderation.

DETERMINING YOUR OWN
METABOLIC TYPE

Rate how well the statements apply to you, on a 0–5 scale.

0 = It *never* applies.

1 = It *rarely* applies.

2 = It *sometimes* applies.

3 = It *often* applies.

4 = It *almost always* applies.

5 = It *always* applies.

SCORE

1. I hardly ever lose my temper. ——

2. I often get hungry quickly, even after a relatively big meal. ——

3. I love to eat and look forward to each meal. ——

4. I really don't like to exercise, and have to feel highly motivated to do it. ——

5. If I eat a light breakfast, consisting mostly of fruit, I like to have a mid-morning snack. ——

6. I would rather work a longer day at a slower pace than a shorter day at a more hectic pace. ——

7. I have to be careful about not letting my blood sugar get too low, because that makes me run out of energy. ——

8. I seem to gain weight more easily than most people. ——

9. I rarely experience the condition of cold hands and feet. ——

10. When I get hungry, I tend to mostly desire sweet or starchy foods. ——

11. I usually don't develop digestive problems, such as heartburn or gas, unless I eat rich, acidic, or reactive foods. ——

12. Skipping a meal affects me strongly. ——

13. My mood is usually stable unless I get very hungry or am under stress. ——

14. I'm not very fond of sour or salty snacks. ——

15. I tend to react relatively calmly to sudden stressors, such as unexpected noises. ——

16. I'm not a morning person, and often need a cup of coffee to get going. ——

17. I usually don't worry about things I can't control. ——

18. My skin tends to be relatively clear, moist, and soft. ——

19. I tend to have problems with sleep, such as insomnia, frequent waking, or fatigue when I awaken in the morning. ——

20.   I like to think things over carefully before I make decisions.   ——

      Add all of your scores together, for a total score.   ——

                                                                    TOTAL SCORE

Here is what your total score indicates:

TOTAL SCORE	METABOLIC TYPE
0–10	You are a vegetarian type, who thrives on a non-meat diet.
10–40	You are a Predominantly Vegetarian Type, who needs only small amounts of animal proteins (meats).
40–70	You are a Mixed Vegetarian–Carnivore Type, who should eat a small amount of meat (approximately one serving daily of beef, fowl, fish, or pork).
70–90	You are a Predominantly Carnivore Type, who should eat a moderate amount of meat (about two servings daily).
90–100	You are a Carnivore Type, who thrives on a relatively high consumption of animal protein (several servings daily).

When you do eat beef, limit your portion to approximately the size of a deck of cards, and eat mostly lean beef. Chicken is significantly less fattening than beef if you remove the skin and eat primarily white meat. Fish is generally far lower in calories than beef or chicken, and is the healthiest type of animal product for most people. I highly recommend fish for people who need animal protein. It's delicious, low in calories, packed with protein and nutrients, full of healthy oils, and satisfying. Be careful not to smother it in tartar sauce, though, because tartar sauce made from mayonnaise can be very fattening.

Exercise

You will probably never have the kind of body you want if you do not exercise. *Diet alone will not do it.* Without exercise, your body will never be firm, toned, and well-defined, even if you achieve your ideal weight.

A few of my patients who refused to exercise did reach their goal weights, but still didn't like how they looked. They were not very overweight, but their bodies were still flabby, puffy in places, and dimpled with cellulite. Their skin seemed to hang on them like a suit that didn't fit, and they just didn't have that shining spark of vitality that only exercise can ignite. Even these patients, though, were better off than *most* patients who refused to exercise. As a rule, when people have failed to exercise, they have failed to reach the weight they want.

In a way, patients are *lucky* if they can't lose weight without exercising, because that motivates them to do it – and then they reap the many varied rewards that exercise offers. When patients *can* lose weight without exercising, it ultimately works against them. For example, I had a food reaction patient a few years ago, Lila, who was about 20 pounds overweight and reached her goal weight without exercising. She was 48 years old and had been sedentary most of her life. Unfortunately, though, she looked much older than 48, even after she'd lost her extra weight. Her skin was slack and without lustre, and she was often tired and depressed. Her arms weren't fat, but the flesh under her upper arm was loose and floppy. I tried to talk her into exercising, but she told me she didn't need to. She was wrong. She badly needed exercise. There's much more to having an attractive body than just being able to fit into a small dress size.

A more typical patient who refused to exercise was Rick. He'd been an athlete in college and seemed to think that gave him a free pass on ever again having to work out. Rick lost most of the 30 pounds that he'd hoped to, but he kept the weight off for only a few months.

Without the balancing effect of exercise, the False Fat Diet is notably less effective. The False Fat Diet was designed as a comprehensive, complete programme, and when patients try to pick and choose just the parts of the programme that they like, as Rick did, they seriously undermine the entire programme. The False Fat Diet is a *health-promoting programme* with the motto of: 'If you strive for thin, you'll never win. Strive for health, and thin will follow.' Rick just strived for thin – and he didn't win.

* * *

Exercise has four *primary* effects that fight fat, and several *secondary* effects.

The primary effects are:

1. Exercise burns calories. A fast walk or slow jog for 30 minutes burns about 300 calories. If you do this every day, you'll burn about 2,100 calories each week. This is enough to oxidize two-thirds of a pound of fat. Therefore, if you exercise 30 minutes each day, you'll burn the equivalent of about 35 pounds of fat each year.

2. Exercise increases metabolic rate. Exercise can change a slow, inefficient metabolism into a faster metabolism, which burns fat even during inactivity. Every time you exercise, your metabolism stays revved up for several hours. This effect can burn almost as many calories as exercise itself.

3. Exercise adds muscle, and muscle burns extra calories. The normal metabolic actions of muscle tissue require extra calories for energy, even when the muscles aren't being used. This is one of the primary reasons that it's easier for men to stay thin than it is for women. Men naturally have more muscle mass than women, and because of this, they burn approximately 10–20 per cent more calories at rest than women do.

4. Exercise helps control insulin levels – and high insulin levels increase fat storage. Exercise can even help to control blood sugar levels without the help of insulin.

As you can see, these four factors are every bit as important as caloric restriction.

Besides these four primary factors, exercise exerts several secondary, indirect factors that help control weight. For some people, these indirect factors are even more important than the four direct factors. For example, exercise often decreases depression, which can be a significant factor in weight gain. In the early 1990s, I had a patient who suffered from depression, and who responded to it with food binges and subsequent weight gain. When she started to exercise, though, her depression lifted. This is not uncommon. Several studies have indicated that exercise is as effective for depression as antidepressants and counselling, because it increases levels of the neurotransmitters that dispel depression. When my patient's depression cleared up, her food binges stopped, and she became slender and fit. On a few occasions she suspended her exercise programme, but when she did, she became depressed again. For her, exercise was very much like an effective pharmaceutical drug, because it improved the balance of her neurotransmitters.

The secondary benefits of exercise are:

1. Exercise increases energy, and energy is one of the best weapons against fat because it keeps us active. Exercise increases energy mostly by improving circulation and increasing production of stimulating neurotransmitters and hormones. One of the hormones increased by exercise is testosterone, which is energizing for both men and women and which helps build muscle mass.

2. Exercise helps control appetite, primarily by increasing output of energizing neurotransmitters and hormones. You've probably noticed that when you're hungry, you can kill your appetite temporarily by exercising.

3. Exercise alleviates depression by stimulating the production of the neurotransmitters serotonin, dopamine, and norepinephrine. This is extremely important, because many people overeat when they're depressed. In one study, a group of college students with depression who exercised improved significantly more than a control group who received conventional treatment. Exercise also decreases anxiety by triggering a tranquilizer effect that lasts for up to four hours after the exercise is over.

4. Exercise decreases illness, and illness is a frequent cause of weight gain, since it often imposes inactivity and it also prompts some people to overeat. Exercise appears to decrease both major and minor illnesses. In one study, people who exercised missed 18 per cent fewer work days than people who didn't. Other studies indicate that exercise reduces the risk of stroke by 400 per cent, the risk of cancers of the reproductive organs by 250 per cent, the risk of breast cancer by 200 per cent, and the risk of colon cancer by 67 per cent. Exercise even appears to be a significant factor in the prevention of Alzheimer's disease.

5. Exercise improves function of the lymphatic system, one of the body's primary systems for removing toxins from the body. When the lymphatic system is congested, people don't feel well and are more prone to food reactions, and therefore are more prone to weight gain.

6. Exercise improves general quality of life, which helps motivate people to live healthy lifestyles. When people have a pleasant life and feel content, they are far less likely to make the mistake of living to eat, instead of eating to live. When they have an unpleasant quality of life, they often grasp at anything that might feel good, such as overeating. Exercise improves quality of life in many ways, including several ways that I've already mentioned, such as decreasing illness and dispelling depression. It definitely makes people *feel* better and *look* better. It even makes people smarter; numerous studies show that it powerfully boosts cognitive function.

As you begin your Balance Programme, you should gradually begin to integrate exercise into your False Fat Diet. Don't push yourself into a sudden, strenuous regimen, though, because crash exercising is just as foolish as crash dieting. If you are in relatively poor physical condition, start with less intense activities, such as walking for 10 to 15 minutes. As you become increasingly fit, add both *time* and *intensity* to your workout.

Within a month or two, you should aim to be exercising for 7 to 10 hours each week, or one to one and a half hours each day. This amount of exercise may sound excessive, but it's not. Over the past 2½ million years of evolution, the human body was genetically programmed to require *at least* that much exercise. This genetic programming is as inescapable as the genetic programming that determined your metabolic type. Like it or not, you're stuck with this need for exercise, just as you're stuck with the need for vitamin C or fresh air. In fact, your ancestors were physically active for most of the day, instead of just an hour or an hour and a half. As recently as the early 1900s, the majority of people in America were very active for about 5 to 10 hours every day. At that time, 40 per cent of all Americans lived on farms, and 80 per cent of all farm work was done with human labour. Most people who did not live on farms were still very active, working hard in factories, walking to work, and doing innumerable chores at home. Obesity was so uncommon back then that it was considered a sign of success.

The 60 to 90 minutes of exercise that you will do each day need not be exhausting. Actually, exercise burns fat best when it is moderate; jogging for example, burns fat more efficiently than sprinting.

Exercise can be so mild that you may not even recognize it as exercise. For example, if you go for a pleasant walk, that's exercise. If you play catch with your child, that's exercise. The main thing is to get on your feet and start moving. *Just don't be sedentary.* Turn off the TV. Get off the couch.

Ideally, though, your exercise programme should be centred around a 30- to 40-minute period of aerobic exercise, which should be strenuous enough to make you sweat. Even this relatively intense period of exercise, though, need not make you breathless. As you do your aerobics, you should be able to maintain a normal conversation.

To increase your fitness, your heart rate should increase by about 75–100 per cent over your resting heart rate. For most people, this will consist of about 115 to 135 beats per minute, depending upon age and fitness level.

If you exercise harder than this, your body will be more likely to burn stored blood sugar than fat. It is helpful, though, to occasionally do bursts of very strenuous activity to increase the strength of your heart, and muscles. But don't overdo it. If you push yourself too hard, you'll end up hating your exercise – just as you'll end up hating your diet if you try to starve yourself. Be moderate. Achieve balance. Think about the long term, not the short term.

In addition to your centrepiece of aerobic exercise, you should also do about 15 minutes of stretching and about 15 minutes of strength training with weights.

Stretching is critical for maintaining flexibility, and flexibility seems to have an almost magical effect upon the body. It appears to help preserve optimum function of the circulatory system, nervous system, skeletal system, and muscles. In fact, one of the tenets of yoga is 'You're as young as your spine is flexible.'

A BALANCED EXERCISE PROGRAMME

Stretching (10–15 minutes per day)	for	**Flexibility**
+		
Weights (10–15 minutes (every other day)	for	**Strength**
+		
Aerobics (30–40 minutes per day)	for	**Endurance**

It all adds up to **energy, relaxation** and **feeling great.**

I once saw a dramatic example of the youth-preserving effects of exercise in general, and flexibility in particular, in an elderly man who had a generally unhealthy lifestyle. He smoked, drank beer, and ate carelessly. But he had a three-acre mini-farm and did all the work on it himself, even in his seventies. He was extremely fit and healthy, and was so agile that every year, on his birthday, he performed an amazing feat of flexibility. He would hold a straight pole, such as a broom-stick or yardstick, behind his back with both hands, and then jump over the stick, without letting go, so that it ended up in front of him. (Try this sometime. It's practically impossible.) When he was 76, though, he slipped off a roof and shattered his heel. He stopped exercising and was dead in about 18 months.

Your stretching can consist of yoga or any simple exercise that gently stretches muscles, tendons, and ligaments. It's wise to stretch just before you begin your aerobic exercise, to help avoid injury and muscle strain. You should also stretch just after exercising.

After you have eliminated reactive foods from your diet, you may find that you have much more flexibility, because your joints may become healthier. Many people overcome joint stiffness and arthritis-like symptoms on the False Fat

Diet, since food reactions and general toxicity commonly cause stiffness in joints.

Besides stretching, you should also do about 10 to 15 minutes of weight work every day, or at least every other day. This is the best way to strengthen your muscles. Some people hate weight training, because it *can* be hard, especially if you try to lift as much as possible. This is not necessary, however. You can achieve a remarkable degree of muscle definition and strength by lifting very light weights. Many people only need to work out with a light set of 2-pound to 5-pound dumbbells. Of course, you'll have to do a higher number of repetitions with light or moderate weights, but even a high number will be relatively easy. If you use light or moderate weights, you won't experience the gut-wrenching 'grunt and groan' labour that's often associated with weight training. Lifting light weights is so easy that most people enjoy it – especially when they see the fast and dramatic benefits it achieves.

As you integrate exercise into your lifestyle, don't get hung up on how much you can lift or how far you can run. That's the kind of self-critical, competitive attitude that will eventually doom your exercise programme. If you impose artificial expectations on yourself, you'll eventually either fail or become resentful of your own self-imposed authority.

Don't *work* at exercise. *Play* with it. Work is something we all hope to someday retire from. Play is something that we hope will last forever.

You should never force yourself to exercise. Have fun. Just force yourself to get off the couch.

Stress Management

A great many of my patients do not really know what stress actually is. They think that it's an outside force causing them to feel tense. But that's not stress – that's a stressor. Stress is a person's *negative reaction* to a stressor.

For the most part, people have a negative reaction to stressors when they feel that their stressors are greater than their ability to deal with them. When they feel like this, they see their stressors as *threats*. On the other hand, if they think they *can* handle their stressors, they usually see them as *challenges* and generally enjoy grappling with them.

If you now feel as if your life is full of *threats*, instead of *challenges*, you are experiencing stress. If your degree of stress is severe, it's going to be quite difficult for you to live a balanced, healthy lifestyle free from compulsion, including the compulsion to overeat.

To succeed, you must overcome this stress.

On occasion, I've had patients who initially mastered the physical elements of the False Fat Diet – such as exercise and the avoidance of reactive foods – but who ultimately failed to keep their weight off because of stress. They just couldn't cope with the stressors in their lives, and this eventually ruined their diets. They began to engage in stress eating, and eventually felt too emotionally exhausted to maintain a regular programme of exercise.

For example, I had a 29-year-old patient named Darlene, who initially did very well on her diet. She lost about 18 pounds in four months. But the weight loss didn't last.

Darlene had credit card debt which she worried about far too much. Every minor financial setback made her feel threatened and sent her into a state of anxiety. When she felt anxious, she 'stuffed down' her anxiety with food. She avoided eating reactive foods, but she ate too many calories.

Darlene made the classic mistake that most often creates stress. She perceived her financial situation as a threat to her well-being, instead of a challenge. She eventually paid off her credit card debt, but she never achieved balance in her lifestyle, and she slowly regained her weight.

At about the same time that I was treating Darlene, I was also working with another weight-control patient, Thomas, who had even more debt. His small company had gone out of business, saddling him with a lot of debt. However, Thomas had excellent coping skills and just didn't let the debt get him down. He perceived paying it off as the biggest challenge of his life and attacked the problem with gusto. It took him much longer to become debt-free than it did Darlene, but it never encroached upon his lifestyle and never destroyed his diet.

More than anything else, it's our *perceptions* that cause stress.

There are a few fundamental ways to help perceive stressors as challenges, instead of threats. If you work these methods into your life, you'll probably feel a lot less stress and will enjoy a much healthier, more balanced lifestyle. The three fundamental coping skills that I most often recommend are *control, support,* and *release*.

Control is vitally important; feeling as if you're in control of a stressor is the best way to make it feel like a challenge, instead of a threat.

There are a number of ways to feel in control. One of the best is simply to realize that you can *never* control every outside force, but that you can almost *always* control how you react to those forces internally. The next time you have a stressor that feels beyond your control, focus on changing the way you *feel* about it.

Another great way to stay in control of your life is simply to tell people how you really feel about some problem that they may be causing you. Don't aggressively *blame* them, or they'll get defensive. Just tell them you've got a problem and ask politely for their help. You'll be amazed at how much people will want to co-operate with you when you're honest and straightforward.

It's also important to give a lot of thought to what you *most* want, and stop worrying about controlling the little things that don't matter much. Figure out what your bottom-line desires are and put your energy into achieving them. In essence, don't sweat the small stuff.

Lastly, don't be afraid to fail. The path to every major achievement is littered with small setbacks.

Support is also an excellent stress-buster, because having a support system of friends and family helps people feel far more confident about dealing with their stressors. When people have that terrible, lonely feeling of 'me against the world,' every minor stressor can feel like a threat. The support of other people, though, makes people feel protected.

Often, people think that not asking for help makes them stronger. In regard to health and well-being, though, this isn't true. Being overly self-reliant makes people far more prone to illness. One study, for example, showed that people who had no support system of good friends or family were three times more likely to die from illness than people who felt supported.

Even talking to strangers about your problems can help. A study of people who told strangers about their problems showed that these people had significantly lower levels of stress hormones than people who kept their problems to themselves.

Having a pet can also help. Many studies have shown that people with pets are less prone to stress, and have notably less incidence of stress-related illness than people who don't have pets.

Release is also vital for keeping stressors from becoming stress. When you feel stressed, let it out. If you hold in your reactions to stressors, the stressors may begin to feel far more oppressive than they really are. But if you let yourself release the tension that stressors may cause, the tension will be far less likely to mount up and turn into full-blown, chronic stress.

One of the best ways to release stress is with physical activity. The human body is naturally designed to react to stress with the fight-or-flight response, characterized by increased heart rate and increased energy to the muscles. Therefore, it makes sense to burn off this extra energy with activity. If you just sit on your feeling of physical agitation, your body will suffer. People who internalize stress, instead of releasing it, often develop problems such as ulcers and heart disease.

Another great form of release is to vent your frustration verbally. You can let go of stress by talking, crying, or yelling. Just be careful not to direct your verbal venting at another person, or you'll just make your problems worse by creating conflict. Be sensitive and treat people with respect. Venting is just as effective when you're alone.

That's the best possible advice I can offer about overcoming stress. This advice was gleaned from a large number of the best current books about stress, as well as from the experiences I've had in my own clinical practice and the advice I've received from other health professionals.

If you make the effort to integrate this advice into your life, you'll probably be far less vulnerable than ever before to the forces that made you overeat due to stress.

As you can see, the Balance Programme is simply good sense and good science. The hard part isn't understanding it – it's *doing* it.

In the past, achieving a balanced lifestyle might have been practically impossible for you, because food reactions were constantly wrecking the balance in your life by triggering your food cravings, draining your energy, and ruining your mood. *But those days are over.*

Now you have the best opportunity in your life to achieve true balance. Make the most of it! The more you do it, the easier it will get!

This is the end. In this book, I've told you more about weight control than I am ever able to tell any patient during an individual series of consultations.

If you've been reading carefully, you probably now have more knowledge about food reactions and weight gain than do many doctors. Knowledge is power. Thus, knowledge about food is *power over food*.

No-one can ever take this knowledge away from you – and no-one can take this power. It's yours to use for the rest of your life. This knowledge will make the rest of your life easier. You'll no longer be fighting in the dark against forces you don't understand.

I congratulate you on gaining this knowledge and this power. I know that some of this material was technical, but you stuck with it. That shows how much you want to succeed.

Now that you have the knowledge to make this success possible, nothing is going to stop you. Your new life has already begun.

SAMPLE MENU PLAN FOR
THE BALANCE PROGRAMME

YOUR OWN INDIVIDUALIZED BALANCE PROGRAMME DIET will naturally emerge from your elimination diet as you continue to avoid the foods you react to. Your long-term Balance Programme Diet will consist, quite simply, of *all the healthy, nutritious foods that do not cause you to react*.

Of course, if you have determined your food reactions with a blood test, you'll have a head start on knowing which foods to avoid. Nonetheless, people who do a blood test should still be very alert for reactions, because frequently blood tests are not 100 per cent accurate.

Your Balance Programme Diet will serve you well for the rest of your life. From time to time, you may need to adjust it somewhat, because food reactions tend to come and go.

The most sensible approach is just to pay attention to how various foods affect you. After you eat something, ask yourself: 'How did that make me feel?'

The Balance Programme Diet can begin *anytime after you have cleansed your body and then determined your food reactions*. As a rule, this is approximately 3 weeks after beginning the False Fat Diet. By this time, you may have determined most or all of your reactions. You will also have progressed through the Cleansing Phase and False Fat Week.

The following sample menu for the Balance Programme Diet *consists of about 2,300–2,400 calories per day*. This number is appropriate only for the *average* person, though – and it's extremely possible that you are not average. If you are tall or large-framed or very active, you may need to eat *more* calories. If you're short or small-framed or inactive, you may need to eat *fewer* calories.

Furthermore, in your first few weeks or months on the False Fat Diet, if you want to keep losing adipose tissue, you may need to eat somewhat *less* than 2,300–2,400 calories. Remember, about 500 calories a day calculates to one pound a week (3,500 calories). Therefore, if you maintain your weight with 2,500 daily calories, you will drop about one pound weekly on 2,000 calories, given the same activity level. After you've reached your goal weight, though, you may be able to eat the 2,300–2,400 calorie diet, or even more without gaining weight.

Ultimately, though, you should not depend on *any* mathematical formula of calorie consumption or energy expenditure for weight control. Instead, you should simply pay close attention to how your body feels and looks. If you start to gain weight, *cut back on food or exercise more*, or do both. If you start to get too thin or too low on energy, *add* some foods to your diet, especially vital and energizing foods like fresh juices, vegetables, and nuts.

The following menu guideline is less restrictive than the elimination diet menu plans, but is still generally free from the most commonly reactive foods. However, if you are reactive to a food in this menu plan, replace it with another food or another, similar recipe. And overall, try to rotate your foods as best as you can to reduce new reactions. It is wise to skip at least one day between eating the same foods, while the classic allergy avoidance diet focuses on a 4-day rotation programme.

SAMPLE MENU
THE BALANCE PROGRAMME DIET
DAY 1

Breakfast
- Fruit salad, 3–5 varieties, with yogurt dressing (or apple juice or other sauce, if you avoid dairy products), and 5–10 cashews or almonds
- Rice cake, with 1 tsp apple butter

- Hot herbal or green tea

Snack
- Almonds or almond milk (225 ml) or an apple

Lunch
- Grilled chicken breast, with onion and pineapple slices (cold or hot)
- Rye bread (1 slice), with 1 tsp non-dairy butter (or butter if tolerated)
- Green salad, with 1 tbsp Avocado Dressing (see page 283)

Snack
- Frozen fruit juice bar or apple or pear
- Iced herbal tea

Dinner
- Baked or sautéed Red Snapper on Black Bean Relish (see page 301) or fish or choice
- Herbed Couscous Salad (see page 338)
- Braised or steamed asparagus with garlic and pepper
- Sliced tomatoes, with dill, pepper and salt

Snack
- Blackberry pie (see non-wheat pie crust, page 346) or a simpler apple and date

Day 2

Breakfast
- Hot cereal (rice, oatmeal, buckwheat, or any non-reactive grain), with 1 tbsp honey or maple syrup and 1 tsp non-dairy butter or flaxseed oil with sliced banana, apple or fruit of choice.
- Hot herbal tea

Snack
- Corn bread (4-inch square), with 1 tsp non-dairy butter

Lunch
- Rich Veggie Soup (see page 329) or Broccoli Soup (see page 330)
- Rice cake, with almond butter
- Green salad with 1 tbsp Italian dressing or vinaigrette

Snack
- Walnuts or cashews (7–10)
- Vegetable juice

Dinner
- Roasted Sirloin of Beef with Herbed Baby Potatoes (see page 313), or vegetarian entree (Blackened Tofu Steaks, page 316)
- Green salad with sliced avocado and tomato, with Basil Balsamic Vinaigrette (see page 331)

Snack
- Ice cream (non-dairy), sprinkled with crushed walnuts

Day 3

Breakfast
- Pancakes (from a non-wheat mix) (4 pancakes), with 1–2 tbsp maple syrup, 1 tsp non-dairy butter, and 2–3 tbsp fruit compote
- Hot herbal tea

Snack
- Frozen banana, dipped in carob or chocolate powder, coated with crushed almonds, or plain banana

Lunch
- Turkey salad (turkey strips on a bed of lettuce, tomatoes, sliced cucumbers, shredded carrots, and other fresh salad vegetables), topped with 2 tbsp Avocado Dressing (see page 332) or a few slices avocado with some lemon and olive oil
- Toasted spelt bread, with 1 tsp non-dairy butter
- Iced herbal tea

Snack
- Carrot sticks (5–6)
- Carrot juice (225 ml)

Dinner
- Barbecued chicken, with tomato-based barbecue sauce or baked with mushrooms, olive and garlic (2 pieces)
- Baked potato, with 1 tbsp non-dairy butter, salt, and tamari
- Mushrooms sautéed in olive oil and fresh garlic
- Green salad, with 1 tbsp vinaigrette

Snack
- Cashew or Almond Butter Cookies (2) (see page 346)
- Hot nut milk (170 ml)

Day 4

Breakfast
- Melon (e.g., honeydew, cantaloupe) (¼ melon) (wait 20 minutes before you eat other food)
- Rice cake (1–2) with 1 tbsp cashew butter or natural peanut butter, and 1–2 tsp all-fruit spread
- Hot herbal tea

Snack
- Banana Bread (see page 345)
- Milk (non-dairy) (225 ml)

Lunch
- Spiced Butternut Squash Bisque (420 ml) (see page 328)
- Bread (non-wheat) (1 slice), with 1 tsp non-dairy or almond butter
- Green salad, with 1 tbsp oil and vinegar dressing
- Iced herbal tea

Snack
- Apple (1)
- Almonds (8–10)

Dinner
- Stone-Ground Mustard Rubbed Rack of Lamb with Roasted Garlic Potato Hash (see page 311), or substitute a vegetarian or fish entree or Fusilli with Fresh Tomatoes and Basil Sauce (see page 316)
- Braised broccoli, with chopped red onion, and basil
- Green salad, with 1 tbsp Basil Balsamic Vinaigrette (see page 331)

Snack
- Ice cream (non-dairy) with 1 tsp natural chocolate sauce (optional)

Day 5

Breakfast
- Waffles (from non-wheat mix) (2 waffles), with 1–2 tbsp maple syrup and 1–2 tsp butter or butter substitute, sprinkled with 5–7 crushed nuts of your choice or a slice banana
- Hot herbal tea

Snack
- An apple or other fruit, or 1–2 rice cakes with 1 tbsp natural chunky peanut butter and 1–2 tsp all-fruit spread
- Hot mint tea

Lunch
- Beef barley soup (420 ml), or vegetable soup (see Rich Veggie Soup, page 329)
- Green salad, with 1 tbsp Avocado Dressing (see page 332) or other dressing.
- Bread (from spelt, or other non-reactive flour), with 1 tsp non-dairy butter

Snack
- Courgette Cake (1 piece) (see page 345)

Dinner
- Roast duck (or chicken) with orange or apricot sauce, or Pasta with Courgettes (see page 317)
- New potatoes, boiled with pearl onions and parsley (don't have potatoes if you have pasta)
- Greek salad, with feta cheese (optional) with olive oil and lemon dressing

Snack
- Cherry Cobbler (see page 348), or 1 apple and 2 dates
- Hot herbal tea

Day 6

Breakfast
- Cold cereal (non-wheat, if reactive), with milk (non-dairy, if reactive), 1–2 date sugar or honey, and fruit slices
- Hot herbal tea

Snack
- Hot cider
- Toasted hazelnuts (10)

Lunch
- Sautéed chicken and asparagus with mushrooms, seasoned with salt, garlic, and coarse black pepper (optional)
- Toast (non-wheat, if reactive), with 1 tsp non-dairy butter
- Green salad, with 1 tbsp Italian dressing
- Iced herbal tea

Snack
- Orange, apple, or banana

Dinner
- Quinoa and Prawn or Bay Shrimp Salad with Lemon Pepper Vinaigrette (see page 303)
- Salad greens and Beetroot with Orange Vinaigrette (see page 321)
- Hot mint tea

Snack
- Brownie (from non-wheat mix), topped with 1 scoop of non-dairy ice cream

Day 7

Breakfast
- Fruit smoothie (blended with yogurt, if non-reactive, or banana and rice milk)
- Rice cake (1), with 1 tbsp cashew butter or natural peanut butter
- Hot herbal tea

Snack
- Honey and Chilli Roasted Hazelnuts (35 g) (see page 340)

Lunch
- Rainbow Rice (see page 326)
- Baked butternut squash (¼ squash) with olive oil and honey glaze
- Strawberry Yogurt Freeze (see page 344)

Dinner
- Etouffade de Boeuf Bourguignonne (see page 314) or Sea Bass en Papillotte (see page 309) or vegetarian entree, such as Tofu Brochettes (see page 317) or Pasta with Courgettes (see page 317)
- Garden Tomatoes with Balsamic Vinaigrette (see page 319)
- Mushrooms sautéed in tamari, olive oil, and black or red pepper
- Mashed potatoes

Snack
- Chocolate ice cream (non-dairy), sprinkled with crushed almonds or a piece of fruit if still full from dinner

PART THREE

WHAT TO EAT

This part has two sections:

- *The Food Reaction Reference Guide*, a simple set of lists that will help you decide the foods you should avoid and the foods you should eat.
- *The False Fat Diet Recipes*, a special collection of some of the finest non-reactive recipes ever assembled.

This part of the book will give you the details you need to succeed. This is a reference resource, so you don't need to read through it in order. Just flip through it, and find the facts you need to know.

Happy hunting.

FOOD REACTION REFERENCE GUIDE

FOLLOWING IS A SERIES OF LISTS THAT WILL HELP YOU determine what to eat, and what not to eat. The first series of lists covers the most commonly reactive foods and the food products in which they are often hidden. After that you'll find lists of food families, lists of substitutes for wheat, dairy, and sugar, special information about avoiding yeast overgrowth, and other pertinent information.

Don't try to memorize any of these lists. There's no need to. Just consult them when you need them. They're here for your convenience.

The Most Commonly Reactive Foods

The Sensitive Seven
1. Dairy products
2. Wheat
3. Corn
4. Eggs
5. Soya
6. Peanuts
7. Sugar

The Other Usual Suspects
Gluten (present in wheat, rye, barley, oats, spelt and kamut)
Rye
Oats
Shrimp and other shellfish (crab)
Chocolate
Yeast
Tomatoes
Potatoes
Aspartame

Citrus fruits
Monosodium glutamate (MSG)
Additives, including dyes,
    sulphites, and other
    preservatives

Coffee
Beer and wine
Cocktail mixes, such
    margaritas

Occasionally Reactive Foods

Bacon and other pork
    products
Cinnamon
Mustard
Grapes and raisins
Berries, especially strawberries
Onions
Nuts
Beef
Peas
Coconut
Vinegar
Bananas
Celery

Various spices, including
cloves, curry, and turmeric
Green and red peppers
Quinoa
Pineapple
Cherries
Mushrooms
Plums
Barley
Melon
Chicken
Kidney beans
Black pepper

The Good Guys: Foods that are Seldom Reactive

Rice
Pears
Lamb
Kale
Salmon and other ocean fish
    such as halibut or sole
Trout
Turkey
Rabbit
Sweet potatoes
Honey

Cabbage
Carrots
Cauliflower
Broccoli
Beetroot
Apricots
Cranberries
Squash
Olive oil, olives
Herbal teas
Tapioca

Sources of the Sensitive Seven

Following are various foods, dishes, and food products that contain the Sensitive Seven most commonly reactive foodstuffs. If you are reactive to a Sensitive Seven food, you should avoid anything that contains it.

Wheat

The following contain at least some wheat. Most breads contain wheat, even if they are labelled as rye bread or oat bread. Buy breads labelled 'wheat free.'

White flour and bread
Whole wheat flour and bread
Graham flour and bread
Cornflour and bread
Rye flour and bread
Pumpernickel flour and bread
Many cereals, including:
   Cream of wheat cereals
   Bran cereals
   Shredded wheat cereals
   Grape-nut cereals
   Puffed wheat cereals
   Wheat flake cereals
   Granola cereals
   Cornflake cereals
   Crispy rice cereals
Matzos
Cakes (most)
Ice cream cones
Cookies/Biscuits
Candy bars (some)
Vermicelli
Noodles
Dumplings
Pies with standard crust
Doughnuts

Gravies
Bouillon
Pancakes
Swiss steak
Waffles
Turnovers
Some salad dressings
Creamed soups, including chowders
Batter-coated vegetables
Hot dogs
Bologna
Coffee substitutes
Stuffings in meats (e.g., turkey stuffing)
Croutons
Breadcrumbs
Malted milk
Gin
Ovaltine
Whisky (some)
Pretzels
Sausages
Chilli
Au gratin potatoes
Liverwurst

Macaroni   Beer or malt liquor
Chocolate (read label)   Rolls

Various forms of wheat, listed on food labels, may include farina, semolina, wheat germ, durum, couscous, and bran.

Corn

The following may contain at least some corn, cornmeal, corn syrup or cornflour.

Many baking mixes, including pancake and doughnut mixes

Corn syrup (in hundreds of packaged and processed foods)

Cornflour

Prepared meats, including
   Bacon
   Sausages
   Bologna
   Hot dogs
   Cured ham
   Batter-coated meats

Margarine

Ice cream (with corn syrup)

Jelly and jam (with corn syrup)

Gelatin desserts (some)

Ale, beer, gin, whisky

French dressing

Crackers (some)

Crisps (corn crisps)

Frostings (some)

Foods fried in corn oil

Grape juice (with corn syrup), and other juices with corn syrup

Graham crackers

Icing

Creamed soups

Vegetable soups (most)

Syrup (containing corn syrup)

Tortillas

Vinegar (distilled)

Sherbet (with corn syrup)

Sauces (with corn syrup or corn oil)

Popcorn

Fritters

Cream puffs

Carbonated soft drinks (with corn syrup)

Many cereals, including:
   Cornflake cereals
   Round oat cereals
   Cornmeal cereals
   Puffed corn cereals

Ketchup (with corn syrup)

Shrimp sauce (with corn syrup)

Cookies (some)

Cheese (some)

Candy (many sweets use corn syrup)

Cake (some)

Chow mein (with cornflour)

Cream pies (some)
Salad dressings (with corn oil
  or syrup)
Puddings (some)
Peanut butter (some)

Egg nog
Chop suey (with cornflour)
Enchiladas
Burritos
Tamales

Various forms of corn listed on food labels include corn syrup, cornflour, corn oil, and cornmeal.

Eggs
The following may contain at least some egg. Be especially wary of eggs in baked goods and desserts.

Waffles
Pancakes
French toast
Salad dressing (some)
Mayonnaise
Tartar sauce
Hollandaise sauce
Meat loaf
Batters for frying
Bouillon cubes or powder
Meringue
Spaghetti
Soups (some, including noodle
  soups)
Breads (many)
Cake (most)
Icing (most)
Soufflés
Pretzels

Pudding
Fritters
Sherbets (many)
Sausages
Custard
Cookies/Biscuits (most)
Macaroni
Ice cream
Marshmallows
Sauces (some)
Noodles
Pie fillings (some)
Omelettes
Muffins
Candy/Sweets (some)
Dumplings
Doughnuts
Croquettes

Various forms of eggs listed on food labels include the protein allergens ovomucin, albumin, ovomucoid, livetin, vitellin, and ovovitellin.

Soya

The following may contain at least some soya. Be alert for foods containing soya sauce or tamari.

Miso
Processed cheese
Soya sauce
Tamari
Worcestershire sauce
Sausage and bologna (some
Salad dressings and mayonnaise (some)
Coffee substitutes (some)
Bean curd
Soya sprouts (in Chinese restaurants)
Soya milk
Hamburger bulking agents
Protein powder and protein supplements
Sherbet (some
Hard candy/sweets (some)
Tofu
Margarine (many)
Caramels (some
Lecithin supplements
Crackers (some)

Various forms of soya listed on food labels include soya oil, lecithin, tamari, soya protein isolate, and soya flour.

Milk and Dairy Products

The following often contain at least some milk. Milk is also present in many baked goods.

Butter
Buttermilk
Yogurt
Malted milk
Milkshakes
Ice cream
Pancakes, waffles, French toast
Biscuits
Cookies/Biscuits (many)
Creamed foods
White sauce
Salad dressing (cheeses)
Mashed potatoes
Bologna
Margarine
Cake (most)
Bread (some)
Creamed soups and chowders
Omelettes
Candy/sweets (some)
Gravy (some)
Soufflés
Ovaltine
Cheese
Chocolate (except bitter chocolate)
Cream cheese
Whipped cream

Various forms of milk listed on food labels may include whey, casein, lactose, curds, lactalbumin, dried milk solids, sodium caseinate, calcium caseinate, and potassium caseinate.

Sugar

The following may contain at least some sugar.

Cereals, including most cold breakfast cereals, such as:
Cornflakes
Crispy rice
Bran flakes
Almost all 'children's' cereals, such as frosted cornflakes
Chocolate syrup
Prepared meats, packaged and frozen
Flavoured yogurts
Processed cheese sauce
Peanut butter (many)
Ketchup
Canned soup
Salad dressings (many)
Cookies/Biscuits (most)
Cake
Candy/Sweets
Ice cream
Jelly, jam
Canned fruits (most)
Fruit juices (many)
Rum
Custard
Fizzy drinks (unless diet)
Biscuits
Liqueurs
Syrups (most)
Bread (some)
Desserts (most)
Canned vegetables (many)
Hot dogs

Various forms of sugar listed on food labels include molasses, corn syrup, rice sugar, succinate, turbinado sugar, brown sugar, cane sugar, beet sugar, sucrose, and glucose.

Peanuts

The following may contain at least some peanuts.

Any food cooked in peanut oil (especially common in Chinese restaurants)
Peanut butter
Certain Asian dishes, such as Pad Thai salad, Kung Pao chicken, and curries and other sauces
Peanut brittle
Peanut butter cookies
Candy/Sweets

Food Families

Every food belongs to a family of similar foods. For example, turkey, chicken, and duck are all in the poultry family. If you are reactive to a certain food, you might also be reactive to its family members. If you have an *especially strong* reaction to a certain food, you will be more likely to react to other foods in that food's family.

Some people find that they must avoid entire families of foods. Other people with food reactions find that they must avoid only one or two members of the same food family. Many others with food reactions, however, do not react at all to other members of a food family.

In general, people tolerate foods better if they do not eat various foods from the same family day after day, *every single day*. For example, if a person eats prunes (from the plum family) on Monday, he or she should usually try to avoid other members of the plum family on Tuesday, Wednesday, or Thursday. Thus, it would be a mistake to eat cherries on Tuesday, peaches on Wednesday, and nectarines on Thursday since all these fruits are in the plum family.

It's wise to wait at least a couple of days before eating another food from the same family. In other words, rotate food families as well as individual foods. This will not only decrease existing food reactions, but will also help prevent new food reactions.

Following are the families of foods.

Dairy Food Family   Cow's milk, and all foods derived from cow's milk, such as cheese, yogurt, and cottage cheese (butter tends to be somewhat less reactive, because it is relatively low in milk proteins; it's pure fat)

Poultry Family   Chicken, turkey, capon, grouse, duck, pheasant, goose, and partridge

Mollusc Family   Clam, oyster, scallop, mussel, squid, and abalone

Crustacean Family   Crab, shrimp, lobster and crayfish

Fish Family   Trout, tuna, halibut, red snapper, sole, salmon, sardine, haddock, whitefish, flounder, and herring (these finned fish have a similar protein that may cause cross-reactions)

Plum Family Plum, prune, cherry, almond, nectarine, apricot, and peach

Citrus Family Grapefruit, lemon, lime, tangerine, kumquat, and orange

Apple Family Apple, pear, and quince

Rose Family Strawberry, blackberry, loganberry, and raspberry

Heath Family Blueberry and cranberry

Banana Family Arrowroot, banana, and plantain

Papaya Family Papaya

Grape Family Grape, raisin, and buckthorn tea

Pineapple Family Pineapple

Gluten Grain Family Wheat, rye, oats, and barley

Corn Family Corn and popcorn

Rice Family White rice, brown rice, basmati, and Patna rice

Buckwheat Family Buckwheat, rhubarb, and sorrel

Walnut Family Butternut, hickory nut, walnut, and pecan

Sunflower Family Jerusalem artichoke, safflower, and sunflower

Legume Family Beans and peas, alfalfa sprouts, green bean, lentils, black-eyed bean, peanut, licorice, acacia, and senna

Mustard Family Mustard, cabbage, spring greens, cauliflower, broccoli, Brussels sprouts, turnip, kale, kohlrabi, radish, horseradish, and watercress (the *cruciferous* members, of this family are cabbage, cauliflower, broccoli, Brussels sprouts, and kohlrabi)

Composite Flower Family Lettuce (leaf, head), endive, chicory, artichoke, and dandelion

Lily Family Asparagus, onion, garlic, chive, green onion, leek, spring onion, shallot, and aloe vera

Parsley Family Parsley, parsnip, carrot, celery, caraway, anise, dill, fennel, and coriander

Nightshade/Potato Family Potato, tomato, aubergine, peppers (bell, red, green, chilli, cayenne), tomatillo, pimento, and tobacco

Morning Glory Family Sweet potato and yam

Goosefoot Family Beetroot, spinach, chard and Swiss chard

Gourd Family   Cantaloupe, melon, cucumber, pumpkin, and summer and winter squash
Laurel Family   Avocado, cinnamon, and bay leaf
Olive Family   Green olive and black olive
Fungi Family   Mushrooms and brewer's and baker's yeast
Chocolate Family   Chocolate and cocoa
Cane Family   Cane sugar, molasses, and sorghum
Honey Family   Bee pollen, royal jelly, and honey

Substitutes for Reactive Staples

Many people must avoid reactive foods that are staples in their diets, particularly wheat, cow's milk and sugar. A number of excellent substitutes are available.

Following are brief descriptions of these substitutes.

Wheat Substitutes

Many varieties of flour may be used in place of wheat flour. Following are some of the most popular wheat flour substitutes. Many of these grains may also be eaten directly (as 'whole grains'), rather than used as flour, by cooking them (at a slow simmer) with two parts water to one part grain.

If you react to wheat, you may also react to spelt and kamut, which are similar to wheat, or to oats, rye, and barley, which contain gluten.

Spelt is an ancient form of wheat that is widely used for baking. It is in the same family as wheat, so sometimes it is not tolerated by people with wheat reactions. Also, it contains gluten, which causes reactions in some people. Baked goods made from spelt tend to be more crumbly than those made from wheat, so extra oil may be needed. Spelt is good for pancakes, pasta, and a wide variety of foods that usually contain wheat.

Kamut (pronounced 'kuh-*moot*') is related to wheat, but for some people it is a good wheat substitute for baking. It is more cohesive than many other wheat substitutes and is therefore suitable for making pasta. It has more nutrients than wheat, and does contain gluten.

Rice is a staple throughout most of the world, and produces a richly textured flour that can be excellent for baking. Some people find the texture too gritty, but it can work well in cookies and brownies.

Amaranth flour is gluten-free and is fine for baking. It is available in some packaged products, such as crackers. Amaranth tastes best if you buy it from a shop that refrigerates it and if you continue to refrigerate it at home. It mixes well with other foods and browns quickly as a breading. When baking with it, try using 25 per cent amaranth combined with 75 per cent rice flour (or oat flour).

Quinoa (pronounced '*keen*-wa') is a light, pleasant whole grain and flour that makes fluffy pastries, cakes and pancakes. It's low in gluten and easy to digest. A staple of the Incas, it is extremely nutritious and has more protein than any other grain. It's good for mixing into casseroles and other dishes.

Arrowroot is a fine white powder that resembles cornflour. It's great as a thickening agent in soups or cooked dishes, in place of wheat flour or cornflour. It has very little flavour, so it won't disturb the taste of the dishes in which you use it. For baking, use 25 per cent arrowroot, combined with 75 per cent of other non-wheat flours.

Buckwheat sounds as if it's a form of wheat, but it's not. It's actually a seed that is related to rhubarb. Popular for pancakes, it has a distinctive flavour. It can be used in noodles and is generally well tolerated by people who react to wheat.

Teff is an African grain, now more available, that is used for flour. It can be used in most baked goods, and is also often added to soups, stews and puddings. It has a rather sweet taste and a slightly rough texture.

Tapioca is well known as a pudding ingredient and can also be used as a thickener.

Millet is a high-protein grain that has a rather bland flavour. It is not ideal for baking because it's too crumbly. It can be good in casseroles or mixed with vegetables. It's a little like couscous.

Rye is a popular grain for bread, although most rye breads contain wheat. Bread made solely from rye is very dense, but tastes good to most people. It does contain gluten.

Oats are used to make a flour that is rich, heavy, and suitable for baking. Plain oats can also be added to casseroles or stews, instead of wheat. Oat flour is one of the best non-wheat baking flours, and can constitute 75 per cent to 100 per cent of the flour in a baking recipe. It's often used for cookies/biscuits and pancakes, and can be blended into soups to make milk-free 'cream' soups. It contains gluten.

Barley is commonly used in soups, but can also be made into a light white flour that is excellent for baking, or for adding to other dishes. It makes a good pie crust. It contains gluten and can take longer to cook than other grains.

Dairy Product Substitutes

Goat's milk can generally be tolerated by people who react to cow's milk. Some people, however, react to both goat's milk and cow's milk. Goat's milk tends to have a stronger, more distinctive flavour than the more bland cow's milk. It can be used for virtually anything that cow's milk is used for. The fat globules in goat's milk are smaller than those in cow's milk, and this makes goat's milk easier to digest. Many grocery stores and most health shops stock goat's milk. Fresh goat's milk is somewhat harder to find than dry, powdered goat's milk. It can be better for infants than other milk substitutes.

Soya milk is a popular milk substitute that does not have the heavier, more distinctive flavour found in goat's milk. A variety of types are available, such as vanilla-flavoured soya milk or chocolate soya milk. Soya milk can be used in almost all the ways that cow's milk is used. The various commercial brands have a wide variety of tastes, so you may want to try several brands to find the one you like best. I recommend organic soya milk, to reduce exposure to genetically engineered soya beans.

Rice milk is fairly similar to soya milk and is appropriate for people who react to both soya and dairy products. It is available at practically all health food shops.

Nut milk is somewhat less commercially available than goat's milk, soya milk, or rice milk, but various brands can be found at some health food shops. Nut milk is creamy and satisfying, but it does not taste as much like cow's milk as other milks do. Many people make their own nut milk by blending 90 to 120 g of almonds, cashews or hazelnuts with twice that amount of water, ¼ teaspoon of vanilla, and 1 teaspoon of honey or maple syrup. Toasted nuts usually lend a richer flavour than raw nuts.

Oat milk has recently become available and is generally thicker and richer than some of the other 'milks.'

Soya ice cream is surprisingly delicious. It has a slightly different taste than milk-based ice cream, but many people like this taste as much as that of standard ice cream. Soya ice cream is sweet, rich, and smooth in texture. Like regular ice cream, however, it's high in calories, so it must be eaten in moderation. Many of my patients, though, find it easy to eat soya ice cream in moderation, because it doesn't trigger the food cravings that standard ice cream often does. Soya ice cream is available in almost all health food stores and many grocery shops.

Rice ice cream is similar to soya ice cream and just as good. It's sweet, creamy, and filling, and it tastes substantially like regular ice cream. It's good by itself or as a topping for desserts. Like soya ice cream, rice ice cream can be high in calories, so it must be eaten in moderation even though it is lower in fat.

Sorbet, sherbet, and fruit ices are all good ice cream substitutes. A wide variety of flavours are available. However, sometimes these products contain some milk, so it's wise to ask if a brand is dairy-free before buying it. Most brands may contain corn syrup or sugar.

Non-dairy margarines are available at virtually all grocery shops. Many of the low-calorie brands use soya instead of milk. Non-dairy brands include Weight Watchers. These products tend to be less rich, creamy and sweet than real butter, but they are also lower in calories than real butter. Many margarines, though, including some of the low-calorie brands, still contain saturated fat and should be used in strict moderation. Many margarines also contain yellow dye. Most other types of margarine are hydrogenated, and this makes them particularly unhealthy. Avoid all hydrogenated margarines. For cooking, it is best to not use butter substitutes, but to use oils, such as olive oil or sunflower oil.

Non-dairy yogurts, cheeses, and sour cream are available, and some of them are tasty and satisfying. Because individual tastes vary so much, it is often hard for me to predict which of these non-dairy products patients will like, so I generally advise people to simply experiment with various non-dairy products to see which ones they enjoy. Examples of these types of products include tofu sour cream, soya cheese, soya yogurt, and certain cheeses made from seeds and nuts. Virtually all health food shops carry a variety of these products.

Sugar Substitutes

Honey is generally less reactive than cane sugar, which comes from a grass related to wheat, or beet sugar, which comes from a vegetable. Honey is about twice as sweet as sugar, so if you're cooking with it, you can usually use half as much honey as you would sugar. Honey is high in calories, so don't overdo it.

Maple syrup is a good natural sweetener, but it is approximately 60 per cent sucrose and should therefore be used sparingly. Some maple syrups, however, contain corn syrup or cane sugar, and some are just sugared syrup with maple flavour. Pure maple syrups are free from added sugar, but may have been processed with formaldehyde; to avoid this chemical, buy maple syrup imported from Canada, which does not allow the use of formaldehyde in the extraction process.

Rice syrup is a good alternative for people who react to cane or beet sugar. It is a potent sweetener, however, and can therefore destabilize blood sugar levels. Even so, it has less of this effect than sugar, honey, or maple syrup. Rice syrup is somewhat less sweet than most other sugar substitutes, but is still high in calories and should be used in moderation.

Date sugar is more nutritionally complete than other sweeteners, because it is made from whole, dried dates. It has a pleasant, rich taste and is high in fibre. It doesn't dissolve, but is a good topping. Like virtually all sweeteners, it's high in calories.

Raw sugar, turbinado sugar, and molasses are all derived from cane sugar, and should generally be avoided, or used in very small quantities. They are less refined than white sugar, but have similar metabolic effects. Blackstrap molasses actually has some nutrients from the sugar cane, including iron.

Artificial sweeteners, including aspartame and saccharin, may be acceptable for some people, but are disastrous for others, due to their relatively high degree of reactivity. Aspartame, in particular, cannot be adequately metabolized by a relatively large number of people; it often causes headaches and other food reaction symptoms. In fact, 75 per cent of all FDA non-drug complaints are about aspartame. Because of this, and because the long-term effects of these sweeteners are unknown, I generally do not recommend them.

The Anti-Yeast Diet

The following foods contain yeast or yeast-like substances, or encourage the growth of yeast. They should be avoided or eaten in very limited amounts by people who are prone to candida yeast overgrowth. Candida is very common, so be wary of these foods and alert for candida symptoms. For other details and treatments of candida, see Chapters 4 and 5.

Primary Yeast-increasing Foods
- The worse offenders are foods containing *both* sweeteners (sugar, honey, jam, etc.), *and* yeast (baked goods, etc.). For example, breads, cakes, biscuits, cookies, pastries, pancakes, waffles, etc.
- Foods containing sweeteners, such as candy, pie, pudding, ice cream, etc.
- Foods containing yeast, such as breads, crackers, rolls, beer, etc.

Secondary Yeast-increasing Foods

These are foods that stimulate and support yeast growth.

Beer, especially fermented with yeast

Wine and other fermented beverages, including brandy, rum, whisky, and vodka

Cheese (fermented)

Mushrooms

Sour cream

Buttermilk

Ginger ale

Malted products, including candy, cereals, and malted milk

Vinegar, and vinegar foods, including:

Pickles

Ketchup

Sauerkraut

Salad dressings

Barbecue sauce

Olives

Mustard

Dried fruits

Fruit juices, especially citrus

Teas

Antibiotics, steroids, and birth control pills are major causal factors in yeast overgrowth. Be alert for yeast overgrowth symptoms whenever you take any antibiotic, including:

• Penicillins, ampicillins, tetracyclines, and sulpher drugs
• Cephalosporin drugs, such as Keflex
• New classes of strong antibiotics, such as the fluorquinolones and macrolides, which includes Zithromax

Household and environmental moulds are also significant contributors to candida yeast colonization. Take steps to clear them out whenever possible.

If you believe you may suffer from yeast colonization, please review the previous material describing this condition. Also, be sure to take adequate amounts of *probiotics*, such as acidophilus and bifodobacteria. Probiotics are present in cultured yogurts, and can also be ingested in powdered or encapsulated form if you are reactive to yogurt or want higher concentrations.

An Anti-Hypoglycemia Programme

Diet

- Avoid sugars, refined flour products, candies, and other sweetened foods, sodas, alcohol, fruit juices, and dried fruits
- Eat plenty of protein foods: fish, poultry, nuts, seeds, legumes, etc.
- When you consume simple carbohydrate foods or starches such as potatoes or rice (which provide quick-absorbing sugars), eat some protein or oil to slow down the sugar absorption.
- Eat regularly throughout the day, at least every 2 to 3 hours. However, a pure carbohydrate snack, like a fruit, should be followed by some other food within the hour.

Supplements

- B-complex, 25–50 mg, once or twice daily, after breakfast and lunch.
- B_5 (pantothenic acid), 250–500 mg, twice daily, after breakfast and lunch.
- Vitamin C, 500–1,000 mg, 2–3 times daily, after breakfast, lunch and at bedtime.
- Chromium, 100–200 mcg, twice daily, after breakfast and 3 p.m. (after lunch is also OK).

Others

- L-glutamine (for sugar or alcohol cravings), 500 mg 1–2 caps twice daily, after breakfast and dinner, or for cravings.
- Ginseng may be helpful to strengthen the body's systems of balance. Try 250–500 mg, once or twice daily, all before lunch.
- Licorice root supports the adrenals and helps reduce hypoglycemia; 1–2 capsules, twice, daily. Also available as a liquid extract.

Some people prefer a GTF formula (Glucose Tolerance Factor), which contains other ingredients besides chromium, such as niacin, that helps the body utilize sugars.

Medications That May Cause Water Retention

Female hormones
Estrogens, such as Premarin
Progestins, such as Provera

Anti-inflammatories
NSAIDs (nonsteroidal anti-inflammatory drugs) such as ibuprofen, naproxen, Feldene, etc.

Steroids
Anti-inflammatory, anti-allergic and anti-immunologic effects from drugs including prednisone, prednisolone, triamcinolone, dexamethasone, etc.

Most blood pressure medications (anti-hypertensives)
Beta-blockers, such as Inderal
ACE inhibitors
Calcium channel blockers
Vasodilators

Antidepressants
Tricyclics
SSRIs (Selective Serotonin Reuptake Inhibitors), such as Prozac

Antibiotics
Cephalosporins
Acyclovirs

Other Factors That May Cause Water Retention

- Protein deficiency
- Vitamin B_6 deficiency
- Magnesium deficiency

- Excessive caffeine or alcohol consumption, or withdrawal from caffeine or alcohol
- Sugar and salt consumption
- White wheat flour consumption
- Consumption of additives or preservatives

Reactive Food Combinations

Author and clinician Jacqueline Krohn, M.D., has identified various *combinations* of foods that *increase the risk of reactivity*, due to their synergistic chemical compositions, and has described these combinations in *Allergy Relief and Prevention*. Even if you do not react to these foods when you eat them individually, you may react if you eat them together. Thus, it may help to pay attention also when you eat foods in these combinations.

Worst Combinations

Corn	+	Banana
Egg	+	Apple
Beef	+	Yeast
Cane Sugar	+	Orange
Milk	+	Mint
Pork	+	Black Pepper

Other Unwise Combinations

Wheat	+	Tea
Chicken	+	Pork
Chocolate	+	Coffee
Milk	+	Chocolate
Cola	+	Chocolate
Cola	+	Coffee

Inhalant Allergies That Make Food Reactions Worse

Dr Jacqueline Krohn and other physicians have noted an increase in reactions when patients simultaneously *eat certain foods* and *inhale certain allergens* (or suffer from *specific physical conditions*, such as viral infections). Following are various combinations that appear to increase reactive response. The reactivity of these combinations has not been proven by controlled studies, and probably differs among people. Look at these combinations interactions as information that may help you assess your health and symptoms.

Inhalant Allergen or Physical Condition		Food
Grass pollens	+	Beans, peas, soya, wheat, corn, barley, rye, oats, rice, millet, cooking oils
Dust	+	Oysters, clams, scallops, nuts
Cedar or juniper pollen	+	Beef, yeast
Cottonwood pollen	+	Lettuce
Elm pollen	+	Milk, mint
Oak pollen	+	Eggs, apples
Pecan, hickory pollen	+	Corn, bananas
Ragweed	+	Eggs, dairy products, mint, melons, bananas, lettuce
Sage, mugwort	+	Potatoes, tomatoes, celery
Poison ivy	+	Pork, black pepper
Viral infections	+	Milk, mint, onions, chocolate, nuts
Cystic breast disease	+	Coffee, chocolate, cola
Candida yeast overgrowth	+	Yeast, mushrooms, sugar, vinegar, and other fermented foods

The Most Common Allergenic Chemicals

Environmental substances that cause allergies or sensitivities can *exacerbate food reactions*. Following are the chemicals that most frequently cause allergy-like reactions. Exposure to these substances can increase vulnerability to food reactions.

Chemical	Source
Petrochemicals	Car exhaust, gas or oil furnaces
Formaldehyde	New articles, including new clothing, carpets, paint, cars, or homes; hair gel; wood smoke
Chlorine	Tap water, swimming pools and hot tubs, bleach, household cleaners
Phenol	Perfumes and colognes, newspapers, glue, wood smoke
Ethanol	Car exhaust, perfume, household cleaners, wood smoke
Fluoride	Tap water, toothpaste, fluoride treatments
Benzyl alcohol	Solvents, perfume, artificial flavours
Glycerin	Makeup, soap, lotion, furniture polish

Food Additives That Can Cause Reactions

Sometimes patients mistakenly think they are reactive to foods when they are actually reactive to additives in these foods. Be wary of the following items, which may be listed on food labels.

Additive	Found in
Nitrites and nitrates	Bacon, hot dogs, sausage, bologna
Sulphites	Dried fruits, fresh fruits and vegetables, lettuce, pre-packaged foods and restaurant foods
Sorbic acid	Cheese, icing, dried fruit, dips
Dyes (especially yellow dye #5)	Hundreds of processed coloured foods
Parabens	Jelly, fizzy drinks, pastry, beer, cake, salad dressing
Benzoic acid	Fizzy drinks, fruit juice, margarine, apple cider
Monosodium glutamate (MSG). MSG may also be present in glutamate, hydrolyzed protein, sodium caseinate, calcium caseinate, or yeast extract	Bouillon, Chinese restaurant dishes, chicken broth or flavouring, canned soups, soup mixes, and many other foods
EDTA	Margarine, salad dressing, frozen dinners, and other processed foods
Aspartame	Artificially sweetened foods, sodas
Propyl gallate	Frozen dinners, gravy mix, turkey sausage
Alginates	Ice cream, salad dressing, cheese spread, frozen dinners
Bromates	Baked goods, breadcrumbs, refrigerated dough

Alternate Sources of Calcium

People who react to dairy products may ensure adequate calcium intake with calcium supplementation, or by eating abundant amounts of the following calcium-rich foods.

By comparison to the following foods, 225 ml of whole cow's milk contains 288 mg of calcium.

Food	Milligrams of Calcium
Wild rice (190 g)	30 mg
Spring greens (190 g)	48 mg
Kidney beans (190 g)	50 mg
Green beans (190 g)	58 mg
Sunflower seeds (45 g)	65 mg
Pumpkin seeds (45 g)	71 mg
Chickpeas (190 g)	80 mg
Pinto beans (190 g)	82 mg
Artichoke (190 g)	94 mg
Kale (190 g)	94 mg
Okra (190 g)	100 mg
Swiss chard (70 g)	102 mg
Hazelnuts (45 g)	103 mg
Mustard greens (190 g)	104 mg
Turnip greens (190 g)	106 mg
Sesame seeds or tahini (45 g)	110 mg
Haricot beans (190 g)	128 mg
Blackstrap molasses (15 ml)	137 mg
Almonds (45 g)	150 mg
Lamb (125 g)	232 mg
Sardines (with bones)	240 mg
Broccoli (2 stalks)	250 mg
Tofu (190 g)	258 mg
Sesame butter (60 g)	281 mg
Soya beans (190 g)	460 mg

Other calcium-containing foods include dried apricots and figs, Brazil and other nuts, carob, parsley, and others.

RECISES

H ERE ARE SOME TERRIFIC RECIPES THAT WILL HELP MAKE
your False Fat Diet delicious, satisfying, and interesting.
Many of these are world-class recipes created by French chef
Philippe Boulot, one of the most highly acclaimed and in-
ventive chefs in America who has won a number of national
awards, including recognition as chef of the Restaurant of the
Year by *Esquire* magazine.

Being able to offer you recipes by a famous French chef
clearly indicates, I believe, the uniqueness of the False Fat
Diet. It shows that *success on this diet does not depend upon
deprivation*. You need never again try to live on a 'starvation'
regimen of bland, unsatisfying foods. This diet relies upon
improving *quality* of food, rather than severely restricting
quantity.

Therefore, Chef Boulot has assembled a spectacular array of
recipes, most of which are devoid of commonly reactive foods.
Other supportive recipes come from my previous books, recipe
designer Eleanora Manzolini, and Cameron Stauth with the
help of his mother, Lorraine Stauth.

Chef Boulot has found that a large and ever-increasing
number of patrons of fine dining are now aware of their food
reactions, and insist upon eating dishes that do not contain
frequently reactive foods, such as wheat, dairy products, corn,
or eggs. Therefore, he has learned to adapt his Normandy-
inspired cooking style to the demands of the new breed of
health-savvy gourmands.

Many of these recipes, such as the animal protein and
vegetable dishes are naturally free of reactive foods. They

consist of simple, wholesome ingredients – combined and seasoned brilliantly – that rarely cause reactions. Other recipes are for dishes that often do cause reactions when prepared conventionally, but the offending ingredients have been replaced with healthy substitutes. Because of this careful substitution, you will be able to eat most of these recipes as part of a normal, realistic diet – one you'll be able to stick with. Do be aware that a very few of the recipes do contain some of the Sensitive Seven reactive foods. If you have determined that you *are* reactive to these foods, you'll probably want to avoid these recipes or, where possible, substitute ingredients. Also, those of you watching your salt intake should avoid the salt or use a salt substitute in these recipes. And for those of you familiar with the principles of food combining from my previous books, although these principles may not be as obvious in this book's menus, which focus on food reactions, they are still at work here.

Some of the gourmet recipes will require time and effort, and will appeal to epicures who love to cook, and entertain. Others were specifically designed for the '5-minute chefs' who need to prepare food on the run.

As you settle into your False Fat Diet, you'll probably want to broaden your food preparation repertoire by purchasing a variety of the excellent cookbooks that have been written especially for people with food reactions. My favourites include *Allergy Cooking with Ease* and *The Dairy Free Cookbook*. For access to these cookbooks and others, see Resources and Referrals.

You'll notice that several of these recipes are for beef, pork, or lamb, all of which tend to be relatively low in reactivity. However, I personally do not eat these animal products and have not recommended them in my other books. I am primarily concerned about the chemicals to which animals are often exposed, and also the saturated fat that these meats contain. Both of these factors appear to contribute to certain cancers and to cardiovascular disease. Therefore, you may substitute poultry, fish, or vegetarian dishes for these meats. If you do eat beef, pork or lamb, it's wise to buy organic produce (at least antibiotic- and steroid-free), and to eat them in moderate amounts.

Although our recipes will add zest and culinary richness to your diet, remember that most of your meals probably won't require any recipes at all. Because the False Fat Diet revolves around whole, simple foods, most of your meals will probably consist of ordinary – albeit delicious – whole foods: a piece of nicely seasoned fish; a salad made from juicy, ripe ingredients; a fresh, hot vegetable; and some steamed rice with your favourite seasonings. This is the type of meal anyone can make in just a few minutes. It's healthy, easy and delicious. We have also added some simple recipes for preparing vegetables, fish and poultry.

Ultimately, I think you'll find that the most richly rewarding foods for your palate will be those that are the most simple, fresh and wholesome. This will be especially true after your food cravings fade. Almost all true aficionados of fine food – including, not incidentally, Chef Boulot – find that their deepest appreciation of food lies in the innate quality of the whole food itself, rather than in the complexity of its preparation.

Simple whole foods are not only the most revealing of flavour, but are also the easiest to prepare, the least expensive, and the least likely to cause reactions. In short, when it comes to good food, the simpler the better.

Enjoy the recipes!

Entrees

Fish or Poultry with Vegetables

Begin with the appropriate amounts of fish or poultry for the number of people you wish to serve. Use the fish of your choice – snapper, salmon, halibut, sea bass, or others – or use chicken or turkey breasts. Add the sliced or diced vegetables of your choice, with onions, garlic, carrots and mushrooms being good selections. Since the poultry can dry more easily, you can cut up an onion and put it under the breasts, or moisten a little more with white wine (the alcohol evaporates with cooking). Olive oil, lemon, salt or soya sauce, and other seasonings can be used.

Two Methods of Preparation

1. Baking dish or parchment paper (en papillote)
Place the fish or poultry in a large oven-proof baking dish with cover or parchment paper. Add olive oil and lemon (for fish) and seasonings and then the vegetables. Cover and place in a preheated oven at 350°F, 175°C. Bake for 30 to 45 minutes, or until dish is done. Serve with a fresh salad or some cooked rice.

2. Sauté or pan-sear
You can marinate the strips of poultry or fish in some olive oil, tamari or salt, lemon, and seasonings. Or you crust the fish with a mixture of sea salt, pepper, and grated lemon peel, ideally from organic lemons. To a large iron skillet or wok over medium-high heat, add a little olive oil, broth, or water, and then add small amounts of water as needed. Sauté the fish or poultry on both sides, and add the vegetables as you go, the firmer ones first. Cover if you wish for 5 to 10 minutes to allow the dish to cook throughout and to keep it moist. You can add some water or broth, or keep open if you like it a bit drier.

Flavouring Options
Oriental – soy, ginger, and cayenne
Mediterranean – olive oil, garlic, thyme, rosemary, and majoram
Mexican – coriander, onion, tomato, and chilli or cayenne pepper

Potato-Crusted Salmon
(SERVES 4)

4–6 large potatoes
3 tbsp melted butter, or olive oil
Salt and pepper to taste
4 175 g salmon fillets

Preheat oven to 375°F, 175°C. Peel and cut the potatoes into matchstick-size pieces. Drizzle 2½ tablespoons of butter or olive oil on potatoes, enough to coat them. Season with salt and freshly ground black pepper.

Season the salmon fillets. On medium to medium-high heat, add remaining ½ tablespoon butter or olive oil to non-stick sauté pan. Cover bottom of pan with potatoes. Place salmon flesh side down on the potatoes. Add more potatoes to the top of the fish. Cook until the potatoes begin to crust and brown. Turn and cook 2 or more minutes. Remove and place on a well-oiled baking sheet. Finish cooking in the oven, about 10–20 minutes more, until done.

Red Snapper on Black Bean Relish
(SERVES 4)

Relish
225 g dried black beans
4 spring onions
2 tomatoes
1 tbsp fresh coriander or parsley
2 tbsp olive oil
1 tbsp diced red pepper
1 tbsp diced green pepper
1 tbsp diced yellow or red pepper
¼ cup balsamic vinegar
1 tbsp lime juice
Salt and pepper to taste

Sauce (optional)
6 strands saffron
1 tbsp white wine or vegetable stock
1 egg yolk, or substitute
1 tbsp stone-ground mustard
170 ml olive oil
45 g mashed potatoes
Salt and pepper to taste

Snapper
4 red snapper or other type of fish fillets
Salt and pepper (optional)
1–2 tbsp olive oil

Wash the beans and place in a large saucepan. Cover with cold water and bring to a boil. Remove from heat and let sit for an hour, covered. Return to the heat and simmer until tender.

Trim and slice spring onions thinly. Remove skin from the tomatoes and dice. Remove leaves and chop coriander or parsley. Dice the peppers.

When beans are tender, drain and chill. Combine all the ingredients for the relish. Allow to sit at least overnight for best flavour.

To make the sauce, in a medium-sized bowl, mix the saffron with the white wine. Whisk in the egg yolks and mustard. Gradually add olive oil to yolks. Add the mashed potatoes. Season with salt and pepper.

Remove all small bones from the fish fillets. Season with salt and pepper. Sauté in the olive oil in a large frying pan over a medium heat, skin side down at first, until crispy and brown.

To serve, cover the serving plate with black bean relish. Crisscross a design with the sauce. Place the snapper on top.

Quinoa and Bay Shrimp/Prawn Salad with Lemon Pepper Vinaigrette
(SERVES 4)

    180 g quinoa
    170 ml extra virgin olive oil
    1 tsp garlic, minced
    2 tsp coriander, fresh, chopped
    90 g pine nuts, toasted
    Salt and pepper
    1–2 lemons (56 ml juice and grated peel)
    540–720 g mixed greens
    270–360 g bay shrimp/prawn, cooked and rinsed
    2 chillis (dried)
    6 garlic cloves, peeled
    2 tbsp lime juice, or white wine vinegar
    45–90 g parsley leaves

Thoroughly wash the quinoa. In a medium-sized saucepan, bring 450–560 ml cups of salted water to a boil and add quinoa.

Reduce heat to medium-low and simmer, covered, until liquid is absorbed – approximately 10 to 15 minutes. Quinoa should be translucent and cooked through. Place container in ice water immediately to cool it and stop the cooking process. Coat with 2 tablespoons oil while fluffing with a fork. Add lemon juice and fold in minced garlic, coriander, and pine nuts. Season to taste with salt and pepper.

Make the lemon pepper vinaigrette by combining 56 ml lemon juice and grated peel with 6–7 tablespoons olive oil. Season with salt and pepper. Toss the mixed greens with approximately 1 to 2 tablespoons of vinaigrette, and toss some of the vinaigrette with the bay shrimp/prawn, to taste.

In a dish or mould, layer the quinoa mixture alternately with the lemon pepper bay shrimp/prawn. Chill until ready to serve.

In a small bowl, cover chillis with boiling water. Steep for about 10 minutes, or until soft and tender. Combine chillis with the whole garlic cloves in a processor or blender. Gradually add 2 tablespoons olive oil and 2 tablespoons lime juice. Purée until mixture is very fine and emulsified. You may have to thin with water. Season with a little salt and pepper. Do the same thing with the parsley: purée, gradually add the remaining oil, and season to taste.

To serve, remove the quinoa from the fish or mould, and place it on a plate. Place a small handful of tossed mixed greens next to the quinoa. Garnish the top of it with the chilli vinaigrette and parsley oil.

Chèvre/Goat Cheese and Smoked Salmon in Grape Leaves
(SERVES 4–6)

350 g chèvre (goat cheese)
225 g cold smoked salmon (preferably nitrite-free) cut into thin strips
1 tsp minced garlic
Salt and pepper to taste (the salmon is already salty)

56 ml olive oil
1 jar grape leaves

In a medium-sized mixing bowl, combine the chèvre, smoked salmon, and garlic. Beat until evenly combined and season with salt and pepper.

Brush a muffin tin with olive oil and line the muffin cups with grape leaves. Fill each with the cheese and salmon mixture. Fold the grape leaves over and press firmly.

Warm them briefly in a 425°F, 200°C oven and serve.

Lobster Baked Potato
(SERVES 4)

4 potatoes
4 lobsters or 450–675 g lobster meat
110 ml olive oil
56 ml milk or substitute
2 tsp chopped fresh tarragon
Salt and pepper
2 tbsp sherry or red wine vinegar
80 ml olive oil
4 handfuls baby spinach (540 g)

Bake the potatoes in a 400°F, 200°C oven until done, about 40 minutes to 1 hour. Steam the lobsters. Separate the meat from the shells and set aside. Roughly chop the shells. Boil the shells in the olive oil. Strain and reserve the oil.

Slit open the potatoes and scoop out the flesh into a large mixing bowl. Reserve the skins. Mash the potatoes with the milk, tarragon and enough of the lobster oil to flavour it. Put the mash back into the skins. Top with the sliced lobster meat and salt and pepper to taste.

Mix together the sherry, olive oil, and salt and pepper to make a vinaigrette. Add a tablespoon of the lobster oil. Toss the spinach in the dressing.

Serve each lobster baked potato on a bed of dressed spinach.

Grilled Salmon on a Bed of
Braised Lentils with Baby Artichokes
(SERVES 4)

½ tbsp canola oil
¼ onion, peeled and finely diced
1 carrot, finely diced
1 stalk celery, finely diced
180 g lentils, rinsed
3 sprigs fresh thyme
½ bay leaf
Vegetable stock (preferably) or water
Salt and pepper
90 g peeled and diced tomato
12 baby artichokes, washed
1 lemon, halved
½ tbsp olive oil
1 small onion, julienned
1 roasted red pepper, julienned
Freshly grated Parmesan cheese (optional)
4 salmon fillets (175–200 g each)

In a large saucepan, heat oil over medium heat. Add the onion, carrot, celery, lentils, thyme sprigs, and bay leaf to the saucepan and add enough vegetable stock to cover. Bring liquid to a boil, then reduce heat and simmer until lentils are tender but not mushy. Add more liquid during cooking if necessary. Drain the lentils, if any liquid is left over, when they are cooked. Remove from heat and season to taste with salt and pepper. Let cool. Fold in the tomato.

Heat a large pot of salted water to a boil. Trim the tough outer leaves from the outside of the artichokes and cut the tops off, leaving a flat top. Rub with lemon. Cook the artichokes in the water until tender (pierce with a fork). Drain and set aside. Heat the olive oil in a large sauté pan. Add the onion and cook over medium heat until soft. Add the red peppers and artichokes to the pan and sauté lightly. Season with salt and pepper. Sprinkle grated Parmesan over the top and place the whole pan into a 400°F, 200°C oven or under the grill until the Parmesan melts, glazing the vegetables with cheese.

Season the salmon fillets with salt and pepper. Cook about 2 minutes per side in a heavy non-stick skillet over high heat to desired doneness. To serve, put a bed of lentils in centre of the plate. Arrange 3 artichokes per plate, and place some of the onions and red peppers around the edge of the plate. Place the salmon on the lentils and top with a garnish of lentils.

Seared Sea Scallop and Tiger Prawn Salad with Curry Vinaigrette
(SERVES 4)

Curry Vinaigrette
¾ tsp Dijon mustard
30 ml sherry vinegar
½ tsp curry powder
3 tbsp canola oil (or peanut oil, if non-reactive)
3 tbsp olive oil
Salt and pepper

Salad
540 g baby spinach
½ tbsp sherry or red wine vinegar
1½ tbsp olive oil
350 g tiger prawns (approximately 12)
225 g sea scallops (approximately 8)
1½ tsp canola oil (or peanut oil, if non-reactive)
30 ml bottled clam juice or vegetable broth
30 ml dry white wine
Coriander leaves

Combine mustard, vinegar, and curry powder in a small mixing bowl. Gradually add oils with a whisk. Adjust seasoning with salt and pepper.

Wash baby spinach. Combine sherry or red wine vinegar and oil together. Season with salt and pepper.

Rinse the seafood well under running cool water and pat dry with paper towels. Remove shell/skin and legs from the prawns but leave the tails on. Slice the scallops in half crosswise, so that each scallop becomes two thinner scallops

Heat 1 teaspoon of the canola oil in a large frying pan over a high heat. When it begins to smoke, add half of the scallops. Sear each side until lightly brown, approximately 15 seconds on each side. Remove the seared scallops from the pan to a plate. Set aside and keep warm. Repeat the process with another teaspoon of oil and remainder of scallops.

Using the same pan, heat the last teaspoon of oil and sauté the prawns for about a minute over a high heat. Be sure to shake the pan, so that prawns are cooked on all sides. Add the clam juice and white wine and season with salt and pepper. Cover the pan and let the prawns steam for 2 minutes. The prawns should be pink in colour. Drain liquid from pan.

Toss baby spinach in sherry vinaigrette and heap in the centre of the plate. Arrange the prawns and scallops to the side. Garnish with a drizzle of curry vinaigrette and fresh coriander leaves.

Prawns with Lentil Salad
(SERVES 4)

12 prawns (3 per person)

Parsley Sauce
2 bunches parsley leaves
110 ml olive oil
Salt and pepper

Lentil Salad
225 g lentils
1 small onion, quartered
1 bay leaf
Chicken or vegetable stock or water
1 small red onion, finely diced
2 tomatoes, finely diced
2 tsp basil
2 tsp balsamic vinegar
2 tsp olive oil
Salt and pepper to taste

Grill the prawns and set aside.

Clean the parsley leaves. In a blender, purée the parsley and gradually add olive oil. Season.

In saucepan, combine the lentils, onion, bay leaf, salt and pepper. Cover the beans with stock or water. Cook until tender. Drain and discard onions and bay leaf.

Combine the cooked lentils with the red onion, tomato, basil, vinegar, oil, and salt and pepper. Serve with grilled prawns and garnish the plate with parsley sauce.

Sea Bass en Papillote
(SERVES 4)

4 sea bass fillets
1 tbsp olive oil
Sea salt and pepper to taste
½ onion, or 2 shallots
1 lemon or lime
Few sprigs fresh thyme

Brush the fish with oil and season with salt and pepper. Place on a piece of parchment large enough to contain the fish and make a package. Place slices of onion and lemon on top of the fish together with the thyme. Lift the two sides of the parchment paper to form a pouch and crumple shut at the top. Try to close the paper as tightly as possible. The paper will trap the steam and juices inside, cooking the fish and keeping it moist. (You can use two pieces of parchment, one to lay the fish on and the other to make a lid, crimping the two pieces together at the sides.)

Bake at 400°F, 200°C for 20 minutes.

Snapper Mexicana
(SERVES 4)

1 tbsp olive oil
4 medium snapper fillets, or 2 large cut in half
Seat salt to taste
360 g salsa

Heat oil in a saucepan and sauté the snapper for a few minutes on each side. Season with salt. Pour the salsa over the fillets and cover. Allow to simmer a few more minutes, and serve.

VARIATION: For a more elegant version, use a tropical fruit salsa, found in some natural food shops. Or make your own (see below).

Tropical Fruit Salsa
(SERVES 4)

1 medium mango, cut in small chunks
½ medium papaya, cut in small chunks
1 lime, juiced
1 garlic clove, minced
½ medium onion, cut in squares
45 g fresh coriander, minced
1 small hot chilli pepper, minced
Sea salt to taste

Combine all ingredients in a medium-sized mixing bowl.

Grilled Swordfish with Pineapple Mustard
(SERVES 4)

1 tbsp tamari, or ½ tsp sea salt
1 tbsp lemon juice
1 tbsp grated fresh ginger
4 swordfish steaks
180 g pineapple chunks
1 tbsp whole grain (stone-ground) mustard

Combine the tamari and lemon juice in a small bowl. Squeeze the juice from the grated fresh ginger through a cheesecloth or garlic press into the bowl. Dribble this mixture over the fish steaks and grill for 5 minutes. Turn the fish over, dribble sauce over the other side, and grill another 5 minutes or more, depending on the thickness of steaks. The fish is done when it is opaque and flakes easily.

In a blender or food processor, purée the pineapple with the mustard. When the fish is done, remove from the oven and spread a tablespoon of the pineapple mixture on top of each steak.

Navarin of Lamb
(SERVES 4)

1.2 kg diced lamb shoulder
110 ml olive oil
1½ onions, chopped
1½ tbsp wheat flour, or substitute
1½ tbsp tomato puree
2 cloves garlic
Bouquet garni (thyme, rosemary, bay leaf,
    parsley)
675 g red potatoes, halved
225 g baby onions, peeled
1½ tbsp chopped parsley

In a large saucepan, sauté the diced lamb in hot olive oil, then add the chopped onions. Sprinkle with flour, then add the tomato purée. Add the garlic and bouquet garni and cover with water. Cook until tender. Add the potatoes and cook until tender. Sauté the baby onions separately with a little oil until they are brown, and add them to the finished stew. sprinkle the stew with chopped parsley and serve.

VARIATION: Poultry may be substituted for the lamb. Dice 900g–1.35 kg of chicken or turkey and cook as directed for the lamb.

Stone-Ground Mustard Rubbed Rack of Lamb
with Roasted Garlic Potato Hash
(SERVES 4)

Lamb
675 g lamb, bone in
90 g stone-ground mustard mixed with
    1 tablespoon fresh tarragon, 2 minced cloves
    garlic, and 2 minced shallots

Potato Hash
5 medium-sized potatoes
1–2 tbsp olive oil
Provençal herbs (rosemary, thyme,
    marjoram, etc.)
Salt and pepper
1 onion, chopped
3 garlic cloves, minced

Rub the rack of lamb with most of mustard mixture. Barbecue or cook in a 450°F, 230°C oven for 20 minutes. Rub the remaining mustard mixture on the lamb after 10 minutes. Keep a close eye on the lamb, because the fat can cause flare-ups.

Peel and dice the potatoes and sauté in olive oil until lightly golden. Add the other ingredients and cook until tender or, if using an ovenproof pan, finish in a 375°F, 190°C oven, turning the mixture now and then so it cooks evenly.

Serve the lamb over potato hash.

Maple and Orange Marinated Pork Loin
(SERVES 4)

56 ml olive oil
225 ml orange juice
1 clove garlic, minced
1 tbsp lemon juice
½ tsp ground ginger
½ tbsp dry mustard
¼ tsp salt
1½ tbsp tamari sauce (if reactive to soya, skip)
30 ml maple syrup
25 g orange marmalade (sugar-free, if reactive)
Pork loin (900g–1.2 kg), boned, trimmed of skin
    and excess fat

In a medium-sized mixing bowl, slowly whisk the oil into the orange juice. Add remaining ingredients for marinade and mix thoroughly. Place the loin in a pan just large enough to hold it. Pour marinade over loin and marinate, refrigerated, for 3 hours to overnight. During marination, stir the marinade occasionally and turn the roast. Remove from the refrigerator about an hour before cooking. Preheat over to 450°F, 230°C. Place the roast on a rack in a shallow pan just large enough to hold the roast. Reserve marinade and set aside. Place the roast in oven and reduce the heat to 325°F, 160°C. Cook uncovered for approximately 1 to 1½ hours, until the juices run clear. Allow the roast to rest 15 to 30 minutes before carving.

Place reserved marinade in a saucepan, bring to a boil, lower to a simmer, and reduce amount by one-third. If desired, thicken sauce by adding cornflour or a cornflour substitute, such as arrowroot powder.

Roasted Sirloin of Beef
with Herbed Baby Potatoes
(SERVES 4)

1 onion, chopped
1 carrot, chopped
1 celery stalk, chopped
450 g baby red potatoes
1 clove garlic, minced
1 shallot, sliced
½ sprig rosemary
Olive oil
Salt and pepper to taste
1 sirloin (900 g), trimmed of excess fat

Preheat the oven to 350°F, 180°C. In a shallow roasting pan, toss together all the vegetables with the garlic, shallot, rosemary, olive oil, and salt and pepper. Season the sirloin with salt, pepper and thyme and place it fat side up on top of the vegetables. Roast, uncovered, for about 1½ hours for rare meat, longer for medium or well done. Let the meat rest 10 minutes before carving.Rewarm the vegetables while the meat rests.

VARIATION: Poultry may be substituted for the sirloin. Use 4 pieces of turkey or chicken breast. Cooking time will be about 45 minutes to 1 hour.

Etouffade de Boeuf Bourguignonne
(SERVES 4)

900 g diced top sirloin
90 g diced carrots
90 g diced onions
1 bottle red wine (if non-reactive)
2 tbsp butter or butter substitute or olive oil
2 tbsp flour, or wheat flour substitute
Salt and pepper to taste
3 cloves garlic
1 sprig rosemary
1 sprig thyme
1 bay leaf

Marinate the meat and vegetables in the red wine for 24 hours, then drain, reserving the liquid. Over medium heat, sauté the meat and vegetables in butter until golden brown. Sprinkle lightly with the flour and toss to coat evenly. Cover with the reserved red wine, season with salt and pepper, and add the garlic, rosemary, thyme and bay leaf. Bring to a boil, reduce the heat, and summer until the meat is tender, stirring occasionally to prevent the bottom of the pan from burning. If the liquid dries too quickly, add more red wine. Adjust seasoning before serving. Serve over fresh pasta, grain or rice.

VARIATION: 900 g–1.3 kg of turkey breasts, chicken breasts or other chicken pieces may be substituted for the sirloin.

Braised Rabbit or Chicken 'au Muscadet'
(SERVES 4)

900 g rabbit or chicken, cut into pieces
Salt and pepper to taste
3 tbsp flour or wheat-flour substitute
2 tbsp olive oil
1 onion, diced
1 carrot, diced
1 celery stalk, diced
180 g whole button mushrooms

1 sprig thyme
1 sprig rosemary
Dash parsley
3 cloves garlic
1 bottle white wine (if non-reactive)

Season the rabbit (or chicken) with salt and pepper, coat with flour, and in a medium-sized frying pan sauté in the oil over a medium heat. When browned, add the onion, carrot, celery, mushrooms, thyme, rosemary, parsley, and garlic. Cover with white wine, bring to a boil, stirring occasionally so the sauce does not stick to the bottom of the pan. Simmer 40 minutes, stirring occasionally. Adjust seasoning to taste.

Stuffed Bell Peppers
(SERVES 4)

4 bell peppers
2 tsp sesame oil
1 clove garlic, minced
180 g tempeh, crumbled, or 180g cooked beans
    (cannelini, haricot or adzuki)
360 g cooked rice
2 green onions, chopped finely including green
    part
2 tbsp fresh coriander, chopped, or
    1 tsp coriander powder
1–2 tbsp salsa (optional)
Sea salt to taste

Preheat oven to 400°F, 200°C.

Cut the tops off peppers and set aside. Scoop out seeds and white part and discard. Rinse peppers and turn over on wooden board to drain.

Heat oil (or water for lower fat) in a large frying pan and sauté garlic and tempeh (or beans) until golden brown. Add the rice, green onions, coriander and salsa and mix well. Salt to taste and fill peppers with the mixture. Place peppers in the oven-proof dish, put the tops back on them and bake for 30 minutes.

A sauce can be made to cover the peppers before baking them. Either top simply with 60–100 g of grated Monterey Jack cheese, or blend 100 g of tofu with 1 tablespoon tamari, 1 teaspoon tahini, and 2–3 tablespoons of water, depending on the consistency desired.

Fusilli with Fresh Tomatoes and Basil Sauce
(SERVES 4)

5–8 tomatoes, ripe but firm
450 g fusilli or other short pasta
1–2 cloves garlic
1 bunch basil
A few sprigs fresh parsley
Seat salt to taste
225 ml olive oil

Cut the tomatoes into wedges if small, or chop into 1-inch squares if large. Cook pasta according to instructions on package. In a food processor or blender, purée the garlic, basil, and parsley with the salt and olive oil.

Drain the pasta and toss with basil sauce to taste. Add tomatoes and toss. Excellent warm or cold.

VARIATION: Can also add more vegetables, such as sliced or baby carrots, red or yellow peppers, or courgettes to make a pasta primavera with basil.

Blackened Tofu Steaks
(SERVES 4)

1 block tofu
2 tbsp tamari
3 tbsp mirin (sweet cooking sake) or sherry
1 tsp grated ginger, or
    1 tbsp fresh ginger and press the juice

Cut tofu block into 4 slices. Place tamari, mirin, and ginger into a pan with the tofu slices. Cook slowly over medium to low heat, turning the steaks occasionally, until all liquid is absorbed and steaks are golden brown on both sides.

Serve with rice or mashed potatoes and veggies.

Tofu Brochettes
(SERVES 4)

Seasonal vegetables, such as broccoli, bell pepper,
    mushrooms, potatoes, shallots, or small onions
1 block tofu
3–4 cloves garlic, minced
1 tbsp olive oil
1 tbsp tamari or salt
1 tsp grated ginger

Cut vegetables into bite-sized chunks. Cut tofu into bite-sized cubes. Place tofu and vegetables onto skewers. Combine the garlic, olive oil, tamari, and ginger and brush the skewers. Grill or barbecue, turning over a few times and brushing with marinade occasionally to avoid drying. Serve over herbed rice.

Pasta with Courgettes
(SERVES 4)

900 g courgettes
1 medium onion
1 clove garlic
Olive oil
Sea salt to taste
450 g short pasta (wheat, rice, or quinoa pasta)
Grated Parmesan cheese (optional)

Slice the courgettes very fine, chop onion, and mince garlic. Heat the oil in a frying pan and sauté onion, garlic and courgettes until golden brown. Season with salt. Bring salted water to a boil and cook pasta according to the instructions on the packet.

Drain pasta but reserve water. Toss pasta with the courgettes, adding more oil if necessary, or some of the pasta water, if desired. Sprinkle with Parmesan cheese to taste.

Vegetables and Grains

Seasonal Vegetable Medleys

Three Methods of Preparation

1. Steaming

Chop the vegetables to appropriate sizes. Place in the steamer tray first the veggies that take the most time to steam — potatoes; roots, such as carrots or beetroot; and cauliflower or hard squashes. After 5 to 10 minutes add the ingredients that require less time, such as onions, courgettes, or the stems of chard. Finally, just before you turn off the heat, add any leafy greens to the top. Serve with a splash of olive oil and any seasoning you can handle, such as sea salt, garlic salt, or cayenne pepper.

2. Water Sauté

Start with a hot frying pan or wok, then add just a splash of olive oil and the first layer of vegetables (as above, the ones that need the most time to prepare). As the veggies cook, add small amount of water (stock or a little wine can be used for added flavour). As you progress over the 10 to 15 minutes it takes to make this dish, add additional vegetables, saving the greens for last. You can also add a little more oil for flavour along with seasonings before consumption.

Choose four to six of the vegetable options for your seasonal dishes.

3. Roasting

Preheat oven to 350°F, 180°C. Cut up vegetables into bite-sized pieces or strips and place in baking dish. Bake most vegetables for 20–30 minutes, then raise heat to grill. Turn veggies after a few minutes when they start to brown. Remove when done to taste. Top with a splash of olive oil and seasonings of your choice.

Buy them as fresh as possible and organic or grow them when possible for the best possible nutrition and taste.

Spring Medley

Asparagus, baby carrots, chard, spinach, spring garlic or green onions, leeks, beetroot, Brussels sprouts, greens (mustard or sorrel), and artichokes.

Summer Medley
Green beans, courgettes, beetroot, new potatoes, yellow and other soft squashes, peppers, aubergine, corn, and sugar snap peas.

Autumn Medley
Hard squashes (acorn, butternut, etc.), cauliflower, bell peppers, broccoli, carrots, celery, spinach, potatoes, okra, fresh corn, and Jerusalem artichokes.

Winter Medley
Onions, kale, cabbage, leeks, bok choy, Jerusalem artichokes, potatoes, chard, broccoli, cauliflower, and sweet potato.

Garden Tomatoes with Balsamic Vinaigrette
(SERVES 4)

> 450 g tomatoes (about 4 medium)
> 2 tbsp balsamic vinegar
> 56 ml olive oil
> ½ tsp salt
> ½ tsp ground pepper
> ½ tsp fresh basil leaves (optional)

Wash, core, and cut the tomatoes into thick slices or wedges and place in a shallow bowl. Whisk together the vinegar, oil, salt, and pepper. Dress the tomatoes with the vinaigrette. If you're adding the basil, do so now. Use whole picked leaves that have been rinsed, or tear the leaves into small pieces. Toss the tomatoes gently and set aside to marinate, refrigerated, before serving.

Oven-Cured Tomato and Aubergine Caviar Napoleon with Basil Essence
(SERVES 4)

Oven-Cured Tomatoes
2 tomatoes, medium
¼ tsp cumin
¼ tsp coriander
¼ tsp white pepper
½ tsp crushed garlic
Salt and pepper
Olive oil

Aubergine Caviar
2 medium aubergines
110 ml extra virgin olive oil
1 onion, diced
1 red pepper, diced
1 yellow pepper, diced
3 cloves garlic, crushed
45 g parsley, chopped
25 g thyme
25 g basil
Salt and pepper

Basil Oil
225 g basil, cleaned and dried
450 ml olive oil

Slice the tomatoes ⅛ inch thick. Place greaseproof paper on a baking sheet. Combine spices, salt and pepper and spread on paper. Lay the tomatoes on top of the spices and brush with olive oil. Bake in a warm oven for 2 hours, or until dried. Allow to cool.

Rub the aubergines' skins with olive oil. Place in a roasting pan and cook in a 400°F, 200°C oven for 45 minutes, until very soft all the way through. Allow to cool, then cut in half. Spoon contents of aubergines into a bowl and discard the skins. Chop the aubergines into small, evenly sized pieces. In a medium frying pan, heat 3 teaspoons olive oil. Sauté onions, peppers, and garlic. Add the aubergines. Transfer the mixture to an ovenproof dish and bake for 40 minutes in a 370°F, 190°C oven. Remove from oven and cool. Stir in chopped herbs and salt and pepper to taste.

Puree basil and gradually add the olive oil.

In a serving dish alternate the aubergine caviar with the tomatoes until it is 3 layers high, and garnish with basil oil.

Beetroot with Orange Vinaigrette
(SERVES 4)

450–900 g fresh raw beetroot, small ones if possible
56 ml orange juice
80 ml canola oil
25 g grated orange peel
1 pinch salt
45g chopped, toasted walnuts (optional)

Scrub the beetroot and cook it in water in a medium-sized saucepan, simmering until tender when pierced. Drain and cool. Peel and slice or cut into wedges. When ready to serve, combine the orange juice, oil, grated orange peel, and salt in a small mixing bowl. Drizzle sauce over the beetroot. Sprinkle with the toasted walnuts if desired, and serve immediately.

Stuffed Baked Acorn or Butternut Squash
(SERVES 4)

2 medium acorn or butternut squashes
180 g crumbled corn bread
110 ml chicken or vegetable broth
½ tsp sage
Salt and pepper to taste

Cut the squashes in half and remove seeds. Preheat oven to 375°F, 190°C. Place in shallow baking dish, cut side down, and bake for about 30 minutes, or until soft. While squashes are baking, in a small mixing bowl combine corn breadcrumbs with the chicken or vegetable broth and sage. After the squash has baked about 30 minutes, remove from oven, turn right side up, and salt and pepper. Spoon the stuffing into the centres and place the filled squash halves in a casserole dish to which you have added about 110 ml of hot water. Cover. Return to the oven and bake another 30 minutes, removing the cover during the last 10 minutes to brown the centre stuffing.

Honey Minted Carrots
(SERVES 2–4)

1 tbsp minced fresh mint
6 medium-sized carrots, sliced
1 tbsp honey

In a small saucepan, add the mint to the water and cook the carrots until tender. Drain, add honey, and shake pan over the heat until the carrots are honey coated.

Baked Mushrooms
(SERVES 4)

450 g fresh mushrooms
1 tbsp butter, melted, or olive oil
1 tbsp lemon juice
1 tsp dill
1 tsp diced parsley
Dash of garlic powder, if desired
Salt and pepper

Wash the mushrooms, pat dry, and place in a greased baking dish with a cover. Brush with butter and sprinkle with the lemon juice, dill, parsley, garlic powder, salt, and pepper. Cover and bake at 350°F, 180°C for about 25 minutes, or until mushrooms are tender.

Twice-Baked Potatoes
(SERVES 4)

4 baking potatoes
56 ml butter or olive oil
110 ml milk substitute, such as soya milk or
   rice milk
Salt and pepper
Garlic powder

Bake the potatoes in a 400°F, 200°C oven for 40 minutes to 1 hour. When cool enough, lay them on their sides, and cut off the upper half of each. Scoop the insides into a large bowl. Add the other ingredients and whip with a mixer until fluffy. Return this mixture to the four potato jackets, add a topping, if desired, and bake them again for about 10 minutes, or until the tops are golden brown. For toppings, consider bread-crumbs, chopped nuts, or diced spring onions.

Peas Pulão with Rice
(SERVES 4–6)

360 g uncooked rice
1 tbsp butter or olive oil
1 onion, sliced very thin
½ tsp cumin seed
2 cinnamon sticks
2 tsp crushed cardamom (or ½ tsp powdered)
3 bay leaves
2 whole cloves
180 g fresh or frozen peas
1 tsp salt

In a bowl, soak the rice in water for 30 minutes. Drain. In a medium-sized saucepan, heat the butter and sauté onions till golden. Add the spices and continue sautéing for a minute or so. Add the peas and stir-fry for about 5 minutes. Add 900 ml water and salt. When the mixture reaches a boil, add the soaked rice, stir well, cover and cook until done, about 20 minutes. Remove cinnamon sticks before serving.

Polenta
(SERVES 4)

1.35 ml water
½–1 tsp sea salt
360 g polenta

In a large saucepan, bring the water and salt to a boil. Slowly
add polenta while stirring constantly with a whisk, until well
mixed. Lower flame to minimum, cover pot, and simmer until
polenta has thickened, about 40 minutes. Stir occasionally to
avoid burning the bottom. Transfer the polenta to a glass loaf
pan and let set for 5 minutes. Cut into squares, and serve with
a sauce of your choice.

Leftover polenta can be grilled, sautéed or fried and served
with veggies, meat or fish. It can also be treated like pizza by
putting tomatoes or tomato sauce, herbs, and cheese on top
and baking until cheese melts.

Mexican Quinoa with Spinach
(SERVES 4–6)

1½ tbsp canola oil
1 medium onion, diced
2 cloves garlic, minced
1 jalapeño pepper, minced
1 tsp ground cumin
1 tsp ground coriander
180 g quinoa
1 bell pepper, seeded and diced
450 ml vegetable stock or water
Sea salt to taste
360 g fresh spinach, chopped
2 tbsp minced fresh parsley

In a large saucepan, heat the oil and sauté the onion, garlic,
and jalapeño pepper with the cumin and coriander, until
onion is translucent and garlic slightly golden. Add the
quinoa, bell pepper, stock, and salt; cover and simmer for 10
minutes. Add the spinach, cover, and simmer 5 to 10 more

minutes, or until all liquid is absorbed. Adjust seasoning, stir in parsley and serve.

Colourful Quinoa Salad
with Raspberry Yogurt Dressing
(SERVES 4–6)

2 medium tomatoes, cut into ¼-inch cubes
180 g endive, sliced into ¼-inch slices
½ green pepper, seeded and diced
360 g cooked quinoa
1 tbsp parsley, minced
45 g raisins
4 spring onions, finely sliced
Raspberry Yogurt Dressing (recipe follows)

Combine all the ingredients in a large bowl.

Raspberry Yogurt Dressing

110 ml olive or canola oil
3 tbsp raspberry vinegar
110 ml low-fat yogurt or goat yogurt
½ tsp honey
½ tsp mustard

Mix all ingredients in a bowl or a blender and pour over salad.

Breakfast Rice
(SERVES 4)

180 g raisins
1 tbsp lemon rind, grated
1 cinnamon stick, or ½ tsp ground
225 ml apple juice
675 g cooked rice
90 g walnuts or almonds, coarsely chopped and
    lightly roasted

In a medium saucepan, simmer the raisins, lemon rind, and cinnamon stick in juice for a few minutes, until the raisins are plump. Add the rice, simmer a few more minutes, turn off heat, add the walnuts or almonds, and let stand, covered, for 10 minutes or longer before serving.

Rainbow Rice
(SERVES 6–8)

90 g chopped onion
90 g chopped red pepper
90 g chopped carrot
90 g chopped yellow squash
90 g chopped courgettes
90 g chopped purple (red) cabbage (or beetroot
   or aubergine)
45 g chopped green onions
2 tbsp sunflower or sesame oil (or olive or canola)
110 ml water
2 tsp soya sauce, or to taste (or salt if off soya)
675 g cooked rice
180 g chopped parsley
Cayenne to taste (optional)

In a large skillet, sauté the vegetables in oil in this order: onion, pepper, carrot, squashes, cabbage (or aubergine or beetroot), and green onions, adding water and soya sauce and stirring. Add the cooked rice in batches, stir into vegetables, and heat gently for 5–10 minutes. Leave covered and serve warm. Before serving, add parsley (and cayenne if desired). Good with a tofu or miso-tahini dressing. This is a good cold salad as well.

Rice Milanese
(SERVES 4)

¼ tsp saffron
675 ml chicken or vegetable broth
2 tbsp butter or substitute (olive oil)
90 g finely chopped onion
180 g uncooked rice (arborio is best)
110 ml white wine (optional)
1 tsp salt

Place the saffron threads and the stock in a small saucepan and simmer until dispersed. Keep hot. Melt the butter or heat oil in a medium-sized saucepan. Add the onion and sauté until golden. Add the rice, stirring frequently for a few minutes, until fully coated and heated. Add the wine and stir until combined. Add hot stock a cup at a time, stirring constantly, until rice is al dente and creamy. You can also add stock all at once, cover tightly and simmer for 20–30 minutes. Season with the salt.

Rice Creole
(SERVES 4)

180 g uncooked long-grain brown rice
  or basmati
450 ml water
1 tsp salt
1 tsp freshly ground or coarse-ground black
  pepper
1 tbsp minced hot green chilli pepper
1 tbsp whipped butter or olive oil
1 tomato, cut in wedges

In a medium-sized saucepan, cook the rice in water until tender, following directions on the package. Drain. Add the remaining ingredients except the tomato. Garnish with tomato wedges and serve with poultry or fish.

Chinese Fried Rice
(SERVES 4)

90 g finely diced chicken
2 tbsp safflower oil
90 g sliced mushrooms
675 g cooked rice
1 green onion, finely chopped
2 tbsp soya sauce
Other vegetables to taste, chopped
1 egg, well beaten (can use just egg white
   or eliminate)

In a frying pan over medium heat, cook the chicken in the oil
for 2 to 3 minutes. Add the mushrooms, rice, onion, and soya
sauce. Feel free to add more chopped vegetables, such as
celery, carrot, and courgettes, if you want to have a more filling and nutritious yet low-calorie dish. Reduce the heat to low
and cook for about 10 minutes, stirring almost constantly. Add
the egg and stir-fry for another 5 minutes.

Soups

Spiced Butternut Squash Bisque
(SERVES 4)

1 large onion (coarsely chopped)
2 cloves garlic, chopped
1 tbsp curry powder
1½ tbsp unsalted butter, or butter substitute,
   like safflower oil
675 g butternut squash, peeled and seeded
1.2 l chicken stock, or vegetable stock
Salt and pepper
45 g coarsely chopped hazelnuts

In a medium-sized stockpot or large saucepan, sauté the
onion, garlic and curry powder in the butter over medium
heat. Cut the squash into 1-inch chunks. After approximately

5 minutes, or when the onion is tender and translucent, add the squash and stock to the pot. Bring to a simmer and simmer until squash is very tender, approximately 30–40 minutes. Puree in a blender or food processor. Season with salt and pepper. Serve with a garnish of toasted hazelnuts.

Gazpacho
(SERVES 2)

180 g celery, chopped
90 g chopped red onions
5 whole tomatoes, diced
1½ cucumbers, diced
½ bunch coriander, chopped
Tomato juice
Juice of 2 limes
Tabasco or cayenne pepper to taste
Salt and pepper to taste

In a blender, puree the vegetables and coriander, adding enough tomato juice to keep it moving in the blender. Leave it coarse; it should have some texture. Pour into a mixing bowl. Thin to desired consistency with more tomato juice. Season with lime juice, Tabasco or cayenne, and salt and pepper. Chill and serve cold.

Rich Veggie Soup
(SERVES 4–6)

450 g potatoes (5 small or medium), peeled
    and quartered
900 ml water
¼ tsp black pepper or 1/8 tsp cayenne
½ tsp dried basil
½ tsp cumin
3 tbsp sesame oil
½–1 tsp salt
1 small onion, chopped

2 cloves garlic, chopped
90 g tomato, diced
90 g several of the following vegetables:
   carrot, celery, green pepper, courgettes,
   broccoli, cauliflower, beetroot
90 g chopped green onions

In a large stockpot, combine the potatoes and water and boil for 15 to 20 minutes. Add the seasonings, oil, and salt. Place the chopped vegetables into the pot, cover, and cook over low heat for 10 to 20 minutes, until veggies are tender. Sprinkle with green onions.

Old-Fashioned Potato Soup
(SERVES 4)

4 medium potatoes, cooked, then mashed or
   sieved
225 ml liquid in which potatoes were cooked
225 ml skimmed milk, or milk substitute
1 tbsp whipped butter, or butter substitute, or
   dollop of yogurt if non-reactive
Salt and pepper to taste
2 tsp chopped onions
Paprika

In a medium saucepan, combine the potato liquid and milk, add cooked mashed potatoes and heat until simmering. Add butter, salt, and pepper. Add ½ teaspoon chopped onion to each bowl, pour soup over, and sprinkle with paprika.

Broccoli Soup
(SERVES 4)

400 g vegetable or chicken broth
450 ml water
450 g broccoli, trimmed and chopped
180 g sliced carrots
1 onion, sliced and separated into rings

1 tsp salt
1 tsp coarsely ground back pepper (optional)

Combine broth and water in a medium-sized saucepan. Bring to the boil and add remaining ingredients. Simmer for about 30 minutes, or until the vegetables are tender. For a creamier soup, blend briefly.

Split Pea or Haricot Bean Soup
(SERVES 6)

360 g dried split peas or haricot beans
1 minced onion
2 stalks celery, minced
1 carrot, finely diced
Salt and pepper
Fresh parsley

Soak peas or beans in water to cover overnight. Drain. In a stockpot, cover the peas or beans with 1.70 l fresh water, add vegetables, and cook slowly: if using peas, for 1 hour; if beans, for 3 hours, or until beans are tender and liquid is cooked down to consistency you prefer. Season with salt, pepper, and a touch of chopped parsley.

If you prefer a smooth pea soup, run the vegetable mixture through a sieve or place in a blender.

Both soups are excellent with corn bread sticks, or rice crackers if you are sensitive to corn and wheat.

Sauces and Dressings

Basil Balsamic Vinaigrette
(SERVES 6)

One medium bunch fresh basil
170 ml olive oil
56 ml balsamic vinegar
Salt and pepper to taste

Put the basil leaves in blender and add olive oil. The oil should just cover the leaves. Blend until smooth.

Whisk basil oil into balsamic vinegar. Add salt and pepper to taste.

Avocado Dressing
(SERVES 4)

2 medium avocados, stones and skins removed
Juice of 1 lemon
1 tsp salt or tamari to taste
110 ml water
⅛ tsp cayenne pepper
1 clove garlic

Puree all ingredients in a blender and toss with salad.

Green Onion Dressing
(SERVES 4–6)

360 g chopped green onions
1–2 tsp chopped garlic
½ tsp black or white pepper, or
    ¼ tsp cayenne pepper
1 tbsp soya sauce, or salt to taste
2–3 tsp sugar or 1–2 tsp honey
2 tsp whole grain mustard
80 ml apple cider vinegar
225 ml olive oil

Place all ingredients in the blender except the oil and blend until smooth. Slowly add the olive oil. Adjust seasonings.

A creamy version of this dressing can be made by adding one or two eggs, more like a light mayonnaise. But the dressing will be smooth and tasty if it is well blended.

Sweet and Sour Sauce
(SERVES 4–6)

420 ml water
225 ml rice syrup
4 tsp tamari (skip if sensitive to soya), or
    ½ tsp salt
2 tbsp rice vinegar
1 tbsp tahini
½ tsp fresh ginger, grated
1 tbsp kudzu or arrowroot powder, diluted
    in 2 tbsp cold water
2 green onions, finely chopped

In a saucepan, combine the water, rice syrup, tamari, vinegar, tahini, and ginger and bring to a boil. Add the diluted kudzu and stir until sauce thickens. Add green onions. Serve over vegetable or grain dishes.

Dairy-Free Pesto Sauce
(MAKES ABOUT 225 ML)

1 bunch fresh basil or spinach (or mixture of
    both), cleaned and with stems removed
1 tbsp light miso (use 1 tbsp sea salt if sensitive
    to soya)
1 clove garlic
90 g pine nuts and/or walnuts
4 tbsp olive oil
Handful of parsley (optional), chopped

Puree all ingredients well in a blender or food processor. Some fresh parsley can be added to the blender to enhance the green. If too thick, dilute with a little water. This dairyless pesto can be used for pastas or grain vegetable dishes. A more traditional (and fattening) pesto sauce will use grated Romano and more olive oil.

Egg-Free Mayonnaise (Tofunaise)
(SERVES 4)

1 block tofu (175–225 g)
1 tbsp brown rice or red wine vinegar
½ tsp salt, or to taste
½ tsp ground coriander
1 tsp Dijon mustard (optional)
2 tbsp olive oil

Puree all ingredients in a blender.

Bean Spreads
(MAKES 450 ML)

Basics
360 g beans, cooked, mashed
2 tbsp olive oil
Juice of 1 small lemon
1 clove garlic, pressed
½ onion, chopped
Cumin to taste
Salt to taste

Herbs and Seasoning Options
2 tbsp green or chilli pepper, chopped
1–2 tbsp parsley, minced
1 tbsp green onions, chopped
½ tsp cumin
½–1 tsp chilli powder
1 tsp dried basil, or 1 tbsp fresh chopped basil
½ tsp oregano
½ tsp coriander
¼ tsp dried thyme, or 1 tsp fresh thyme
1 tsp mustard
1–2 tbsp red wine vinegar
1–2 tbsp sesame tahini

You may use chickpeas, cannellini beans, split peas, black-eyed beans, pintos, kidney beans, or black beans. Besides using one of these beans, this recipe can be made with a variety of tastes, using many different ingredients. To make a dip, add a little more water, lemon juice and some oil.

In a small bowl blend the beans with the oil, lemon, garlic, and onion, then add cumin and salt and 2–3 other herbs and seasonings selected from the list of choices. Add any other ingredients of choice. Use as sandwich spread, or serve with crackers and vegetable sticks; celery and cucumber are good choices. As a sandwich with sliced tomato and sprouts or lettuce, or on a rice cake, it provides a nutritious meal.

Butter-Free Veggie Spread
(MAKES 1 SMALL BOWL)

> 720 g sliced carrots, apples, onions, or squash
> 110 ml water
> 1 pinch sea salt
> 1 tbsp kudzu or arrowroot powder, dissolved
>   in 3 tbsp water
> 1–2 tbsp sesame tahini

Place the carrots, apples, onions or squash in a pressure cooker with water and salt. Bring to pressure, turn down and simmer for 10 minutes. (If you don't have a pressure cooker, steam or boil for 20 minutes.) Puree carrots in blender, with 110 ml liquid from pressure-cooking or steaming. Dissolve kudzu or arrowroot in cool water, mix with carrot puree, and reheat. Stir until it bubbles (kudzu must be heated thoroughly to thicken). For a buttery flavour, stir in sesame tahini.

Use courgettes, broccoli, or cauliflower – or apple, squash, or pear – or a mixture of apple with any of the above veggies. Also, onion butter is very good.

Salads

Beijing Pea Pod Salad
(SERVES 4)

180 g snow peas
180 g Chinese cabbage
45 g bamboo shoots
4 water chestnuts
4 mushrooms
1 tbsp lemon juice
2 tsp soya sauce or ½ tsp salt
½ tsp dry mustard
Cherry tomatoes

In a saucepan, cook the snow pea pods in boiling salted water just until tender. Shred the Chinese cabbage and drain canned bamboo shoots. Slice the water chestnuts and mushrooms. In a large salad bowl combine the drained, chilled pea pods with the other vegetables. In a small bowl, combine the lemon juice, soya sauce, and mustard. Pour the dressing over the vegetables and toss well. Garnish with cherry tomatoes.

Cider Slaw
(SERVES 4–6)

540 g shredded cabbage
2 apples, cored and chopped
225 ml apple cider or juice
1 tbsp cornflour or arrowroot powder
1 tbsp honey
Lettuce leaves

In a large salad bowl, toss the cabbage and apples to combine. Use about 3 tablespoons of the cider to make a smooth paste with the cornflour. In a saucepan, heat the remainder of the cider to boiling, add honey, stir in the cornflour paste, and cook until thickened and clear. Cool and pour over the cabbage and apples. Mix well and serve on lettuce leaves.

Warm Red Cabbage Salad
(SERVES 4–6)

1 head red cabbage
1 small onion, sliced
90 g sweet peas
5 tbsp olive oil
2 tbsp rice or balsamic vinegar
1 tbsp ume vinegar or sea salt to taste
90 g roasted walnuts (optional)
50–110 g feta cheese, crumbled (optional)

Cut the cabbage into 4 quarters, then slice into ¼-inch strips. In a large saucepan, steam until soft, 3 to 5 minutes.

In a frying pan, sauté the onion until limp and transparent and add to cabbage together with peas.

Combine olive oil, rice vinegar, and ume vinegar or sea salt and toss with the cabbage. Sprinkle roasted walnuts and feta on top and serve warm.

Watercress Salad with Pears and Goat Cheese
(SERVES 4)

2 bunches watercress
Balsamic vinaigrette, or other dressing,
   enough to dress salad lightly
2 ripe pears, sliced (like Comice, Red Anjou,
   Bosc – whatever you like, as long as they're
   ripe)
90 g crumbled, soft fresh goat cheese

Trim and wash the watercress. Dry in a salad spinner. In a large bowl, toss the cress with the vinaigrette. Serve on plates topped with a few slices of ripe pear and sprinkled with the crumbled goat cheese.

Spinach Salad with
Mushrooms and Sesame Dressing
(SERVES 4)

3 bunches spinach leaves (tender baby leaves
   are best)
12 white button mushrooms
3 spring onions
Sesame Oil Dressing (recipe follows)

Clean the spinach thoroughly, removing stems. Spin dry in a
salad spinner. Wash and dry the mushrooms. Slice thinly.
Clean the spring onions and slice into long thin slivers.

Toss spinach, mushrooms, spring onions, and dressing
together lightly. Serve.

Sesame Oil Dressing

110 ml rice wine vinegar
2 tsp salt
1 tsp pepper
2 tbsp sugar, or 1 tbsp honey
110 ml sesame oil

In a small mixing bowl, combine the vinegar, salt, pepper, and
sugar. Add the oil and shake well or mix before using. Store in
refrigerator.

Herbed Couscous Salad
(SERVES 4)

360 ml whole wheat couscous
675 ml boiling water
45 g chopped black olives
45 g capers
1 red bell pepper, diced
1 stalk celery, diced
2 green onions, sliced thinly
180 g parsley, minced

56 ml olive oil
2 tsp ume vinegar (or 1 tbsp lemon juice with
    ½ tsp sea salt), or to taste
¼ tsp cayenne pepper
Lettuce leaves
Cherry tomatoes

Place the couscous in a large bowl and pour boiling water over it. Cover and let sit for 10 minutes. Fluff with a fork. Add olives, capers, vegetables, and parsley and toss with the olive oil, ume vinegar and cayenne. Serve over a bed of lettuce garnished with cherry tomatoes.

Wilted Spinach Salad
(SERVES 4–6)

3 large bunches spinach cleaned, dried,
    coarsely chopped
1 red onion, sliced into rings
1 red bell pepper, chopped
6 tbsp olive oil
2 tbsp balsamic vinegar
sea salt to taste
180 g crumbled feta cheese (optional)
90 g roasted walnut pieces (optional)

Place the spinach in a saucepan or frying pan over medium flame and stir just until limp; it should be bright green. Combine with the onion rings and pepper, and toss with oil, vinegar, and salt to taste. Sprinkle the feta and walnut pieces on top and serve warm.

Mexican Salad Bowl
(SERVES 4–6)

3 tbsp fresh lemon juice

2 tsp mustard

1 tbsp ume vinegar (or apple cider and sea salt)
    or to taste

3 tbsp tahini

4 tbsp water

2 heads butter or other green lettuce, shredded

2 green onions, sliced fine

1 cucumber, grated

1 bunch red radishes, grated

720 g cooked black beans

1 tsp ground coriander (optional)

In a small bowl, whisk the lemon juice, mustard, vinegar, tahini, and water together to make the dressing. (For a more Mexican dressing, use 3 tablespoons salsa, 1 tablespoon sesame oil, and ½ teaspoon salt or 1 teaspoon tamari.) Assemble all other ingredients in a salad bowl and toss with dressing.

Desserts

Honey and Chilli Roasted Hazelnuts
(SERVES 10)

900 g whole shelled hazelnuts (filberts)

1 tsp ground cumin

1 tsp ground coriander

1 tsp paprika

¼ tsp cayenne

2 tbsp honey

Salt to taste

In a shallow baking dish, roast the hazelnuts in a preheated 400°F, 200°C oven for 7 to 10 minutes, stirring frequently. Add the spices, honey, and salt to taste. Roast for 5 minutes more, stirring occasionally. Remove from the oven, allow to cool, and adjust the seasonings. When fully cool, break up the larger clumps of nuts and store in an airtight container.

Honey Sundae
(SERVES 1)

½ nectarine or peach, sliced (or other available
    fruit)
½ banana, sliced
45 g seasonal fruit (blackberry, cherry, peach, etc.)
180 g soya or rice ice cream
5–10 cashews (or other nut)
½ tsp cinnamon
1 tsp honey

Add the sliced fruit to the ice cream and sprinkle with nuts and cinnamon. Drizzle honey over top.

Chocolate Pudding
(SERVES 2–3)

1 cake (175 g) silken tofu
¼–½ tsp gelatin (plain) or agar-agar
½ tbsp water
25 g semi-sweet chocolate, or 45 g cocoa powder
½–1 tbsp vanilla
3 tbsp honey

Puree the tofu in a blender. In a saucepan, combine the gelatin with water and let it stand for 5 minutes. Warm it to help the gelatin dissolve. Add the creamy tofu and the other ingredients. If the chocolate is not in powder form, melt it. Heat to thicken. If it's not sweet enough, add more honey.

Pour into individual ramekins or into a mould and allow to set for at least an hour in the refrigerator.

Cashew Torte
(SERVES 4)

2 tsp grated orange peel
2 tbsp honey
1 tbsp water
2 eggs, separated (optional or substitute)
90 g ground cashews
⅜ tsp baking powder
30 ml orange juice
45 g ground raw sunflower seeds

In a saucepan, combine the grated orange peel, 1 tablespoon of the honey, and all the water; then bring to a boil, reduce the heat immediately, and let simmer for 3 minutes. Allow to cool.

In a mixing bowl, beat the egg whites until stiff. In another mixing bowl, beat the egg yolks.

Mix the cashews and baking powder.

To the egg yolks, add the remaining tablespoon of honey, the orange juice, the cashews and the sunflower seeds, and then the egg whites. Mix well.

Oil a 9-inch cake tin. To make sure the torte won't stick, line the tin with oiled brown paper. Fill and bake at 375°F, 190°C for 25 minutes, or until the top is cooked and the centre is firm.

Cool it somewhat before removing from the tin.

Fruit Sorbet
(SERVES 4–6)

900 ml fresh orange juice
3 tbsp maple syrup
2 tbsp grated orange rind
360 g fresh or frozen strawberries or raspberries, chopped
Fresh mint sprigs
Orange slices

Blend the first four ingredients together in food processor or blender. Transfer to a bowl and freeze for 2 to 3 hours, until solid. Break into large chunks and blend again until creamy and smooth. Return to the bowl and freeze again for about 30 minutes. Serve in individual parfait glasses garnished with a sprig of mint and a slice of orange.

Pumpkin Pie with Oat Crust
(MAKES 1 PIE)

Crust
135 g rolled oats
½ tsp salt
60 g ground almonds
135 g whole wheat pastry flour
3 tbsp maple syrup
½ tsp vanilla
2½ tbsp water

Filling
360 g pureed pumpkin
420 ml soya milk
80 ml maple syrup
1 tsp cinnamon
½ tsp ginger
½ tsp salt
½ tsp allspice
⅛ tsp ground clove
3 tbsp oat flour, toasted in dry pan

To prepare the crust, combine the dry ingredients in a food processor. In a mixing bowl, combine the wet ingredients. Add the wet ingredients to the food processor and pulse to combine. Pat into an oiled pie plate.

Preheat oven to 350°F, 180°C.

To prepare the filling, mix all ingredients well or blend in a food processor. Put into pie crust and bake for 40 minutes.

Yogurt Freezes
(SERVES 2–4)

There are many choices for these frozen yogurt treats. Many fruits will work well. Either mash the fruit and add the yogurt, or puree the fruit in the blender with a little honey or pure maple syrup, and add water or lemon juice for a tangy taste. Use plain regular, low-fat, or non-fat yogurt. Mix the yogurt in with the pureed fruit or blend all together. Add chopped walnuts or almonds, coconut flakes, carob powder, or natural flavourings for variety. Pour the mixture into freezable cups or scoop into Popsicle containers.

Some sample yogurt freezes include:

- **Banana** Mash 2 ripe bananas with ½ teaspoon of honey or maple syrup and ½ teaspoon lemon juice; mix in 180 g of yogurt and freeze. For carob or cocoa banana, mix in 2 tablespoons of carob powder or 1 tablespoon pure cocoa.
- **Banana-Papaya** Mash or blend to puree 1 medium banana with ¼ to ½ fresh papaya and ½ teaspoon lemon juice. Mix in 180 g yogurt.
- **Apple** Puree 180 g fresh apple without skin or use 180 g apple sauce, add 2 teaspoons honey, a pinch of cinnamon, and mix in 180 g yogurt.
- **Strawberry** Puree 270 g strawberries with 1 tablespoon honey and a splash of water. If using frozen, thawed berries, do not add water. Mix in yogurt and freeze.
- **Other berries** or fruits, such as peaches or nectarines, can also be used. Take 180–360 g fresh or fresh frozen fruits, blend with 1 tablespoon honey and 180 g of plain yogurt. Freeze in cups or containers.

Courgette Cake
(MAKES ONE 9 x 13-INCH CAKE)

540 g spelt (or wheat if non-reactive) flour
2 tbsp baking soda
¼ salt (optional)
1 tsp cinnamon
¼ tsp nutmeg
¼ tsp ground cloves
90 g grated unsweetened coconut
360 g grated courgettes
180 g very small piece of fresh pineapple or
    crushed pineapple canned in its own juice,
    drained
280 ml pineapple juice concentrate, thawed
110 ml oil

In a large mixing bowl, combine the flour, baking soda, salt, spices, and coconut. In a small mixing bowl, combine the courgettes, pineapple, pineapple juice, and oil. Stir the liquid ingredients into the dry ingredients until they are just mixed. Pour the batter into an oiled and floured 9 x 13-inch cake tin. Bake at 325°F, 160°C for 50 to 55 minutes, or until the cake is lightly browned and a toothpick inserted in its centre comes out dry.

Banana Bread
(1 LOAF)

540 g spelt flour, or 360 g amaranth flour
    plus 90 g arrowroot
2 tsp baking soda
½ tsp unbuffered vitamin C (ascorbic acid)
    crystals
½ tsp ground cloves (optional)
90 g chopped nuts (optional)
315 g mashed ripe bananas
56 ml oil

In a large mixing bowl, stir together the flour, baking soda, vitamin C crystals (which add a tangy flavour and stabilize the mixture), cloves, and nuts. Combine the mashed bananas and oil and stir them into the dry ingredients until they are completely mixed in, but be careful not to overmix. (The batter will be stiff.) Put the batter into an oiled and floured 9-inch loaf tin and bake at 350°F, 180°C for 55 to 60 minutes, or until the bread is lightly browned and a toothpick inserted in the centre comes out dry. Remove from the oven and allow to cool for 10 minutes. Remove from the tin to cool completely.

Cashew or Almond Butter Cookies
(MAKES 3 DOZEN)

360 g rye or rice flour
½ tsp baking soda
⅛ tsp unbuffered vitamin C crystals
135 g cashew or almond butter
56 ml oil
170 ml maple syrup

In a large mixing bowl, combine the flour, baking soda and vitamin C crystals. In a small mixing bowl, thoroughly combine the cashew butter, oil, and maple syrup. Stir the wet into the dry ingredients. Drop the dough by heaping teaspoonsful onto a ungreased baking sheet. Use an oiled fork to flatten the balls of dough, making an X on top of each with the fork tines. Bake the cookies at 400°F, 200°C for 8 to 10 minutes, or until they are golden brown.

Pie Crust

Amaranth
270 g amaranth flour
135 g arrowroot
½ tsp salt (optional)
110 ml oil
56 ml water

Barley
540 g barley flour
½ tsp salt (optional)
110 ml oil
85 ml water

Oat
540 g oat flour
½ tsp salt (optional)
110 ml oil
56 ml water

Quinoa
360 g quinoa flour
1 tsp baking soda
¼ tsp unbuffered vitamin C crystals
½ tsp salt (optional)
½ tsp cinnamon
110 ml oil
56 to 85 ml water

Rye
450 g rye flour
110 ml oil
56 ml water

Spelt
540 g spelt flour
½ tsp salt (optional)
110 ml oil
80 ml water

Choose one set of ingredients above. In a large bowl, combine the flour(s) with the salt, or, for the quinoa crust, with the baking soda, vitamin C crystals, salt, and cinnamon. Add the oil and blend it in thoroughly with a pastry cutter. Add the water and mix the dough until it begins to stick together, adding an extra 1 to 2 teaspoons of water if necessary. (For the quinoa crust, stir the flour mixture while you are adding the water until you have added enough to make the dough stick together.) Divide the dough in half. For one-crust pies, press each half of the dough into a glass pie dish, gently prick it with a fork, and bake it until the bottom of the crust begins to brown. The baking temperatures and times for each kind of crust are as follows:

Amaranth	15 to 18 minutes at 400°F, 200°C
Barley	15 to 18 minutes at 400°F, 200°C
Oat	15 to 20 minutes at 400°F, 200°C
Quinoa	20 to 25 minutes at 350°F, 180°C
Rye	15 to 20 minutes at 400°F, 200°C
Spelt	18 to 22 minutes at 400°F, 200°C

For a two-crust pie, press half of the dough into the bottom of a glass pie dish. Fill the crust with the filling of your choice. To top the pie, either crumble the second half of the dough and sprinkle it over the filling, or roll out the second half of the dough and place it on to of the pie. This recipe makes two single pie crusts or a more than adequate amount of pastry for a two-crust pie.

Note: The barley crust is the most like a traditional wheat crust in taste and texture.

Cherry Cobbler
(SERVES 6–8)

4 tsp arrowroot or tapioca flour
110 ml apple or pineapple juice concentrate, thawed
720 g pitted fresh cherries, or one 450 g bag frozen unsweetened cherries
1 batch Cobbler Topping (see recipe following)

Stir the arrowroot or tapioca flour into the juice in a saucepan. Add the fruit, bring it to a boil, and simmer it until it is thickened and clear. Put it into a 1.60 l casserole. Make the cobbler topping and put it on top of the fruit. Bake it at 350°F, 180°C for 25 to 35 minutes, or until the topping begins to brown.

Cobbler Topping

Here are a variety of cobbler toppings to mix and match with whatever fruit you choose.

Amaranth

135 g amaranth flour
45 g arrowroot
¾ tsp baking soda
⅛ tsp unbuffered vitamin C crystals
85 ml apple or pineapple juice concentrate, thawed
2 tbsp oil

Barley

158 g barley flour
¾ tsp baking soda
⅛ tsp unbuffered vitamin C crystals
85 ml apple or pineapple juice concentrate, thawed
2 tbsp oil

Quinoa

125 g quinoa flour
2 tbsp tapioca flour
¾ tsp baking soda
⅛ tsp unbuffered vitamin C crystals
85 ml apple or pineapple juice concentrate, thawed
2 tbsp oil

Rye

135 g rye flour
135 g baking soda
⅛ tsp unbuffered vitamin C crystals
85 ml apple or pineapple juice concentrate, thawed
2 tbsp oil

Spelt

158 g spelt flour
¾ tsp baking soda

⅛ tsp unbuffered vitamin C crystals
85 ml apple juice concentrate, thawed
2 tbsp oil

Choose one set of ingredients above. Combine the flour(s), baking soda, and vitamin C crystals in a large bowl. Mix together the juice and oil and stir them into the dry ingredients until they are just mixed in. Put the topping over the fruit mixture in the casserole dish and bake it at 350°F, 180°C for 25 to 35 minutes, or until the topping is slightly browned.

RESOURCES AND REFERRALS

Organizations

The **British Allergy Foundation** advises allergy sufferers to contact their GP in the first instance for referral to an allergy clinic. However, there are a number of private laboratories and homeopathic clinics, some of which advertise on the Internet and will conduct tests direct.

The BAF aims to increase understanding of allergy and to help patients overcome its effects: membership includes a quarterly newsletter, regular booklets on specific allergies, information on local allergy support groups, and product discounts.

BAF
Deepdene House
30 Bellegrove Road
Welling
Kent DA16 3BY
Tel 020 8303 8525
Helpline 020 8303 8583
Email: info@allergyfoundation.com
http://www.allergyfoundation.com

AAA (Action Against Allergy) is an independent charity. Annual subscription (£15) provides information packs, specialist referral, advisory leaflets, and a suppliers list. The regular Allergy Newsletter covers the latest research and offers helpful advice.

PO Box 278
Twickenham
TW1 4QB
Tel: 020 8892 2711
Email: AAA@actionagainstallergy.freeserve.co.uk

The Allergy Research Foundation offers information on allergy and aims to fund research into its causes and prevention.
Middlesex Hospital
Mortimer Street
London W1N 8AA

The British Society for Allergy and Clinical Immunology
66 Weston Park
Thames Ditton
Surrey KT7 0HL
Tel: 020 8398 9240
Fax: 020 8398 2766
http://www.soton.ac.uk/~bsaci

The British Complementary Medical Association
The CMA's mission is to promote ethical professional complementary medicine, and their site offers information on the latest developments in the field.
The Meridian
142a Greenwich High Road
London SE10 8NN
Tel: 0116 282 5511
http://www.the-cma.org.uk

The UK Homeopathic Medical Association
6 Livingstone Road
Gravesend
Kent DA12 5DZ
Tel: 01474 560336
Fax: 01474 327431
Email: info@the-hhma.org
http://www.the-hma.org

The British Homeopathic Association
27a Devonshire Street
London W1N 1RJ
Tel: 020 7935 2163

National Institute of Medical Herbalists
56 Longbrook Street
Exeter EX4 6AH
Tel: 01392 426022
Fax: 01392 498963

The British Naturopathic Association
GCRN
Goswell House
2 Goswell Road
Somerset BA16 0JG
Tel: 01458 840072
Fax: 01458 840075
Email: admin@naturopathy.org.uk
http://www.naturopathy.org.uk

The British Holistic Medical Association
59 Lansdowne Place
Hove
East Sussex BN3 1FL
Tel/fax: 01273 725951
Email: bhma-sec@bhma.org.uk
http://www.bhma-sec.dircon.co.uk

The International Society for Orthomolecular Medicine
Tel: (001) 416 733 2117
http://www.orthomed.org

The Coeliac Society
PO Box 220
High Wycombe
Buckinghamshire HP11 2HY
Tel: 01494 437278
Fax: 01494 474349
http://www.coeliac.co.uk
Email: memsec@coeliac.co.uk

The Vegan Society
Donald Watson House
7 Battle Road
St Leonards-on-Sea
East Sussex TN37 7AA
Tel: 01424 427 393
Fax: 01424 717 064
Email: info@vegansociety.com
http://www.vegansociety.com

The Vegetarian Society
Parkdale
Dunham Road
Altrincham
Cheshire WA14 4QG
Tel: 0161 925 2000
Fax: 0161 926 9182
Email: info@vegsoc.org
http://www.vegsoc.org

Information

OnHealth:com
This website is one of the world's largest health-related sites committed to providing information and resources that promote well-being of the body, mind, and spirit.
http://www.OnHealth.com

The Natural Health Guide
Website containing an index of complementary therapies and practitioners in the UK.
http://www.marches.county.net/health

The Food Allergy Network (US)
Email: fan@worldweb.net
http://www.foodallergy.org

Organic Food.co.uk
The online organic magazine contains a database of organic retailers, a herb listing, chat forums, articles, and news.

Email: info@organicfood.co.uk
http://www.organic food.co.uk

Planet Organic
The London store delivers most of their products nationwide.
42 Westbourne Grove
London W2 5SH
Tel: 020 7221 1345

Inside Story
Subscribe to the Inside Story of Food and Health magazine
worldwide. Their website contains extracts from the magazine, recipes, product review, and links to a wide range of
other websites about food allergies.
http://www.inside-story.com

Products and Services

Biocare
Biocare manufacture and supply a wide range of food supplements for suitable individuals who are either allergic or
intolerant to standard products and includes multi-nutrients,
amino acids, probiotics, vitamins, and minerals.
Lakeside
180 Lifford Lane
King's Norton
Birmingham B30 3NU
Tel: 0121 433 3727
http://www.biocare.co.uk

Higher Nature
Higher Nature is one of the leading vitamin and health
supplement companies in the UK. Their nutrition department
can advise on products best suited to you. Their products can
be found at all good health stores or you can ask for their
catalogue direct.
Burwash Common
East Sussex TN19 7LX
Tel: 01435 882 880

The Healthy House
Products of benefit to chemically sensitive people and to any-
one wishing to reduce pollutants in the home and office.
Cold Harbour
Ruscombe, Stroud
Gloucestershire GL6 6DA
Tel: 01453 752216
Fax: 01453 753533
Email: info@healthy-house.co.uk
http://www.healthy-house.co.uk

The Herbal Factory
A specialist manufacturer of herbal and nutritional supple-
ments selling direct to the public.
Unit 22/26, Addington Business Centre
Vulcan Way
Croydon CR0 9UG
Tel: 080 800 43722
Fax: 1689 843 701
Email: hvitamed@aol.com
http://www.herbal-factory.co.uk

Healthtree
Visit the online shop where you can order health supplements
and peruse their guide.
PO Box 79
Kingston upon Hull, HU1 1RP
Tel: 0800 138 0861
Email: info@healthtree.co.uk
http://www.healthtree.co.uk

Merton Books
Self-help and recipe books for allergy sufferers.
PO Box 279
Twickenham
Middlesex TW1 4XQ
Tel: 020 8892 4949
Fax: 020 8892 4950
Email: mertonbookorders@yahoo.com
http://www.merton-books.co.uk

Health Aid
Offers a wide range of supplements and products.
http://www.healthaid.co.uk

The Allergy Aid Shop
Products and services aimed at allergy sufferers.
83 Pensby Road
Heswall
Wirrall CH60 7RB
Tel/fax: 0151 348 4488
Email: info@allergyaid.co.uk
http://www.allergyaid.co.uk

Allergyfree Direct
Specialist food products.
http://www.allergyfreedirect.co.uk

FoodSensitivity.co.uk
Manufacture remedies to densitise allergic reactions to food.
Food Sensitivity Remedies
PO Box 6, Northleach
Cheltenham
Glos GL54 3YJ
Tel: 01242 890108
Fax: 01242 890514
Email: info@foodsensitivity.co.uk
http://www.foodsensitivity.co.uk

Glutafin
Provide gluten-free products to the UK and Ireland.
Email: glutenfree@nutricia.co.uk
http://www.glutafin.co.uk

Organics direct
Delivers organic vegetarian produce anywhere in the UK mainland.
7 Willow Street
London EC2A 4BH
Tel: 020 7729 2828
Fax: 020 7613 5800
Email: info@organicsdirect.co.uk
http://www.organicsdirect.co.uk

Network Organic is a website dedicated to the concept of organic living and aims to be the UK's leading site for information on the industry.
http://www.networkorganic.com

Cookbooks

Colbin, Annemarie. *The Book of Whole Meals.* Ballantine Books, 1986.

Diamond, Marilyn, *The Fit for Life Cookbook.* Bantam Books, 1991.

Dumke, Nicolette. *Allergy Cooking with Ease.* Starburst Publishers, 1992.

Fenster, Carol. *Special Diet Solutions: Healthy Cooking without Wheat, Gluten, Dairy, Eggs, Yeast or Refined Sugar.* Savory Palate, 1997.

Haas, Elson, and Eleanora Manzolini. *A Cookbook for All Seasons.* Celestial Arts, 2000.

Hurt Jones, Marjorie. *The Allergy Self-Help Cookbook.* Rodale Press, 1992.

Katzen, Mollie. *The Moosewood Cookbook,* revised edition. Ten Speed Press, 1992.

—. *Still Life with Menu.* Ten Speed Press, 1994.

Robertson, Laurel, *et al. The New Laurel's Kitchen.* Ten Speed Press, 1986.

Shulman, Martha Rose. *Fast Vegetarian Feasts.* Doubleday, 1986.

Zukin, Jane. *The Dairy-Free Cookbook.* Prima Publishing, 1998.

Other Books

Barnard, Neal. *Foods that Fight Pain*, Bantam Books, 1999.

Braly, James, and Laura Torbet. *Dr. James Braly's Food Allergy and Nutrition Revolution.* Keats Publishing, 1992.

Brostoff, Jonathan and Gamlin, Linda. *The Complete Guide to Food Allergy and Intolerance*, Bloomsbury, 1998.

Clouatre, Dallas. *Anti-Fat Nutrients.* Pax Pubishing, 1997.

Dumke, Nicolette. *Five Years without Food: the Food Allergy Survival Guide.* Allergy Publications, 1997.

Haas, Elson. *The Detox Diet.* Celestial Arts, 1996.

—. *The Staying Healthy Shopper's Guide.* Clestial Arts, 1999.

—. *Staying Healthy with Nutrition.* Celestial Arts, 1992.

Hobbs, Christopher, and Elson Haas. *Vitamins for Dummies.* IDG Books Worldwide, 2000.

Larson, E., and Jacqueline Krohn. *The Whole Way to Allergy Relief and Prevention*, revised edition, Hartley & Marks, 1997.

Nichols, Trent and Nancy Faass. *Optimal Digestion: New Strategies for Achieving Digestive Health.* Avon, 1999.

Rivera, Rudy and Roger Deutsch. *Your Hidden Food Allergies Are Making You Fat.* Prima Publishing, 1998.

Ross, Julia. *The Diet Cure.* Penguin, 2000.

NOTES

Chapter 1, It's Not Fat

James Braly, M.D. *Dr. Braly's Food Allergy and Nutrition Revolution*. New Canaan, CT: Keats Publishing, 1992.

Luanna Crow, 'Eaten Up with Allergy.' *San Antonio Medical Gazette*, February 15–21, 1996.

J. D. Gryboski. 'Gastrointestinal Milk Allergy in Infants.' *Pediatrics* 40: 354–62 (1967).

W. W. Hamburger. 'Emotional Aspects of Obesity.' *Medical Clinics of North America* 36: 483 (1951).

Mehl McDowell, M.D. 'Appetite Control: An Addiction-Like Component in Overeating and Its Cure.' *Obesity and Bariatric Medicine* 9 (1980).

Rudy Rivera, M.D., and Roger Deutsch. *Your Hidden Food Allergies Are Making You Fat*. Rocklin, CA: Prima Health, 1998.

Fuller, F. Royal, M.D. 'Food Allergy Addiction in a Bariatric Practice.' *Obesity and Bariatric Medicine* 7: 45 (1978)

Douglas H. Sandberg, M.D. 'Gastrointestinal Complaints Related to Diet.' *International Pediatrics* 5 (1990).

Chapter 2. Why You Will Lose False Fat

Timothy D. Brewerton. 'Toward a Unified Theory of Serotonin Dysregulation in Eating and Related Disorders.' *Psychoneuroendocrinology* 6: 561–90 (1995).

M. P. Cleary. 'Current Approaches to Weight Loss.' *The Nutrition Report*, November 1988.

Ellen Cutler, D.C. *Winning the War Against Asthma and Allergies*. Boston: Delmar Publishers, 1998.

'Eat More to Lose More.' *The Edell Health Letter*, February 1993, 1.

A. Golay *et al*. 'Similar Weight Loss with Low or High Carbohydrate Diets.' *American Journal of Clinical Nutrition* 63–2:

174–178 (1996).

Elson Haas, M.D. *Staying Healthy with Nutrition*. Berkeley: Celestial Arts, 1992.

Katzeff and Danforth. 'Decreased Thermic Effect of a Mixed Meal During Overnutrition in Human Obesity.' *American Journal of Clinical Nutrition* 50: 915–921 (1989).

Kenyon and Dowson Lewith. *Allergy and Intolerance*. London: The Merlin Press, 1992.

Nelson Novick, M.D. *You Can Do Something About Your Allergies*. New York: Bantam Books, 1994.

Doris J. Rapp, M.D. *Allergies and Your Family*. New York: Sterling Publishing Co. 1984.

Barry Sears, Ph.D. with Bill Lawren. *The Zone*. New York: ReganBooks, 1995.

Chapter 3. Why You Will Lose True Fat

Steve Carper. *No Milk Today*. New York: Simon & Schuster, 1986.

'Food Intolerance in Patients with Angioedema and Chronic Urticaria.' *European Journal of Allergy and Clinical Immunology* 50 (26) (1995).

George *et al*. 'Effect of Dietary Fat Content on Total and Regional Adiposity in Men and Women.' *International Journal of Obesity* 14: 1085–93 (1990).

M. Eric Gerschwin, M.D. *Taking Charge of Your Child's Allergies*. New York: Berkeley Books, 1998.

Jane Houlton. *The Allergy Survival Guide*. London: Leopard Books, 1995

Jacqueline Krohn, M.D. *Allergy Relief and Prevention*, Point Roberts, WA: Hartley & Marks, 1996.

Alan Pressman, D.C., Ph.D., and Herbert Goodman, M.D., Ph.D. *Treating Asthma, Allergies and Food Sensitivities*. New York: Berkeley Books, 1997.

Dick Thom, D.D.S., N.D. *Coping with Food Intolerances*. Portland, OR: JELD Publications, 1995.

Chapter 4 What Women Need to Know

Anderson *et al*. 'Influence of Menopause on Dietary Treatment of Obesity.' *Journal of Internal Medicine* 173–181 (1990)

W. G. Crook, M.D. *The Yeast Connection: A Medical Breakthrough*. Jackson, TN: Professional, 1984.

Katharina Dalton, M.D., *Once a Month*. Alameda, CA: Hunter House, 1979.

Frank *et al.* 'Weight Loss and Bulimic Eating Behavior.' *Southern Medical Journal:* 457–60 (1991).

Ann Louise Gittleman, M.S. *Super Nutrition for Women.* New York: Bantam, 1991.

Linaya Hahn. *PMS: Solving the Puzzle.* Chicago, IL: Spectrum Press, 1995.

D. C. Jimerson, *et al.* 'Low Serotonin and Dopamine Metabolite concentrations in Cerebrospinal Fluid from Bulimic Patients with Frequent Binge Episodes.' *Archives of General Psychiatry:* 132–138 (1992).

Moses *et al.* 'Fear of Obesity Among Adolescent Girls.' *Pediatrics:* 393–98 (1989).

Ronald N. Norris, M.D., with Colleen Sullivan, *PMS.* New York Berkeley Books, 1983.

Janet Polivy *et al.* 'Food Restriction and Binge Eating.' *Journal of Abnormal Psychology* 2: 409–11 (1994).

Jamie Pope, M.S., R.D., *The Last Five Pounds.* New York: Pocket Books, 1995.

J. S. Schinfeld. 'PMS and Candidiasis: Study Explores Possible Link.' *Female Patient* No. 7: 66–74 (1987).

A. R. Spalter *et al.* 'Thyroid Function in Bulimia Nervosa.' *Biological Psychiatry:* 408–14 (March 15, 1993).

Steege and Blumenthal. 'The Effects of Aerobic Exercise on Premenstrual Symptoms in Middle-Aged Women.' *Journal of Psychosomatic Research* 37–2: 127–133 (1993).

Chapter 5. The Extraordinary Side Benefits

D. Atherton. 'Role of Diet in Treating Atopic Eczema – Elimination Diets Can Be Beneficial.' *British Medical Journal* 297: 1458–1460.

J. M. Bernstein. 'The Role of IgE-Mediated Hypersensitivity in Otitis Media with Effusion.' *Otolaryngology* 89: 874.

J. Brostoff. 'Food Allergies in Migraine.' *Lancet* 1–4 (1980).

M. B. Campbell. 'Neurological Manifestations of Allergic Disease.' *Annals of Allergy* 31: 485–498.

J. Karjalainen. 'A Bovine Albumin Peptide as a Possible Trigger of Insulin-Dependent Diabetes.' *New England Journal of Medicine* 327: 302 (1992).

D. S. Khalsa, M.D., and Cameron Stauth. *The Pain Cure.* New York: Warner Books, 1999.

Gary Null. *No More Allergies.* New York: Villard Books, 1992.

Doris Rapp, M.D. *Allergies and the Hyperactive Child.* New York: Simon & Schuster, 1979.

Rinkel, Randolph, and Zeller. *Food Allergy*. Springfield, IL: Charles C Thomas, 1951.

F. Speer. 'Allergic Tension-Fatigue Syndrome in Children.' *Annals of Allergy* 12: 168–171.

Taylor and Truelove. 'Circulating Antibodies to Milk Protein in Ulcerative Colitis.' *British Medical Journal* 2: 924–929.

Chapter 6. Finding Out Your Own False Fat Foods

Carolee Bateson-Koch, D.C., N.D. *Allergies: Disease in Disguise*. Burnaby, BC, Canada: Alive Books, 1994.

Marj Charlier. 'Cave Man's Life Worth Aping, Doctors Believe.' *The Wall Street Journal*. October 21, 1986, 35.

P. J. Fell, J. Brostoff, and M. Pasula. 'High Correlation of the ALCAT Test Results with Double-Blind Challenge in Food Sensitivity.' Paper presented at the 45th Annual Congress of the American College of Allergy and Immunology, Los Angeles, CA, November 13, 1988.

Ann Louise Gittleman, M.S. *Your Body Knows Best*. New York: Pocket Books, 1996.

Mary James, N.D. 'Toward an Understanding of Allergy and In-Vitro Testing.' *Nature Medicine Journal*. April 1999.

D. Jewett, *et al.* 'A Double-Blind Study of Symptom Provocation to Determine Food Sensitivity.' *Journal of the American Medical Association* 323: 429–433.

Kaats, Pullen, and Parker. 'The Short-Term Efficacy of the ALCAT Test to Facilitate Changes in Body Composition and Self-Reported Disease Symptoms: A Randomized Study.' *The Bariatrician*. Spring 1996.

D. S. Khalsa, M.D., and Cameron Stauth, *Brain Longevity*. New York: Warner Books, 1997.

Barbara Solomon, M.D. 'The ALCAT Test: A Guide and Barometer in the Therapy of Environmental and Food Sensitivities.' *Environmental Medicine* 9, No. 2 (1992).

Chapter 7. The Cleansing Phase

Stephen Astor, M.D. *What's New in Allergy and Asthma*. 4th rev. ed. Two A's, 1996.

Jeff Bland. *Intestinal Toxicity and Inner Cleansing*. New Canaan, CT: Keats Publishing, 1987.

Braverman and Pfeiffer. *The Healing Nutrients*. New Canaan, CT: Keats Publishing, 1986.

Brownell and Rodin. 'Medical, Metabolic and Psychological Effects of Weight Cycling.' *Archives of Internal Medicine* 1326 (1994).

Michael Eades and Mary Eades. *Protein Power.* New York: Bantam Books, 1996.

'Fat, Water, and Fluid Retention.' The American Society of Bariatric Physicians, 1998.

Oz Garcia. *The Balance.* New York ReganBooks, 1998.

Elson Haas, M.D. *The Detox Diet.* Berkeley: Celestial Arts Publishing, 1996.

Kenneth Pelletier, Ph.D. *Think Horses Not Zebras.* New York: Simon & Schuster, 2000.

K. A. Perkins. 'Metabolic Effects of Cigarette Smoking.' *Journal of Applied Physiology* 72: 401–9 (1992)

William Walsh, M.D. *The Food Allergy Book.* St Paul, MN: ACA Publications, 1995.

Merla Zellerbach. *The Allergy Sourcebook.* Chicago: Contemporary Books, 1995.

Chapter 8. False Fat Week

'Biology, Culture, Dietary Changes Conspire to Increase Incidence of Obesity'. *Journal of American Medical Association:* 2157–58 (1986).

Dallas Clouatre, Ph.D. *Anti-Fat Nutrients.* San Francisco: Pax Publishing, 1997.

Robert Crayhon, M.S. *The Carnitine Miracle.* New York: M. Evans & Co., 1998.

William Grimes. 'Self-Denial Takes a Holiday.' *The New York Times.* November 26, 1997, F-1.

Elson Haas, M.D. *A Diet For All Seasons.* Berkeley: Celestial Arts Publishing, 1995.

E. C. Opara *et al.* 'L-glutamine Supplementation of a High-Fat Diet Reduces Body Weight.' *Journal of Nutrition* 126–1: 273–279 (1996).

'A Pill That Burns Calories: New Metabolism Boosters.' *Longevity*, November 1992.

W. P. Pimenta, *et al.* 'The Assessment of Zinc Status by the Zinc Tolerance Test and Thyroid Disease.' *Trace Elements in Medicine* 9 (1): 34–37 (1992)

Julia Ross. *The Diet Cure.* New York: Viking, 1999.

Carol Simontacchi, M.S. *Your Fat Is Not Your Fault.* New York: Jeremy Tarcher/Putnam, 1997.

K. S. Usiskin, *et al.* 'Lack of DHEA in Obese Men.' *International Journal of Obesity* 14: 456–463.

Chapter 9. The Balance Programme

'Biology, Culture, Dietary Changes Conspire to Increase Incidence of Obesity.' *Journal of American Medical Association* 2157–58 (1986).

Peter D'Adamo, with Catherine Whitney. *Eat Right 4 Your Type.* New York: Putnam, 1996.

H. de Vries and D. Gray. 'After-Effects of Exercise Upon Resting Metabolic Rate.' *Res. Q. American Association*, Health Physician, Ed., 34: 314–321 (1963).

Oz Garcia. *The Balance*. New York: ReganBooks, 1998.

Jackie Habgood. *The Hay Diet Made Easy*. Souvenir Press, 1997.

Shad Helmstetter, Ph.D., with Bon Schwartz, Ph.D. *Self-Talk for Weight Loss*. New York: St Martin's Press, 1994.

William Donald Kelley, D.D.S. *The Metabolic Types*. Lake Geneva, WI: Computrition Investments, 1980.

Victoria Moran. *Love Yourself Thin*. New York: Penguin Putnam, 1997.

H. L. Newbold, M.D. *Dr. Newbold's Type A, Type B Weight Loss Book*. New Canaan, CT: Keats Publishing Co., 1991.

Roger Paffenberger *et al*. 'Physical Activity, All-Cause Mortality, and Longevity of College Alumni,' *New England Journal of Medicine* 314: 605–13 (1986).

K. E. Powell *et al*. 'Physical Activity and Chronic Disease.' *American Journal of Clinical Nutrition* 49: 999–1006 (1989).

Barry Sears, Ph.D. *The Anti-Aging Zone*. New York: ReganBooks, 1999.

Cameron Stauth. *The New Approach to Cancer*. New York: T. S. Vernon & Sons, 1982.

Roger Williams. *Biochemical Individuality*. Austin, TX: University of Texas Press, 1956.

William Wollcott. 'Core Premises: The Health Excel System of Metabolic Typing.' Internet www.healthexcel.com

INDEX

acetaldehyde 67
acetylcholine 117, 136, 227
acidophilus 101, 102, 121, 127, 138,
    193, 220, 290
acne 110, 128–9
adrenal glands 29, 45, 57, 97
adrenaline 53, 57, 65, 76, 78, 99, 136
aerobic exercise 207, 256
airborne allergens 54, 110, 115, 131,
    139, 294
ALCAT test (Antigen Leukocyte
    Cellular Antibody Test) 32, 33,
    161
alcohol 51, 60, 61, 118
aldosterone 65, 66, 204
algae 200
alginates 296
alkalinity 198–9
allergic threshold 53, 54, 139, 225
allergy control products 351–8
Allergy Relief and Prevention (Krohn)
    293
aloe vera 192, 195
alpha-galactosidase 224
alpha-lipoic acid 196
amaranth 285
American Heart Association 71
amylase 223
anaphylactic shock 57
aniseed 193
anorexia nervosa 94–5, 110, 127–8
antacids 60, 126

anti-diuretic hormone 65
anti-hypertensives 292
anti-hypoglycemia programme
    290–1
anti-yeast diet 289–90
antibiotics 52, 60, 101, 120, 139, 290,
    292
    herbal 202
antibodies 56, 62, 157, 159
antidepressants 77, 91, 95, 111, 292
antigens 62, 159
antihistamines 140
anxiety 30, 92, 96, 110, 112, 130, 138
arginine 123, 226–7
Argisle, Bethany 245
arrowroot 285
artemesia 123
arthritis 66, 82, 110, 113–15
artificial sweeteners 61, 132, 289
aspartame 61, 132, 289, 296
aspirin 60, 67, 114, 116
asthma 109, 110, 115–16, 134
attention deficit hyperactive
    disorder (ADHD) 110, 133–5
aubergines 114
Avocado Dressing 332

Baked Mushrooms 322
Balance Programme *see* False Fat
    Diet, Balance Programme phase
Banana Bread 345–6
barberry root 192, 195

barley 148, 284, 286
Basil Balsamic Vinaigrette 331–2
Bean Spreads 334–5
beans 61, 224
beer belly 52
Beetroot with Orange Vinaigrette 321
Beijing Pea Pod Salad 336
Bell Jar, The (Plath) 99
benzoic acid 296
berberine 123
beta-carotene 103, 104, 219
betaine hydrochloride 51, 53, 67, 103, 105, 126, 220, 222, 224
bifidobacteria 101, 102, 103, 104, 121, 138, 183, 193, 221, 290
bioflavonoids 220
biotin 220
birth control pills 52, 101, 290
Blackened Tofu Steaks 316–17
bloating and swelling 26–8, 37–8, 63–8
   pre-menstrual syndrome and 97–8
   see also food reactions
blood cleaners 202
blood sugar levels 77, 78
blood tests *see* medical testing
body dysmorphic disorder (BDD) 93–4
body-fat ratio 26, 87, 88
Boulot, Philippe 298, 300
bowel stimulants 202
Braised Rabbit or Chicken 'au Muscadet' 314–15
Breakfast Rice 325–6
Broccoli Soup 330–1
bromates 296
bromelain 220
buckthorn 202
bulimia 94, 110, 127–8
burdock 202
Butter-Free Veggie Spread 335

caffeine 97
calcium 66, 103, 106, 136, 196, 197, 199, 200, 220
   alternate sources of 296–7
Candida albicans 52, 100–4
candidiasis 30, 100–4, 110, 116, 120, 123, 221, 289
caprylic acid 103, 105
carbohydrate craving 78, 81–2, 248
cardiovascular disease 110, 116–17
carnitine 123, 125, 226
cartilage deterioration 113–14
cascara sagrada 192, 195, 202
casein 148
Cashew or Almond Butter Cookies 346
Cashew Torte 342
cayenne pepper 202, 224
cell reactive food tests 160–1
cellular acidosis 66
cellulite 27, 215, 252
chemicals, allergenic 54, 294
Cherry Cobbler 349
Chèvre (Goat Cheese) and Smoked Salmon in Grape Leaves 304–5
chewing 53, 193, 215, 223
childhood obesity 23
Chinese Fried Rice 328
chocolate 61, 89–90, 128, 149
Chocolate Pudding 341
cholecystokinin (CCK) 65, 137, 227
cholesterol 116
choline 117, 227
chondroitin 115
chromium 103, 118, 125, 220, 222, 227–8
chronic ear infections 110, 119–21
chronic fatigue syndrome (CFS) 30, 82, 102, 116, 121–3
chronic pain 110, 123–4
Cider Slaw 336
circulatory immune complex (CIC) 62, 116–17, 159
citrus fruits 115, 153
Cleansing Phase *see* False Fat Diet, Cleansing Phase of
cleavers 202
cobalamin 220

Cobbler Topping 349–50
coenzyme Q$_{10}$ 103, 105, 123, 125,
   220, 221
cognitive disorders 110, 117–18
cognitive function 30
colic 121
colon 191–3
colonic irrigation 194
Colourful Quinoa Salad with
   Raspberry Yogurt Dressing 325
compulsivity 30
copper 103, 220
corn 36, 41, 148, 149, 173, 243, 275,
   278–9
corn syrup 22, 36
cortisol 53, 65, 66, 76, 81, 99–100,
   118, 136
cortisone 60, 101
Courgette Cake 345
cow's milk 119, 120
creatine 131
cysteine 196, 197, 220
cytokines 122

dairy products 41, 43, 44–5, 61, 80,
   137, 148, 173, 275, 280
   substitutes for 286–8
Dairy-Free Pesto Sauce 333
dandelion 194, 196, 202
date sugar 288
delayed food reactions 58–60, 146
delta sleep 130
delta-6-desaturase 82
depression 30, 92, 96, 99, 100, 106,
   109, 110, 130, 138, 253–4
dessert recipes 340–50
Detox Diet, The (Haas) 40, 190, 203
detoxification measures 34, 154–5
   see also False Fat Diet, Cleansing
   Phase of
DHEA 227
diabetes 110, 124–5
diet soda 48
digestion 49–54, 193, 247–8
digestive disorders 23, 110, 113–14,
   125–7

direct cellular reactions 60–2, 118,
   132
diuretics 98, 204
   herbal 202
diverticulitis 191
dong quai 106, 107
dopamine 254
dressings see sauce and dressing
   recipes
dry skin brushing 34

ear infections, chronic 110, 119–21
eating disorders 94–5, 110, 127–8
echinacea 103, 105, 139, 202, 224,
   226
eczema 32, 109, 110, 128–9, 134
EDTA 296
Egg-Free Mayonnaise (Tofunaise)
   334
eggs 22, 41, 61, 80, 134, 148, 149, 173,
   243, 275, 279
eicosanoids 82
elimination diet 24, 41–6, 145–55
   Juice Fast 153–5
      menu plans 164–7
   Limited 147–51
      menu plans 178–84
   Sensitive Seven 149
      menu plans 173–8
   Total 152–3, 164–5
      menu plans 167–73
ELISA test (Enzyme Linked
   Immuno-Sorbent Assay) 157–60
emotional eating 231–4
endocrine system 29, 90
endorphins 75–6, 78, 106
enemas 194, 195, 196
energy 30
   exercise and 254
   premenstrual syndrome and
      99–100
entrees, recipes for 300–17
enzymes 50–1, 126, 137, 220
ephedra (Ma-Huang) 139, 224, 225
essential fatty acids 80, 106, 107, 115,
   125, 129, 192, 195

estrogen 65, 88, 91, 92, 96, 97, 107, 292

Etouffade de Boeuf Bourguignonne 314

eucalyptus oil 140

evening primrose 105, 106

exercise 34, 124, 194
  in Balance Programme phase 240–1, 251–8
  in Cleansing phase 195, 205–11
  premenstrual syndrome and 106

False Fat Diet
  Balance Programme phase 24–5, 28, 35, 237–69
    diet 242–6
    exercise 240–1, 251–8
    expectations 240–2
    menu plan 263–9
    metabolic typing 248–51
    stress management 240, 258–62
  Cleansing Phase of 24, 155–6, 185–212
    expectations 187–90
    gastrointestinal tract cleansing 190–7, 208
    herbal therapy 201–3, 208
    physical therapy 205–11
    sample daily schedule 209–10
    summary of 211–12
    water consumption 203–4, 208
  development of 37–46
  False Fat Week 24, 213–36
    emotional eating 231–4
    enzymes 222–4
    expectations 214–17
    first food challenge 234–6
    herbal therapy 224–6
    learned food fallacies 229–31
    metabolic stimulation 226–8
    supplements for 218–26
    individualization of 35–6
    innovations in 25–36
    overview of 24–5
    recipes see recipes

success of 22
  see also food reactions

False Fat Week see False Fat Diet, False Fat Week

fasting 34, 153–5

fatigue 99

Feingold, Benjamin 133

female hormones 84–6, 92–3, 96, 292

fenfluramine 91

fennel seed 193

fermentation 67, 101, 193, 215

fertility 87

fibre 51, 192

fibromyalgia 30, 92, 129–31, 137

fluconazole (Diflucan) 103, 105

folic acid 220

food additives 295–6

food allergies
  anaphylactic shock and 57
  in history 56
  incidence of 22, 57

food colouring 62, 115, 134, 296

food cravings 19, 24, 28–9, 32, 40, 41, 43–4, 70–4, 137
  causes of 75–9
  checklist for 73–4
  insomnia and 136
  premenstrual syndrome and 89–91

food fallacies, learned 229–31

food families 244–5, 282–4

food reactions
  arthritis and 113–15
  asthma and 115–16
  candida overgrowth and 116
  cardiovascular disease and 116–17
  causing bloating and swelling 63–8
  causing food cravings 73–9
  chronic ear infections and 119–21
  chronic pain and 123–4
  cognitive disorders and 117–18
  diabetes and 124–5
  eating disorders and 127–8
  eczema, acne and hives and 128–9
  fat-creating cycle of 31

fibromyalgia and 129–31
finding *see* elimination diet;
    medical testing
hay fever and 131–2
headache and 132–3
hyperactivity and attention deficit
    disorder and 133–5
hypoglycemia (low blood sugar)
    and 135
incidence of 22
insomnia and 136
irritable bowel syndrome and
    137–8
mood disturbance and 138
reference guide 275–97
risk factors causing 50–4
sinusitis and 138–40
see also food allergies, food
    sensitivities
food sensitivities
    delayed reactions 58–60, 146
    direct cellular reactions 60–2, 118,
        134
    immune complex reactions 62–3,
        113
    incidence of 22, 41
Fruit Sorbet 342–3
Fusilli with Fresh Tomatoes and
    Basil Sauce 316

gamma linolenic acid (GLA) 103,
    105, 220, 221, 222
Garden Tomatoes with Balsamic
    Vinaigrette 319
garlic 103, 105, 121, 139, 202, 224, 226
gas 67, 193, 215, 224
gastrointestinal tract cleansing
    190–7, 208
Gazpacho 329
genetic heritage 246–7
gentian root 224, 225
ginger 106, 107, 193, 202, 224, 225
ginseng 107, 123, 199
glucosamine sulphate 115
glutamine 192, 195, 199, 227
glutathione peroxidase 197

gluten 22, 148, 284–6
goat's milk 286
goldenseal 103, 105, 139, 192, 194,
    195, 196, 202
grapefruit seed extract 103, 105, 123
Green Onion Dressing 332
Grilled Salmon on a Bed of Braised
    Lentils with Baby Artichokes
    306–7
Grilled Swordfish with Pineapple
    Mustard 310–11
guggul 227

hay fever 110, 131–2, 134, 139
headaches 24, 32, 110, 130, 132–3
heartburn 25, 32, 51, 110, 111–12,
    125, 126
herbal therapy 34, 106
    for Cleansing phase 201–3
    for False Fat Week 224–6
Herbed Couscous Salad 338–9
herpes viruses 122
Hippocrates 56
histamine 56, 61, 66, 221
hives 32, 66, 110, 128–9, 134
homeopathic medications 121, 139, 199
honey 288
Honey and Chilli Roasted
    Hazelnuts 340–1
Honey Minted Carrots 322
Honey Sundae 341
hormonal replacement therapy 93
horseradish 224, 225, 226
hospital studies 22
5-HTP (5-hydroxy-tryptophan) 107,
    130–1, 133, 135, 136
human growth hormone (HGH)
    226–7
hunger 69–74, 75, 77
hydrochloric acid (betaine
    hydrochloride) 51, 53, 67, 103,
    105, 126, 220, 222, 224
hyperactivity 110, 133–5
hypoglycemia (low blood sugar) 30,
    79, 81–2, 90, 96–7, 110, 119, 135,
    148, 227

hypoglycemia *(cont)*
  anti-hypoglycemia programme
    290–1
hypothalamus 75, 89
hypothyroidism 95–6, 99

ibuprofen 116
IgA (immunoglobulin A) 59–60
IgE (immunoglobulin E) 40, 56, 59,
  159–62, 242
IgG (immunoglobulin G) 41, 58–9,
  159–62, 242
immune complex food reactions
  62–3, 113
immune system 49–50, 53, 56,
  59–60, 121–2
infections, recurrent 25
inflammatory response 65, 66, 75
insomnia 25, 30, 32, 82, 99, 110, 130,
  135–6
insulin 23, 29, 75, 77, 80, 124–5, 148,
  253
insulin resistance 80
intestinal cleansing 34, 190–7, 208
iodine 103, 220
iron 103, 220
irritable bowel syndrome (IBS) 25,
  30, 32, 82, 109, 110, 130, 137–8,
  191
itraconazole (Sporanox) 103, 105

joint pain 62, 109, 113–15
Juice Fast Elimination Diet 153–5
  menu plans 164–7
juniper berry 106, 107, 202

kamut 284
kava 199
ketoconazole (Nizoral) 103, 105
ketones 26
ketosis 26, 37
Khalsa, Dharma Singh 123
kidneys 62, 203–4
kinesiology testing 163
kinins 56–7
Krohn, Jacqueline 293, 294

lactalbumin 148
lactase 222
lactobacillus acidophilus 101, 102,
  104, 121, 127, 138, 193, 220, 221,
  290
lactose intolerance 45, 222–3
lamisil 105
laxatives 192, 195, 216
leaky gut syndrome 51–2, 67, 101
lecithin 135, 136, 227
lectins 61
leukotrienes 56
licorice root 202, 224, 225
lifestyle 24–5, 72
light therapy 106
Limited Elimination Diet 147–51
  menu plans 178–84
lipase 223
lipotropics 227
liver 103, 105, 194, 196
Lobster Baked Potato 305
low blood sugar (hypoglycemia) 30,
  79, 81–2, 90, 96–7, 110, 119, 135,
  148, 227
  anti-hypoglycemia programme
    290–1
lungs 206–7
lysine 123

Ma-Huang (*Ephedra sinensis*) 139,
  224, 225
magnesium 106, 107, 125, 131, 133,
  136, 199, 200, 201, 220, 221, 222
magnesium malate 131
malic acid 131
manganese 220
Maple and Orange Marinated Pork
  Loin 312–13
maple syrup 288
massage 196, 207–8
mast cells 61, 131, 221
MDRs (Minimum Daily
  Requirements) 200
medical testing 24, 40, 41, 145,
  156–63
  cell reactive food tests 160–1

ELISA test 157–60
kinesiology testing 163
pulse testing 163
scratch tests 161–2
sublingual testing 162–3
meditation 209–11
melatonin 136
menopause 93, 96
menstrual cycle 27, 68, 87
menstruation, painful 130
menthol 140
menu plans
    Balance Programme phase 263–9
    Juice Fast Elimination Diet 164–7
    Limited Elimination Diet 178–84
    Sensitive Seven Elimination Diet
        173–8
    Total Elimination Diet 164–5,
        167–73
metabolic disorders 19, 21, 23,
    29–30, 34, 80–3
    premenstrual syndrome and 95–7
metabolic stimulation 226–8
metabolic typing 33–4, 248–51
Metamucil 192
methane 67
methylsulfonylmethane (MSM) 221,
    222
Mexican Quinoa with Spinach
    324–5
Mexican Salad Bowl 340
migraines 25, 30, 32, 61, 62, 82, 92,
    109, 111, 112, 132–3, 138
milk 22, 119–20, 125, 134, 138,
    147–8, 151, 173, 243, 280
milk thistle 194, 196
millet 285
mitochondria 66, 226
molasses 288–9
molybdenum 221
mood disturbances
    anxiety 30, 92, 96, 110, 112, 130,
        138
    depression 30, 92, 96, 99, 100, 106,
        130, 138, 253–4, 109, 110
    premenstrual syndrome and 91–5

MSG (monosodium glutamate) 22,
    62, 296
mucus reducers 202
mullein leaf 121, 224, 226
mustard 61, 149

Navarin of Lamb 311
nettle leaf 224, 225
neurotransmitters 75, 77, 117, 118,
    253
    serotonin 30, 77, 78, 91–5, 112,
        117, 124, 127, 132, 134, 136,
        137, 254
niacin 196, 206, 219, 221, 222
nicotine 97
nightshade family 114, 153
nitrates and nitrites 62, 132, 296
non-dairy margarines 287–8
non-dairy yogurts, cheeses and sour
    cream 288
norepinephrine 76, 106, 254
nut milk 286
nutritional therapy 102
nystatin 103, 105

oat milk 287
oats 148, 151, 284, 286
obesity 22–3, 71
octopamine 61
Old-Fashioned Potato Soup 330
omega-3 and omega-6 oils 106, 107,
    115, 125, 128–9, 192, 195
oranges 151
Ornish, Dean 234
ornithine 226–7
osteoarthritis 113, 115
ovalbumin 148
Oven-Cured Tomato and
    Aubergine Caviar Napoleon with
    Basil Essence 320–1
overeating 52

PABA 220
pain, chronic 110, 123–4
Pain Cure, The (Stauth) 123–4
Paleolithic Diet 147

pantothenic acid 118, 192, 195, 219
papaya 61
parabens 296
parsley 106, 202
Pasta with Courgettes 317
pau d'arco 103, 105
peach leaf 192, 195
peanuts 41, 61, 149, 151, 173, 243, 281
Peas Pulão with Rice 323
peppermint oil 138, 192, 195
peppers 114
pepsin 126
peptides 61
peristalsis 67, 68
perspiration 206, 215
PGE-2 (prostaglandin E-2) 81
phagocytes 100
phenylalanine 61, 106, 107, 132, 227
phenylethylamine 61, 90
physical detoxification therapy 205–11
Pie Crust 346–8
pineapple 61
pituitary gland 65
Plath, Sylvia 99
PMS see premenstrual syndrome
Polenta 324
pork 61
potassium 98, 198, 200
Potato-Crusted Salmon 301–2
potatoes 114
Prawns with Lentil Salad 308–9
pregnancy 96
premenstrual syndrome (PMS) 30, 65, 85–6, 137
    bloating and swelling and 97–8
    candida and 100–4
    energy and immune dysfunction 99–100
    food cravings and 89–91
    metabolic disorders and 95–7
    mood disturbances and 95
    natural therapy for 103–7
preservatives 116, 133
Preventive Medical Center, Marin, California 37
prickly ash 194, 196, 202
probiotics 102–3, 127, 138, 139, 193–4, 220, 221, 222, 290
processed foods 22, 50, 148, 151
progesterone 92, 97, 107
progestins 292
propolis 202
propyl gallate 296
prostaglandins 221
protease 223
Prozac 77, 91
pseudoephedrine 140, 225
psychology of overeating 228–9
psyllium seed 192, 195
puberty 88, 96
pulse testing 163
Pumpkin Pie with Oat Crust 343
pycnogenol 131
pyridoxal-5-phosphate 220
pyridoxine 106, 107, 131, 196, 220

quercetin 132, 220, 221, 222
quinoa 285
Quinoa and Bay Shrimp/Prawn Salad with Lemon Pepper Vinaigrette 303–4

Rainbow Rice 326
Raspberry Yogurt Dressing 325
RAST test (Radio Allergo-Sorbent Testing) 160
raw sugar 288–9
recipes 298–350
    Avocado Dressing 332
    Baked Mushrooms 322
    Banana Bread 345–6
    Basil Balsamic Vinaigrette 331–2
    Bean Spreads 334–5
    Beetroot with Orange Vinaigrette 321
    Beijing Pea Pod Salad 336
    Blackened Tofu Steaks 316–17
    Braised Rabbit or Chicken 'au Muscadet' 314–15
    Breakfast Rice 325–6

Broccoli Soup 330–1
Butter-Free Veggie Spread 335
Cashew or Almond Butter
   Cookies 346
Cashew Torte 342
Cherry Cobbler 349
Chèvre and Smoked Salmon in
   Grape Leaves 304–5
Chinese Fried Rice 328
Chocolate Pudding 341
Cider Slaw 336
Cobbler Topping 349–50
Colourful Quinoa Salad with
   Raspberry Yogurt Dressing
   325
Courgette Cake 345
Dairy-Free Pesto Sauce 333
Egg-Free Mayonnaise (Tofunaise)
   334
Etouffade de Boeuf
   Bourguignonne 314
Fruit Sorbet 342–3
Fusilli with Fresh Tomatoes and
   Basil Sauce 316
Garden Tomatoes with Balsamic
   Vinaigrette 319
Gazpacho 329
Green Onion Dressing 332
Grilled Salmon on a Bed of
   Braised Lentils with Baby
   Artichokes 306–7
Grilled Swordfish with Pineapple
   Mustard 310–11
Herbed Couscous Salad 338–9
Honey and Chilli Roasted
   Hazelnuts 340–1
Honey Minted Carrots 322
Honey Sundae 341
Lobster Baked Potato 305
Maple and Orange Marinated
   Pork Loin 312–13
Mexican Quinoa with Spinach
   324–5
Mexican Salad Bowl 340
Navarin of Lamb 311
Old-Fashioned Potato Soup 330

Oven-Cured Tomato and
   Aubergine Caviar Napoleon
   with Basil Essence 320–1
Pasta with Courgettes 317
Peas Pulão with Rice 323
Pie Crust 346–8
Polenta 324
Potato-Crusted Salmon 301–2
Prawns with Lentil Salad 308–9
preparation methods 301
Pumpkin Pie with Oat Crust 343
Quinoa and Bay Shrimp/Prawn
   Salad with Lemon Pepper
   Vinaigrette 303–4
Rainbow Rice 326
Raspberry Yogurt Dressing 325
Red Snapper on Black Bean
   Relish 302–3
Rice Creole 327
Rice Milanese 327
Rich Veggie Soup 329–30
Roasted Sirloin of Beef with
   Herbed Baby Potatoes 313
Sea Bass en Papillote 309
Seared Sea Scallop and Tiger
   Prawn Salad and Curry
   Vinaigrette 307–8
Sesame Oil Dressing 338
Snapper Mexicana 309–10
Spiced Butternut Squash Bisque
   328–9
Spinach Salad with Mushrooms
   and Sesame Dressing 338
Split Pea or Haricot Bean Soup
   331
Stone-Ground Mustard Rubbed
   Rack of Lamb with Roasted
   Garlic Potato Hash 311–12
Stuffed Baked Acorn or
   Butternut Squash 321–2
Stuffed Bell Peppers 315–16
Sweet and Sour Sauce 333
Tofu Brochettes 317
Tropical Fruit Salsa 310
Twice-Baked Potatoes 323
Warm Red Cabbage Salad 337

recipes (cont)
  Watercress Salad with Pears and
    Goat Cheese 337
  Wilted Spinach Salad 339
  Yogurt Freezes 344
Red Snapper on Black Bean Relish
  302–3
refined foods 51
resources and referrals 351–9
rhamanosa 105
rheumatoid arthritis 113
rhubarb root 192, 195
riboflavin 133, 219
rice 285
Rice Creole 327
rice ice cream 287
Rice Milanese 327
rice milk 286
rice syrup 288
Rich Veggie Soup 329–30
Ritalin 134
Roasted Sirloin of Beef with Herbed
  Baby Potatoes 313
rotation diets 240, 244
Royal, Fuller 78
rue food family 115
rye 148, 284, 285

saccharin 289
safflower herb 194, 196
salad recipes 336–40
salami 61
salicylates 133
sauce and dressing recipes 331–5
saunas 34, 206
sausage 61
scale weight 72
Sea Bass en Papillote 309
Seared Sea Scallop and Tiger Prawn
  Salad and Curry Vinaigrette 307–8
Sears, Barry 81
seasonal affective disorder 106
selenium 104, 105, 192, 195, 196, 197,
  200, 220
self-respect 69
senna 192, 195, 202

Sensitive Seven Elimination Diet
  151–2
  menu plans 173–8
Sensitive Seven Elimination foods
  see corn; dairy products; eggs;
  peanuts; soy; sugar; wheat
serotonin 30, 77–8, 91–5, 113, 117,
  124, 127, 132, 134, 136, 137, 254
Serzone 112
Sesame Oil Dressing 338
shellfish 61, 153
sherbet 287
Siberian ginseng 199
silicon 220
silymarin 194
sinus problems 25, 82, 110, 138–40
skin cleaners 202
skin rashes 25, 82, 128–9, 134–5
Snapper Mexicana 309–10
sodium 65–7
somatostatin 65
sorbet 287
sorbic acid 296
soup recipes 328–31
soya 41, 107, 119–20, 134, 149, 151,
  173, 243, 275, 280
soya ice cream 287
soya milk 286
special occasions 245–6
spelt 284
Spiced Butternut Squash Bisque
  328–9
Spinach Salad with Mushrooms and
  Sesame Dressing 338
Split Pea or Haricot Bean Soup 331
Spring Master Cleanser 154
starflower seed (borage) 105
starvation response 23, 72, 155, 241
Stauth, Cameron 123–4
Staying Healthy with Nutrition
  (Haas) 40, 201, 219
Staying Healthy with the Seasons
  (Haas) 39
Staying Healthy Shopper's Guide, The
  (Haas) 149
steambaths 206

steroid drugs 52, 63, 290, 292
stomach crunches 194, 195
Stone-Ground Mustard Rubbed
    Rack of Lamb with Roasted
    Garlic Potato Hash 311–12
strawberries 61
stress 34, 52–3, 67, 81
    management 34, 240, 258–62
stretching 256–7
Stuffed Baked Acorn or Butternut
    Squash 321–2
Stuffed Bell Peppers 315–16
sublingual testing 162–3
Sudafed 225
sugar 41, 52, 80, 134, 137, 147–8, 149,
    151, 173, 178, 243, 281
    substitutes 288–9
Sugar Busters diet 23
sulphites 62, 116, 296
sulphur 220
sunflower seeds 61
supplements 34
    for Cleansing Phase 197–201, 208
    for False Fat Week 218–26
    resources for 354–8
Swedish massage 207–8
Sweet and Sour Sauce 333

tapioca 285
tartrazine 115
taurine 68–9
teff 285
testosterone 91
thiamine 219
thirst 64–5
thyroid gland 29, 80
Tofu Brochettes 317
tomatoes 61, 114
Total Elimination Diet 152–3, 164–5
    menu plans 167–73
toxic congestion see False Fat Diet,
    Cleansing Phase of
triglycerides 88
Tropical Fruit Salsa 310
tryptophan 92, 94, 130–1
turbinado sugar 288–9

Twice-Baked Potatoes 323
tyramine 61, 132
tyrosine 227

ulcer drugs 60
University of Michigan in Ann
    Arbor 38
urinary tract infections 32

vaginitis 32
valerian root 199
vegetables and grains
    preparation 318
    recipes 319–31
vegetarianism 248
Vitamin A 103, 129, 139, 195, 196,
    197, 200, 219, 221
Vitamin B_1 (thiamine) 219
Vitamin B_2 (riboflavin) 133, 219
Vitamin B_3 (niacin/ niacinamide)
    196, 219, 221
Vitamin B_5 (pantothenic acid) 118,
    192, 195, 219
Vitamin B_{12} (cobalamin) 220
Vitamin C 104, 117, 118, 129, 132,
    139, 192, 195, 196, 197, 200, 201,
    220, 221, 222
Vitamin D 219
Vitamin E 104, 129, 192, 195, 196,
    197, 200, 219, 221
Vitamin K 219
vitex (chasteberry) 106, 107

Warm Red Cabbage Salad 337
water consumption 203–4, 208
water retention 64–5, 97–8, 106, 204,
    215
    medications causing 292
water weight 26–7, 37, 40, 64–5, 87,
    98, 215
Watercress Salad with Pears and
    Goat Cheese 337
weight training 256, 258
wheat 22, 40, 61, 80, 147–8, 149, 151,
    173, 178, 243, 275, 277–8
    substitutes for 284–6

wheatgrass 194
whey 148
white blood cells 57, 77, 100
Wilted Spinach Salad 339
withdrawal symptoms 24, 29, 44,
    190

yarrow 194, 196, 202

yeast 52, 151, 289–90
yeast infections 100–4, 120
yellow dock 202
Yogurt Freezes 344

zinc 129, 135, 192, 195, 196, 197, 200,
    220, 221
Zone, The (Sears) 81

Grateful acknowledgment is made to the following for permission to reprint or publish recipes:

Celestial Arts Publishing and Eleonora Manzolini: 'Avocado Dressing,' 'Bean Spreads,' 'Breakfast Rice,' 'Butter-Free Veggie Spread,' 'Colourful Quinoa Salad with Raspberry Yogurt Dressing,' 'Egg-Free Mayonnaise,' 'Fruit Sorbet,' 'Grilled Swordfish with Pineapple Mustard,' 'Herbed Couscous Salad,' 'Mexican Quinoa with Spinach,' 'Mexican Sald Bowl,' 'Pesto Sauce,' 'Pumpkin Pie with Oat Crust,' 'Rainbow Rice,' 'Rice Veggie Soup,' 'Stuffed Bell Peppers,' 'Sweet and Sour Sauce,' 'Warm Red Cabbage Salad,' 'Wilted Spinach Salad,' and 'Yogurt Freezes' are reprinted from *Staying Healthy with Nutrition* and *A Diet for All Seasons*, both by Elson Haas, M.D., published by Celestial Arts Publishing.

Eleonora Manzolini: 'Blackened Tofu Steaks,' 'Fusilli with Fresh Tomatoes and Basil Sauce,' 'Pasta with Courgettes,' 'Polenta,' 'Sea Bass en Papillote,' 'Snapper Mexicana with Tropical Fruit Salsa,' and 'Tofu Brochettes.'

Starburst Publishers: 'Banana Bread,' 'Cherry Cobbler,' 'Cashew or Almond Butter Cookies,' 'Pie Crust,' and 'Courgette Cake' are reprinted from *Allergy Cooking with Ease* by Nicolette M. Dumke and William Crook, published by Starburst Publishers.

Philippe Boulot: 'Basil Balsamic Vinaigrete,' 'Beetroot with Orange Vinaigrette,' 'Braised Rabbit or Chicken "au Muscadet",' 'Chèvre (Goat Cheese) and Smoked Salmon in Grape Leaves,' 'Estouffade de Boeuf Bourguignonne,' 'Garden Tomatoes with Balsamic Vinaigrette,' 'Gazpacho,' 'Grilled Salmon on a Bed or Braised Lentils with Baby Artichokes,' 'Honey and Chilli Roasted Hazelnuts,' 'Lobster Baked Potato,' 'Maple and Orange Marinated Pork Loin,' 'Navarin of Lamb,' 'Oven-Cured Tomato and Aubergine Caviar Napoleon with Basil Essence,' 'Potato-Crusted Salmon,' 'Prawns with Lentil Salad,' 'Quinoa and Bay Shrimp/Prawn Salad with Lemon Pepper Vinaigrette,' 'Red Snapper on Black Bean Relish,' 'Roasted Sirloin of Beef with Herbed Baby Potatoes,' 'Seared Sea Scallop and Tiger Prawn Salad with Curry Vinaigrette,' 'Spiced Butternut Squash Bisque,' 'Spinach Salad with Mushrooms and Sesame Dressing,' 'Stone-Ground Mustard Rubbed Rack of Lamb with Roasted Garlic Potato Hash,' 'Stuffed Baked Acorn or Butternut Squash,' 'Twice-Baked Potatoes,' and 'Watercress Salad with Pears and Goat Cheese.'

Cameron Stauth and Lorraine Stauth: 'Baked Mushrooms,' 'Beijing Pea Pod Salad,' 'Broccoli Soup,' 'Cashew Torte,' 'Chinese Fried Rice,' 'Chocolate Pudding,' 'Cider Slaw,' 'Green Onion Dressing,' 'Honey Minted Carrots,' 'Honey Sundae,' 'Old-Fashioned Potato Soup,' 'Peas Pulāo with Rice,' 'Rice Creole,' and 'Rice Milanese.'

Elson M. Haas, M.D.: 'Poultry with Vegetables,' 'Seasonal Vegetable Medleys,' and 'Split Pea or Haricot Bean Soup.'

About the Authors

ELSON M. HAAS, M.D., has been in medical practice for more than twenty-five years and was instrumental in the development of the field that he has termed Integrated Medicine. He is the founder and director of the Preventive Medical Center of Marin, an integrated health care facility in San Rafael, California, where he specializes in family and nutritional medicine, and detoxification. He is also the author of six previous books on health and nutrition: *Staying Healthy with the Seasons, Staying Healthy with Nutrition, A Cookbook for All Seasons, The Detox Diet, The Staying Healthy Shopper's Guide* and *Vitamins for Dummies.*

After his graduation from the University of Michigan Medical School in 1972, Elson received his further training in Northern California, where he has since resided. After his internship, he began additional studies in many health-related fields – nutrition, herbology, Oriental medicine, exercise physiology, body therapies, and mind-body medicine – fulfilling his goal to learn something about health and healing after so many years of studying disease. Over the last two decades, Dr Haas has integrated these many healing disciplines into his family medical practice about which he wrote in his first book, *Staying Healthy with the Seasons,* published in 1981 and now in its 22nd printing.

During the 1980s, Dr Haas designed educational products with associate Bethany Argisle for Health Harvest, Unlimited. Together they created many health-conscious products, such as the Acupuncture and Chakra T-shirts and the popular Sole Sox, anatomical/reflexology socks. These products are still available through Bethany's website, *www.argisle.com*

Dr Haas travels widely, teaches nationally, and appears on numerous American radio shows. He is a professional consultant for many health writers and magazines, including *Natural Health, Women's World* and *Let's Live.* Elson lives on a small family farm in Northern California where he raises food and animals with his wife and their two children.

Contact Dr Elson Haas and sign up for his free newsletter and receive other health information at his website, *www.elsonhaas.com*

CAMERON STAUTH has written about medical subjects since 1972, when he was the first American author to write extensively about alternative therapies for cancer. This work culminated in his first book, *The New Approach to Cancer.*

...er editor in chief of *The Journal of Health Science*, and former editor of a ...y magazine, he has also been a hospital public relations director, network television film producer, and co-founder of a prominent health products firm. His recent book *Brain Longevity*, written with Dharma Singh Khalsa, M.D., was published in eight languages and was an international bestseller. With a wide range of interests, he has written bestsellers on the subjects of business, professional sports, and crime. A former magazine columnist, he has also written on the entertainment industry. *The New York Times* has called him 'a tireless reporter and a talented and graceful writer.' He lives in Portland, Oregon, wth his wife and two children.